Care Ethics and Political Theory

Care Ethics and Political Theory

Edited by
Daniel Engster and Maurice Hamington

OXFORD
UNIVERSITY PRESS

OXFORD
UNIVERSITY PRESS

Great Clarendon Street, Oxford, OX2 6DP,
United Kingdom

Oxford University Press is a department of the University of Oxford.
It furthers the University's objective of excellence in research, scholarship, and education by publishing worldwide. Oxford is a registered trade mark of Oxford University Press in the UK and in certain other countries

First Edition published in 2015
Impression: 1

Published in the United States of America by Oxford University Press
198 Madison Avenue, New York, NY 10016, United States of America

British Library Cataloguing in Publication Data
Data available

Library of Congress Control Number: 2015932776

ISBN 978–0–19–871634–1

Printed and bound by
CPI Group (UK) Ltd, Croydon, CR0 4YY

To Mikki van Zyl, a dedicated care scholar and activist who contributed to this volume, but whose untimely passing did not allow her to see its publication

Acknowledgements

The idea for this book first came up after attending the Western Political Science Association's annual conference in 2012. A number of panels on care ethics were organized at the conference, and it was obvious from the presentations that important and interesting new work was rapidly developing out of the field of care ethics. In 2013, the editors helped to organize a new set of panels on care ethics at the Western Political Science Association conference while soliciting chapters for this volume. In 2014, we were then able to organize a special "conference within a conference" at the Western Political Science Association conference, in which many of the contributors to this book presented and received feedback on their chapters. We would very much like to thank the Western Political Science Association, and especially Elsa Favilla, for helping us to organize this mini-conference and more generally for organizing stimulating annual conferences that do so much to foster the development of new ideas. We encountered so many interesting papers on care ethics at the Western Political Science Association conference that we are only sorry we could not have included more of them in this volume.

Contents

Part III. Care Ethics, Non-Western, and Subaltern Cultures

Part IV. Challenging Dominant Paradigms

List of Contributors

Maxine Eichner is Reef Ivey II Professor of Law at University of North Carolina School of Law. She writes on issues at the intersection of law and political theory, focusing particularly on family relationships, feminist theory, social welfare, and the market. She is the author of *The Supportive State: Families, Government, and America's Political Ideals* (Oxford University Press, 2010). She is also an editor of *Family Law: Cases, Text, Problems*, edited by Ellman, Kurtz, Weithorn, Bix, Czapanskiy, and Eichner (LexisNexis, 2014).

Daniel Engster is an Associate Professor of Political Science at the University of Texas at San Antonio. His books include *The Heart of Justice: Care Ethics and Political Theory* (Oxford University Press, 2007); *Justice, Politics, and the Family*, co-edited with Tamara Metz (Paradigm, 2014); and *Justice, Care, and the Welfare State* (Oxford University Press, 2015). He has published articles on care ethics and animal welfare, public policy and parenting, child poverty, and other issues relating to care ethics, the family, and justice.

Marilyn Friedman works in the areas of ethics, feminist theory, and social and political philosophy. She is the author of numerous journal articles and book chapters in these areas. She has authored several books, including *Autonomy, Gender, Politics* (Oxford University Press, 2003), *What Are Friends For?* (Cornell University Press, 1993), and *Political Correctness: For and Against*, co-authored with Jan Narveson (Rowman and Littlefield, 1995). She has also edited or co-edited several volumes: *Women and Citizenship* (Oxford University Press, 2005), *Feminism and Community* (Temple University Press, 1995), *Mind and Morals* (Bradford/MIT Press, 1995), and *Rights and Reason* (Kluwer, 2000).

Amanda Gouws is Professor of Political Science at the University of Stellenbosch, South Africa. She holds a PhD from the University of Illinois in Urbana-Champaign in the USA. Her specialization is South African Politics and Gender Politics. Her research focuses on women and citizenship, the National Gender Machinery, and representation. She is the editor of *(Un)Thinking Citizenship: Feminist Debates in Contemporary South Africa* (Juta, 2005). In 2007 she was the Edith Keeger Wolf Distinguished Visiting Professor at Northwestern University. In 2012 she received the Wilma Rule Award for the best paper at the International Political Science Association conference in Madrid, Spain, in the category Gender and Politics with the title "Multiculturalism in South Africa: Dislodging the Binary between Universal Human Rights and Culture/Tradition." She was a Commissioner for the South African Commission on Gender Equality.

Ruth Groenhout is Professor of Philosophy and Chair of the Philosophy Department at Calvin College, in Grand Rapids, Michigan, where she has taught for eighteen years. Her publications focus on a range of issues in bioethics and an ethics of care, and include *Connected Lives: Human Nature and an Ethics of Care* (Rowman and Littlefield, 2004); *Transforming Care: A Christian Vision of Nursing Practice* (Wm. B. Eerdmans, 2005); *Bioethics: A Reformed Look at Life and Death Choices* (Faith Alive Christian Resources, 2009), and *Feminism, Faith, Philosophy* (Indiana University Press, 2004). She has written a variety of journal articles on issues ranging from the ethics of public health research, to embodiment and the nurse–client encounter, to virtue theory and feminism. She is currently working on a book that analyzes central structures in the healthcare system from the perspective of an ethics of care.

Maurice Hamington is Director of University Studies and Professor of Philosophy at Portland State University. He has authored four books including *Revealing Philosophy* (Thinking Strings, 2013—an interactive e-textbook), *The Social Philosophy of Jane Addams* (University of Illinois Press, 2009), and *Embodied Care* (University of Illinois Press, 2004). He has edited or co-edited six books including *Contemporary Feminist Pragmatism* with Celia Bardwell-Jones (Routledge, 2012), *Applying Care Ethics to Business* with Maureen Sander-Staudt (Springer, 2011), and *Socializing Care* with Dorothy Miller (Rowman and Littlefield, 2006). His current research and writing address an embodied, performative theory of care and its application.

Virginia Held is Distinguished Professor of Philosophy at the City University of New York, Graduate School, and Professor Emerita at Hunter College. Her books include *The Ethics of Care: Personal, Political, and Global* (Oxford University Press, 2006); *The Public Interest and Individual Interests* (Basic Books, 1970); *Rights and Goods: Justifying Social Action* (Free Press, 1984); *Feminist Morality: Transforming Culture, Society, and Politics* (University of Chicago Press, 1993); and *How Terrorism is Wrong* (Oxford University Press, 2008), as well as several edited collections. In 2001–2 she was President of the Eastern Division of the American Philosophical Association. She has also taught at Yale, Dartmouth, UCLA, and Hamilton, and has five grandchildren.

Eva Feder Kittay is Distinguished Professor of Philosophy and Senior Fellow, Center for Medical Humanities, Compassionate Care, and Bioethics at Stony Brook University. She has authored and edited several books, including *Love's Labor: Women, Equality and Dependency*, and *Cognitive Disability and its Challenge to Moral Philosophy*. She has authored numerous journal articles and book chapters on feminist philosophy, care ethics, and disability theory and philosophy of language. She is a co-winner of the APA and Phi Beta Kappa Leibowitz Award, as well as Guggenheim and NEH Fellowships to complete her *Disabled Minds and Things that Matter: Cognitive Disability and (a Humbler) Philosophy*.

Rita Manning, PhD, is a Professor (and past Chair) of Philosophy at San José State University. She is the author of *Speaking from the Heart: A Feminist Perspective on Ethics* (Rowman and Littlefield, 1992), *Guide to Practical Ethics: Living and Leading with Integrity*, co-authored with Scott Stroud (Westview Press, 2008), and *Social Justice in a Diverse Society*, co-edited with René Trujillo (Mayfield Press, 1996). She has published articles and book chapters in the fields of moral philosophy, applied ethics (business ethics, healthcare ethics, and environmental ethics), philosophy of law, social and political philosophy, feminism, and critical thinking. Her most recent works are "Immigration Detention and the Right to Health Care," in *Global Bioethics and Human Rights: Contemporary Issues*, edited by Wanda Teays et al. (Rowman and Littlefield, 2014) and "Punishing the Innocent: Children of Incarcerated and Detained Parents" (*Criminal Justice Ethics*, 2011).

Nel Noddings is Lee Jacks Professor of Education Emerita, Stanford University. She is a past president of the National Academy of Education, Philosophy of Education Society, and John Dewey Society. In addition to nineteen books, she is the author of more than 200 articles and chapters on various topics, ranging from the ethics of care to mathematical problem solving. Her latest book is *Education and Democracy in the 21st Century* (Teachers College Press, 2013).

Fiona Robinson is Professor of Political Science at Carleton University, Ottawa, Canada; her research and teaching focus on critical, feminist, and ethical theory in global politics. She is the author of *Globalizing Care: Ethics, Feminist Theory and International Relations* (Westview Press, 1999) and *The Ethics of Care: A Feminist Approach to Human Security* (Temple University Press, 2011), and co-editor, with Rianne Mahon, of *Feminist Ethics and Social Politics: Towards a New Global Political Economy of Care* (UBC Press, 2011). In 2014, she was the recipient of the inaugural J. Ann Tickner book prize, which was established in recognition of Professor Tickner's path-breaking scholarship on gender and feminist International Relations, and seeks to recognize the author of a book that helps build practical knowledge to address pressing issues and contribute to a more just and peaceful world.

Maureen Sander-Staudt is an Assistant Professor of Philosophy at Southwest Minnesota State University, where she teaches the philosophy of sex and gender, ethics, and logic. She is the co-editor of *Applying Care Ethics to Business*, with Maurice Hamington (Springer, 2011), and *Maternal Subjects*, with Sheila Lintott (Routledge, 2012). Her journal articles include "The Unhappy Marriage of Care Ethics and Virtue Ethics" (*Hypatia*, 2006) and "Reassembling the Assembly: Care Ethics and Political Agency" (*Journal of Social Philosophy*, 2008). She has written numerous book chapters on topics such as artificial womb technology, hospitality, male lactation, and the comparative moral status of embryos. Her latest writings center around the moral ideal of caring reciprocity.

Michael Slote is UST Professor of Ethics at the University of Miami. He is the author of many articles and books on topics including ethics, philosophy of mind, political philosophy, and philosophy of education. A member of the Royal Irish Academy and former Tanner Lecturer, his most recent books include: *A Sentimentalist Theory of the Mind* (Oxford University Press, 2014); *From Enlightenment to Receptivity* (Oxford University Press, 2013); and *Education and Human Values* (Routledge, 2012). He is currently working on book-length projects in philosophical anthropology and virtue epistemology.

Joan C. Tronto is Professor of Political Science at the University of Minnesota–Twin Cities. She is the author of dozens of essays about the ethics of care as well as *Moral*

Boundaries: A Political Argument for an Ethic of Care (Routledge, 1993) and *Caring Democracy: Markets, Equality, and Justice* (New York University Press, 2013).

Julie Anne White is Associate Professor of Political Science and Director of the Program in Women's, Gender, and Sexuality Studies at Ohio University. She is the author of *Democracy, Justice and the Welfare State: Reconstructing Public Care* (Penn State University Press, 2000). Article-length work has appeared in the *Journal of Politics, Affilia, Law and Social Inquiry*, and *Gender and Politics*. Her current project examines the relationship between the organization of care work and the politics of resentment in the contemporary context.

Mikki van Zyl was a feminist and lifelong gender and social justice activist who had been working as a consultant in the NGO sector. She wrote, lectured, researched, and conducted training on same-sex sexualities, gender activism, homophobia and hate crimes, gender-based violence, HIV and AIDS, ethics of care, diversity, disability, land issues, and participatory action research. Her recent publications included two edited volumes (with Melissa Steyn)—*Performing Queer* (Kwela, 2005) and *The Prize and the Price* (HSRC Press, 2009)—on post-apartheid sexualities in South Africa. She also published short stories and poems in Afrikaans and English. Mikki passed away suddenly in February 2015, just after she completed her PhD at the University of Stellenbosch on gay marriages, citizenship, and belonging. Her loss to the feminist community of scholars is immense.

1

Introduction

Daniel Engster and Maurice Hamington

What contribution does care ethics make to contemporary political analysis? The answer varies, of course, by the practice, policy, or issue being analyzed. Most generally, though, care ethics offers a new orientation to social and political thinking and brings to light a different set of issues. In care ethics, the center of moral action is shifted from interactions among citizens in the public forum and marketplace to personal relationships. Starting at home, as Nel Noddings (2002b) has argued, with the practices and values of good personal care, care ethics challenges us to rethink the nature and purpose of politics and the political vocabulary of justice, freedom, privacy, and the like in terms of what is necessary for promoting and sustaining good personal care. Care ethics ultimately points toward a more relational perspective on social and political problems that eschews simplistic judgments about right or wrong isolated from all context, for a more complete understanding of persons and actions enmeshed in relationships and situated in their environment.

Consider, for example, the contemporary issue of human trafficking. Although accurate statistics are challenging to find, human trafficking is a worldwide tragedy affecting as many as 27 million people in 166 countries and generating $32 billion (US) in profits annually (Polaris Project). Defined as a severe form of exploitation involving labor or sex through the use of force, fraud, or coercion, human trafficking is often referred to as modern-day slavery and a violation of human rights. However, the intricacies of the cases can make moral adjudication very difficult. The following case is emblematic.

On 3 April 2002, Marita Veron was kidnapped in San Miguel de Tucumán, Argentina, where it is believed that she was forced into prostitution. After a decade of pursuit, those accused of kidnapping and enslaving Veron were brought to trial, resulting in an acquittal at first, but, after protests and an intervention by the Argentine president, they were convicted (Bennett 2013). One of the convicted traffickers was Daniela Natalia Milhein, whose personal journey was brought to light in court testimony. Milhein herself had been forced into the sex trade at age 16. Trapped into the industry, Milhein eventually rose to run a sex trafficking ring out of her house. Witness testimony indicated that Milhein did not use physical force but convinced young women that they were in the trade out of personal choice and a desire to be wealthy.

Care ethics approaches issues such as human trafficking, and the Veron case in particular, by asking: how could human relationships have gone so fundamentally wrong? Analyzing human trafficking through the lens of care ethics, Olena Hankivsky notes that many women migrate from their home country in search of a means of caring for their families, only to become exploited in systems of trafficking. We must then begin our analysis from this starting point in care—not at the courtroom trial stage—in order to more fully understand this issue. We must further look beyond individuals in order to understand the choices of these women. The economy and state often fail to provide sufficient support to families in need, driving many women into precarious circumstances in the first place. Hankivsky finds "'repressive' strategies that focus on how to stop migration or that create legal responses to and result in prosecution of traffickers" inadequate (Hankivsky 2011, 160–1). Although Daniela Natalia Milhein is responsible for the pain and suffering she brought to many young women, so too is society responsible for creating conditions that would force a 16-year-old Milhein into the sex industry. The victim/perpetrator dichotomy is problematized and reframed in the context of care. And even though the victims in trafficking cases clearly benefit from being liberated from their captors, liberation for these individuals often means social and economic instability, if not destitution, without social or state support. Lacking education and job training, some victims may even return to lives of prostitution. Long-term and more comprehensive responses are needed to make people and their relationships whole.

Using a care framework, Fiona Robinson similarly situates human trafficking as an outgrowth of systems imbued with masculine bias. She claims that a critical care ethics "seeks to interrogate how and why hegemonic forms of masculinity license men's neglect of caring responsibilities and contribute to the manipulation of images of care and womanhood into images of female subservience and sexual service" (2011, 79). Like Hankivisky, Robinson broadens the responsibility for oppressive behavior but emphasizes particular social constructions of gender. The analysis of Hankivsky and Robinson on human trafficking makes it clear that employing a care approach does not simply mean that a new set of values are brought to bear on this geopolitical issue; rather, care alters the moral landscape in both understanding the issue and formulating an ethical response. It directs us to consider both how issues of care lie behind contemporary problems and how we can better address these problems by providing better care for all.

The richness and potential of care ethics has drawn many theorists from different fields to rethink existing philosophies, practices, and policies. As the human trafficking example demonstrates, care ethics has been applied to a wide variety of questions and issues. An outstanding selection of care theorists and issues is represented in the pages that follow. The introduction provides a context for these chapters. We begin with a definition and overview of the contemporary evolution of care theorizing.

What is Care Ethics?

There is no universally accepted definition of care ethics. Although care theorists' disagreement on this basic matter might seem a weakness, it can also be seen as a sign of care ethics' maturity. There is similarly no one definition of liberalism, libertarianism, socialism, or the capabilities approach, but instead a range of different, sometimes competing understandings. This is the normal course of things. Theories tend to grow through a process of diversification. One thinker finds something lacking in a previous theorist's ideas and puts forth a new theory to correct it. The first theorist responds with a defense of her views and a slight divide enters the field. So it is with care ethics. As evidenced just in this volume, some theorists regard care ethics primarily as a form of virtue ethics; others argue that it should be understood as a form of consequentialism or practice-based theory.

What binds care theories together, as with other schools of thought, is not a doctrinaire commitment to a singular understanding of the theory, but a general endorsement of a number of different themes (for a similar approach, see Held 2006, 9–15). Among the most important of these themes in care ethics are:

1. *A relational approach to morality*. Relational considerations are primary in care ethics. Care theorists suggest that humans are fundamentally relational and interdependent. As Robinson describes, "the relational ontology of care ethics claims that relations of interdependence and dependence are a fundamental feature of our existence" (Robinson 2011, 4).
2. *Responsiveness to the other*. Care is often defined as a response to an expressed need (Noddings 2002b, 53). "What is definitive about care...," Joan Tronto writes (1993, 105), "seems to be a perspective of taking the other's needs as the starting point for what must be done."

At least according to some care theorists (see Kittay in this volume), care is not complete without the other's response. This emphasis on responsiveness has led a number of care theorists to view epistemology as a significant element of care (Dalmiya 2002).

3. *Context matters.* Unlike traditional abstract and universal Western theories of ethics, care ethics values particularism. An authentically caring response is unique and individualized. It requires understanding the particularities of the other's experience, including their history, relative power, relationships, and so forth.
4. *Crossing moral boundaries.* Given its feminist roots, care ethics embraces the dictum that the "personal is political," such that caring should not be a compartmentalized activity of a few people in the private sphere. In her original formulation of a political theory of care, Tronto indicated that at least three moral boundaries needed to be redrawn: the divide between morality and politics, the divide between disinterested ethical theory and particularist approaches, and the divide between public and private life (1993, 6–10). Care challenges the established contours of ethical theory.
5. *Emotions as informative and motivating moral tools.* Breaking with Western moral tradition, care theorists embrace positive roles for emotions in helping to create empathetic connections that promote caring actions. "The ethics of care values emotion rather than rejects it" (Held 2006, 10). Some care theorists (Slote 2007; 2010) have even defined care ethics in terms of the judgments associated with a fully developed sense of empathy.

Different theorists construct their definition of care ethics differently, but all care theorists give at least some attention to these five themes.

A Burgeoning Field of Study

Care ethics has grown over the last three decades from a personal ethical perspective to a full-bodied moral and political theory. Retrospective genealogies have been created that trace aspects of care theory back to moral sentimentalism (Slote 2010; Baier 1987), American pragmatist thought (Hamington 2004), and even Confucianism (Li 1994). American feminist theorists are nonetheless usually credited with the development of care ethics in the early 1980s.[1] Virginia Held places the origins of care ethics in Sara Ruddick's essay "Maternal Thinking" (1980), which explored from a philosophical perspective how mothers think or reason and the values that can be drawn out of this thinking (Held 2006, 26). Most people nonetheless associate the birth of care ethics with Carol Gilligan's *In a Different Voice: Psychological*

Theory and Women's Development (1982). Analyzing conversations with girls and women about moral issues and problems, Gilligan identified an alternative moral voice that she dubbed "care ethics." Abjuring abstract principles that made moral action seem "like a math problem with humans," care ethics by Gilligan's account focused on meeting the needs of others in particular contexts and maintaining relationships with them (1982, 26).

Nel Noddings' *Caring: A Feminine Approach to Ethics and Moral Education* (1984) solidified care ethics' standing as a new ethical theory. As distinct from *In a Different Voice,* which was primarily a work of moral psychology, Noddings' *Caring* offered a broad philosophical definition and defense of care ethics. Noddings constructed a phenomenology of care that emphasized the attentive responsiveness of the care-giver through what she referred to as "engrossment." Noddings, the author or editor of two-dozen books, became the most prolific of the early care theorists.

If the 1980s marked the birth of care ethics in psychology and philosophy, the 1990s witnessed its expansion into political theory. Although early works on care ethics were widely praised and embraced for their revolutionary insights, they were also criticized for their personalized and parochial accounts of care and for essentializing care as a feminine trait. Feminist theorists responded by broadening and clarifying their account of care ethics and carrying it into the realm of political theory. Sara Ruddick's 1989 book, *Maternal Thinking: Toward a Politics of Peace* offered a relational and perspectival approach to morality and politics emphasizing peace and non-violence. In *Feminist Morality: Transforming Culture, Society, and Politics* (1993), Virginia Held drew on some of Ruddick's, Gilligan's, and Noddings' central insights in order to develop a care-inflected feminist philosophy capable of addressing a number of social and political issues. Joan Tronto's *Moral Boundaries: A Political Argument for an Ethic of Care* (1993) more widely and powerfully laid the foundations for care ethics' expansion into political theory. Tronto outlined a broader and by now classic definition of care as "*everything that we do to maintain, continue, and repair our 'world' so that we can live in it as well as possible.* That world includes our bodies, our selves, and our environment, all of which we seek to interweave in a complex, life-sustaining web" (Fisher and Tronto 1991, 40; Tronto 1993, 103). Tronto further divided care into four phases, which have become central to the later analysis of care: 1) "caring about," which involves care recognition; 2) "taking care of," which follows from recognition and is owning or taking responsibility for the need; 3) "care-giving," which is the direct act of giving care; and 4) "care-receiving," which is the responsiveness of the one-caring that completes the feedback loop (Tronto 1993, 105–8). In the final chapter, Tronto offered some initial suggestions for how care ethics might be a tool for political analysis and how care can be framed as a political ideal. Other important works in the early development of care ethics into a political theory include Selma Sevenhuijsen's *Citizenship and the Ethics of Care* (1998), which built upon Tronto's work and extended care ethics into social policy; and Fiona Robinson's *Globalizing Care: Feminist Theory and International Relations* (1999), which applied care ethics to international relations between states as well as cosmopolitan relations among individuals.

By the early 2000s, care ethics was flourishing as a small but growing theory. Philosophers continued to explore the nature of care ethics and its radical implications for our understanding of ourselves and our place in the world (Hamington 2004; Kittay and Feder 2002; Pettersen 2008; Walker 2003; 2006). Although Noddings had published a number of books connecting care theory to education (2002a; 2003; 2007) other educational theorists began to make similar applications (Johnston 2006; Monchinski 2010; Stengel and Tom 2006). Political psychologists used care ethics to explain human behaviors including resistance to injustice (Monroe 1998; 2006). Social scientists used a care framework to compare welfare states and assess welfare policies (Anttonen et al. 2003; Daly and Rake 2003). At least one anthology addressed care and issues of race (Siddle Walker and Snarey 2004). Care ethics was even applied to business ethics (Simola 2007; Hamington and Sander-Staudt 2011). But above all else, the last fifteen years have marked the development of care ethics into a robust political theory. Quite notably, in 2002, Nel Noddings let go of her earlier reservations about the possibility of developing care ethics into a political theory and outlined a broad-ranging account of social policies rooted in an ethics of care. Numerous other works appeared in the following years that developed political theories based on care ethics for both national and international affairs (Hankivsky 2004; Hamington and Miller 2006; Held 2006; Slote 2001; 2007; 2010; Engster 2007; Robinson 2011; Mahon and Robinson 2011; Tronto 2013; Koggel and Orme 2013).

The contemporary care theory movement is young enough that many of the foundational theorists have continued to contribute to its growth during care's turn to the political. In *Joining the Resistance*, Carol Gilligan claims that the "feminist ethic of care is integral to the struggle to release democracy from the grip of patriarchy" (2011, 177). Similarly, Joan Tronto's (2013) and Nel Noddings' (2010) recent works demonstrate innovative applications of care ethics to politics.

Care ethics is regularly held up today as an equal in normative political theory to such theories as Rawlsian liberalism, luck egalitarianism, libertarianism, the capabilities approach, communitarianism, and the like. After roughly a thirty-year gestation and development, care ethics has emerged as an important alternative to politics-as-usual and just in time to help us reconsider some of the new and pressing issues confronting us in our diverse and globalized world.

Why Care Ethics and Political Theory? Why Now?

There are two overlapping reasons motivating this exploration of care ethics and political theory: one is scholarly and the other is social/political. In terms of the scholarly motivation, despite all the progress that care theorists have made toward developing care ethics into a viable political theory, significant disagreements and gaps remain. For example, the central issue of care's relation to justice continues to be a point of debate. How exactly care ethics might guide our thinking about civil freedoms, privacy, jurisprudence, healthcare, and so forth also still remains ambiguous. The essays in this book take on these issues.

The other motivation for this volume is the seeming urgency of developing a new political theory that can usefully guide analysis and action under contemporary conditions. We are at a crucial juncture in world history as many formerly colonized and underdeveloped countries are beginning to undergo significant political and economic reforms. For many of these countries, particularly those with more communal-based cultures and traditions, liberalism has limited value or appeal. Care ethics, however, has readily identifiable roots in these cultures and thus can better engage with them and help to guide them toward a more just future. Contemporary social analyses rooted in individualistic ontologies likewise no longer seem to get things right in our increasingly interrelated and networked society. Care ethics provides here, too, a better way of understanding and coping with the important transitions we are undergoing. As the chapters in this volume should make clear, care ethics offers us an opportunity to reset some of our central assumptions about human beings and politics, and to re-examine the world from a more relational (and potentially more useful) perspective.

Although this book cannot address all the important topics that a new political paradigm should, it gestures toward many of them. By applying care ethics to new topic areas and highlighting its radical potential, we hope this volume can lay the new foundation for the continuing and fuller development of care ethics as a political theory in the future.

The Editors

Although care ethics grew out of women's experience and feminist analysis, it has garnered increasingly widespread intellectual attention from feminist and non-feminist scholars, including greater numbers of men. This development is not without controversy. Some feminist theorists understandably argue that men cannot be feminists or at least must come to the theorizing with significant humility, given that they have not experienced gender discrimination and oppression. The idea that standpoint matters has always been important to feminist theory. Some theorists might worry that care ethics will be coopted and lose its feminist edge. Others might contend that care theory, like feminist theory, obtains a certain level of maturity through widespread application and that more engagement by men and scholars—identified as feminist or not—is a healthy sign of the mainstreaming of some aspects of feminist theory.

Although a number of men, including Lawrence A. Blum, Daniel Engster, Maurice Hamington, Bill Puka, and Michael Slote, have written about care ethics, *Care Ethics and Political Theory* is the first edited volume organized and edited by two men. This development might raise some eyebrows, but it is part of an ongoing intellectual trajectory. More male theorists are accepting the label of feminist and even more are applying the intellectual fruits of various feminist theories. The ultimate test of *Care Ethics and Political Theory* is whether the chapters contained within it contribute to a more robust application and understanding of care, as well as whether the volume advances a feminist agenda of inclusion, social melioration, and challenging identity-based oppression.

Both Daniel Engster and Maurice Hamington view the work of developing and enriching care ethics and its political dimensions as more than an intellectual exercise. For us, this work is not detached analytical work but an effort at changing policies and practices to create a better—a more caring—society.

The Organization of the Book

As befits a volume on care ethics, the chapters in this volume form a crisscrossing web of questions, themes, and arguments that is not easily captured by a standard linear organization of chapters. While we have grouped chapters into four parts organized around general themes, most chapters overlap with one or more chapters from other parts of the book. There are, in fact, any number of creative ways that we might have organized this volume. Readers will find common threads running through the different chapters and parts.

Part I addresses general questions about the relationship between care ethics and justice theories. These chapters not only offer diverse and interesting perspectives on care and justice, but because of the foundational nature of the questions they discuss, they also offer an excellent introduction to care ethics.

The first part begins with an updated account of a long-standing argument. Carol Gilligan (1982, 164–5, 173–4) originally drew the distinction between justice and care, associating justice with rights, rules, and equality, and care with responsibility, meeting needs in context, and equity. Nel Noddings (1984) reinforced this distinction by portraying justice as universal, impartial, and principled, and care as particular, personal, and situational. As care theorists began to translate care ethics into a political theory, however, the usefulness of this original distinction was questioned and theorists began to reconsider the relationship between care ethics and justice theories.

Virginia Held was one of first theorists to explore the relationship between care and justice from a broad moral and political perspective (Held 1995). Quite fittingly, then, Held's chapter, "Care and justice, still" opens this volume. Held argues for maintaining the distinction between care and justice that Gilligan and Noddings originally outlined. Arguing against the general trend of care theorizing in recent years, she contends that we should not attempt to develop theories of justice that include care but instead develop an alternative moral theory of care that has priority over theories of justice. We nonetheless still need justice, Held contends, but care ethics is the broader moral framework within which justice theories should be applied. Held thus devotes much of her chapter to identifying the different domains in which justice might usefully be given prominence.

In his chapter, "Care ethics and liberalism," Michael Slote outlines a position on the care and justice debate nearly the opposite of Held's. If care ethics is to represent a systematic alternative to existing justice theories, Slote argues, it should be able to speak persuasively about all matters, including legal and political issues. Relying on liberal justice principles to guide policy and practice in important domains of life such as law or civil rights represents, from Slote's perspective, an admission of care ethics' inadequacy and results in an inconsistent hybrid philosophy. Not only can care ethics provide a coherent account of political liberties such as religious toleration and free speech, Slote argues, but it actually offers a better approach to these issues than liberalism. Slote's chapter is particularly interesting for the concrete examples he uses to demonstrate his points. By offering practical examples of how care ethics can guide thinking about civil freedoms, Slote supplies the reader with tangible material for assessing the adequacy of his claims, and hence for thinking more deeply about Held's and Slote's different arguments about care and justice.

Eva Kittay's chapter, "A theory of justice as fair terms of social life given our inevitable dependency and our inextricable interdependency," passes over the care and justice debate fairly quickly in order to identify the central features of a care-based theory of justice. Although Kittay agrees with Slote and others that care ethics can form the basis for a theory of justice, she argues that the unique nature of care ethics gives a different focus to a care-based justice theory. Concentrating on the dependencies we all experience and our inextricable interdependence with others, Kittay outlines eight concepts and four main principles of a theory of justice guided by an ethic of care. Especially noteworthy in Kittay's chapter is her discussion of a refined principle of doulia, which further develops one of the main political theoretical concepts originally outlined in her important book *Love's Labor* (1999).

Nel Noddings' "Care ethics and 'caring' organizations" rounds out the first part. In the care and justice debate, Noddings sides with Slote, Kittay, and others who argue that care ethics can provide the foundation of a justice theory. Noddings' concern, however, is not so much with the care and justice debate as with how care ethics can inform justice theories without replicating the shortcomings of traditional justice theories. Drawing a number of important distinctions, Noddings cautions against applying the adjective "caring" to institutions or organizations. Institutions and organizations can care about individuals but not directly care-for them. The proper role of institutions and organizations should be to establish the conditions under which personal caring-for can take place. Much of Noddings' chapter discusses the implications of this idea for policy making, highlighting the different approach that care ethics brings to social policy issues.

The second part of the book, "Applications," opens with Maxine Eichner's chapter, "The supportive state: government, dependency, and responsibility for caretaking," which provides a bridge of sorts between the chapters in Part I and those in Part II. Eichner considers how the role of the state in liberal theory changes once the centrality of dependency in human lives is recognized. As opposed to the views of both Held and Slote, therefore, her argument aims to synthesize liberal political theory and care ethics. Eichner's focus, however, is not on the care and justice debate but on describing a new model for the liberal state: the supportive state. Eichner specifically discusses how a synthesis of liberalism and care ethics changes the way we think about families and the role that the state should play in liberal theory in fostering good care within them.

Marilyn Friedman's chapter, "Privacy, surveillance, and care ethics," applies the themes of justice and care developed in the first part to a society's conflicting needs for privacy and security. Friedman analyzes the current US context to explore whether a society guided by care ethics can support national security efforts associated with surveillance programs and simultaneously uphold privacy rights. Although feminist theorists have sometimes doubted whether care ethics can deal effectively with concepts such as security and privacy, and whether these values should be included in a care ethical framework, Friedman argues affirmatively in both regards. Friedman ultimately does not spell out how states should balance their commitments to security versus privacy under care ethics, but her discussion of these values particularly at the end of her chapter is highly suggestive.

In "Care, normativity, and the law," Rita Manning explores how care ethics can be incorporated into the law and legal reasoning. After briefly reviewing Robin West's and Carrie Menkel-Meadow's arguments for the importance of care ethics in the law, Manning provides a detailed analysis of several important legal decisions in order to demonstrate how care ethics might find a place in judicial decision making. Discussing the important biomedical case of *Moore* v. *Regents of the University of California* regarding informed consent to use bodily tissue for research and ultimately financial gain, Manning demonstrates the superiority of care ethics over deontological and consequentialist legal theories. Care ethics represents, by her account, a necessary corrective to existing frameworks for interpreting and applying the law.

Ruth Groenhout's chapter, "Of medicine and monsters: rationing and an ethics of care," addresses the significant contemporary issue of medical rationing. As many people have pointed out, the rationing of medical resources is inevitable in one form or another. Medical resources may be rationed by the ability of individuals to pay, by national health services, or by some other means, but some limits must be imposed or medical care will consume all our resources. Medical rationing nonetheless presents a particular challenge to care ethics, Groenhout argues, because any denial of potentially beneficial medical services to sick or injured persons seems a failure of care. Here again, then, it might seem that care ethics cannot adequately deal with complex moral and policy issues. Groenhout, however, persuasively refutes this view, arguing that care ethics supports a distinction between personal relationships and institutionalized and professional care, and allows for principled boundaries in professional care that it may not recognize in personal care. Groenhout's distinction between personal and institutional care has resonances with Noddings' distinction between caring-for and caring about in Part I, and further extends thinking about the application of care ethics to political and institutional organizations.

Part III explores the ways in which care ethics can inform and guide moral and political theory in non-Western cultures, and how studying non-Western and subaltern societies can improve upon our understanding of a public ethics of care. In the opening chapter of this part, "Towards a feminist ethics of *ubuntu*: bridging rights and *ubuntu*," Amanda Gouws and Mikki van Zyl argue that neither liberal rights theory nor the indigenous African ethic of *ubuntu* provides an adequate basis for developing an inclusive justice theory in South Africa. Noting the many similarities between *ubuntu* and care ethics, however, Gouws and van Zyl argue that the latter can serve to guide the reform and expansion of the former in a way that provides a basis for justice in South Africa with roots in the indigenous culture. Importantly, Gouws and van Zyl also discuss the relationship between care ethics, *ubuntu*, and a restorative (as opposed to punitive) approach to criminal justice. This last topic provides for an interesting linkage with Manning's discussion of care and jurisprudence, and offers another perspective on how care ethics might inform and change the practice of law.

In "Caring reciprocity as a relational and political ideal in Confucianism and care ethics," Maureen Sander-Staudt explores the relationship between care ethics and Confucianism. Skillfully sorting through the numerous different perspectives that exist on this topic, Sander-Staudt concludes that although care ethics and Confucianism are not fully compatible they are closely related and can usefully learn from each other. Focusing specifically on the concept of reciprocity, she shows that the Confucian ideal of reciprocity can help care theorists to develop a better understanding of this concept and its potential role in a political ethic of care, while care ethics can help to develop a "reconstructed Confucianism" devoid of most of its paternalistic and hierarchical elements and better suited for Chinese life today.

The final chapter in this part, Julie Anne White's "Practicing care at the margins other-mothering as public care," adopts a similar strategy to Sander-Staudt for improving care ethics, while at the same time beckoning toward more radical political conclusions. White looks to the practice of shared childrearing, or "other-mothering," in African-American communities for inspiration in developing a public ethic of care. Other-mothering is particularly valuable in this regard, White argues, because as a grass-roots communal care practice it resists privatization and commodification. White contends that careful attention to this practice can enhance our understanding of a public ethic of care by challenging taken-for-granted understandings of caregiving responsibilities, pluralizing our understanding of care and vulnerability, and perhaps most importantly, helping us to see how care as an intimate practice can be linked to care as political struggle. Importantly, White, like Sander-Staudt, demonstrates that political theorizing about care does not have to exclusively emerge from mainstream Western practices.

The last part of the book, "Challenging Dominant Paradigms," explores the potential for care ethics to overturn existing moral and political paradigms and offer a positive new way forward. In "Care in the state of nature," Daniel Engster draws on evidence from evolutionary theory, biology, ethology, and developmental psychology in order to argue that human beings are innately disposed to care for one another. Engster uses this evidence to challenge classic state of nature and social contract theories that typically portray human beings as isolated, combative, and relatively unsocial. In the real state of nature, Engster argues, human beings would have naturally formed into small communities based on relations of care. However, he also notes that our innate caring dispositions tend to incline us toward parochial care. Re-imagining the state of nature around these communities of care, Engster argues that the main moral and political problem is not so much to generate moral concern and political order out of anarchy as to help individuals to expand their moral and political circles of care to include unfamiliar others. In arguing this way, Engster offers an alternative care-based paradigm for thinking about morality and politics that challenges traditional liberal and statist conceptions.

Joan Tronto's chapter offers up care ethics as a superior framework for thinking about and addressing the challenges of our increasingly interconnected and dynamic world. Tronto's particular focus is on Ulrich Beck's influential account of the risk society. The general contours of Beck's risk society are familiar enough: economic uncertainty, environmental degradation, terrorist threats. But Tronto asks: for whom exactly are these risks new? And are such risks really so out of our control as Beck suggests? Beck's assessment of risks is rooted, by Tronto's account, in a privileged, masculinist, and individualistic worldview. Care ethics, by contrast, provides a better framework for understanding contemporary social changes and how human beings might morally respond to them. From the perspective of care ethics, "risk" is not something that just happens but is something that particular individuals and institutions are responsible for creating. Care ethics also reminds us that risk is something that has always affected all of us—not something new and external to us—and directs us to get along with the important task of finding better ways to cope with it.

Maurice Hamington's chapter, "Politics is not a game the radical potential of care," picks up on some of the themes from Tronto's chapter, highlighting the radical potential of care ethics to reorder our understanding of morality and politics. Hamington argues that care ethics represents a paradigm shift in thinking about morality that is not always appreciated by those who attempt to fit it into existing philosophical categories. Following Noddings and others, Hamington argues that care ethics cannot be captured by principles but is necessarily a performative theory based on iterative acts of care. This alternative approach to ethics has profound implications for morality and politics. As the title of Hamington's chapter indicates, care ethics transforms politics from a game with winners and losers, rules and responsibilities, into a relational endeavor involving authentic contextual engagement with diverse others for the sake of expanding the circle of care.

In "Care ethics, political theory, and the future of feminism," Fiona Robinson explores the ability of care ethics to provide a way forward for feminism. Feminism is in crisis, according to Robinson, due in large part to its failure to adequately deal with the concerns of marginalized and Third World women, post-structuralist critiques of gender and power, and an increasingly pronounced neoliberal influence on women's visions of empowerment. Although some feminists have been suspicious of care ethics, Robinson argues that a critical care ethics can provide the basis for a transnational feminist politics rooted not in fixed notions of gender identity but in the life-sustaining value of care. Care ethics provides a critical lens, by Robinson's account, to challenge existing hierarchies and injustices in interpersonal, national, and global relations, and affect meaningful, if not necessarily revolutionary change, by bringing to the forefront of public debate hard questions about the traditional devaluation of care and its association with gender.

The chapters in this volume offer numerous insights and raise many questions and will, we hope, help to stimulate the next wave of thinking about care ethics and political theory.

Note

1. An independent European tradition of theorizing about caregiving and care work was meanwhile being developed by scholars such as Hilary Graham, Clare Ungerson, and Kari Waerness.

References

Anttonen, Anneli, Jorma Sipila, and John Baldock. 2003. "Patterns of Social Care in Five Industrial Societies: Explaining Diversity." In *The Young, The Old and the State: Social Care Systems in Five Industrial Countries*, edited by Anneli Anttonen, John Baldock, and Jorma Sipila, 167–97. Cheltenham: Edward Elgar.

Baier, Annette. 1987. "Hume, The Women's Moral Theorist?" In *Women and Moral Theory*, edited by Eva Feder Kittay and Diana T. Meyers, 37–55. Lanham, MD: Rowman and Littlefield.

Bennett, Tess. "Court Convicts 10 of 13 Defendants in Marita Verón Case." *The Argentina Independent*, 17 December 2013. <http://www.argentinaindependent.com/currentaffairs/court-convicts-10-of-13-defendants-in-marita-veron-case/>

Dalmiya, Vrinda. 2002. "Why Should a Knower Care?" *Hypatia* 17(1): 34–52.

Daly, Mary, and Katherine Rake. 2003. *Gender and the Welfare State*. Malden, MA: Polity.

Engster, Daniel. 2007. *The Heart of Justice: Care Ethics and Political Theory*. Oxford: Oxford University Press.

Fisher, Berenice, and Joan C. Tronto. 1991. "Toward a Feminist Theory of Caring." In *Circles of Care: Work and Identity in Women's Lives*, edited by Emily Abel and Margaret Nelson, 35–62. Albany, NY: State University of New York Press.

Gilligan, Carol. 1982. *In a Different Voice: Psychological Theory and Women's Development*. Cambridge, MA: Harvard University Press.

Gilligan, Carol. 2011. *Joining the Resistance*. Cambridge: Polity.

Hamington, Maurice. 2004. *Embodied Care: Jane Addams, Maurice Merleau-Ponty, and Feminist Ethics*. Urbana, IL: University of Illinois Press.

Hamington, Maurice, and Dorothy Miller (eds.). 2006. *Socializing Care: Feminist Ethics and Public Issues*. Lanham, Maryland: Rowman and Littlefield.

Hamington, Maurice, and Maureen Sander-Staudt (eds.). 2011. *Applying Care Ethics to Business*. New York: Springer.

Hankivsky, Olena. 2004. *Social Policy and the Ethic of Care*. Vancouver: UBC Press.

Hankivsky, Olena. 2011. "The Dark Side of Care: The Push Factors in Human Trafficking." In *Feminist Ethics and Social Policy*, edited by Rianne Mahon and Fiona Robinson, 145–61. Vancouver: UBC Press.

Held, Virginia. 1993. *Feminist Morality: Transforming Culture, Society and Politics.* Chicago, IL: University of Chicago Press.

Held, Virginia. 1995. "The Meshing of Care and Justice." *Hypatia* 10(2): 128–32.

Held, Virginia. 2006. *The Ethics of Care: Personal, Political, and Global.* New York: Oxford.

Johnston, D. Kay. 2006. *Education for a Caring Society: Classroom Relationships and Moral Action.* New York: Teachers College Press.

Kittay, Eva. 1999. *Love's Labor: Essays on Women, Equality, and Dependency.* New York: Routledge.

Kittay, Eva Feder, and Ellen K. Feder (eds.). 2002. *The Subject of Care: Feminist Perspectives on Dependency.* Lanham, MD: Rowman and Littlefield.

Koggel, Christine, and Joan Orme. 2013. *Care Ethics: New Theories and Applications.* New York: Routledge.

Li, Chenyang. 1994. "The Confucian Concept of *Jen* and the Feminist Ethics of Care: A Comparative Study." *Hypatia* 9(1): 70–89.

Mahon, Rianne, and Fiona Robinson (eds.). 2011. *Feminist Ethics and Social Policy: Towards a New Global Political Economy of Care.* Vancouver: UBC Press.

Monchinski, Tony. 2010. *Education in Hope: Critical Pedagogies and the Ethic of Care.* New York: Peter Lang.

Monroe, Kristen Renwick. 1998. *The Heart of Altruism: Perceptions of a Common Humanity.* Princeton, NJ: Princeton University Press.

Monroe, Kristen Renwick. 2006. *The Hand of Compassion: Portraits of Moral Choice during the Holocaust.* Princeton, NJ: Princeton University Press.

Noddings, Nel. 1984. *Caring: A Feminine Approach to Ethics and Moral Education.* Berkeley, CA: University of California Press.

Noddings, Nel. 2002a. *Educating Moral People: A Caring Alternative to Character Education.* New York: Teachers College Press.

Noddings, Nel. 2002b. *Starting at Home: Caring and Social Policy.* Berkeley, CA: University of California Press.

Noddings, Nel. 2003. *Happiness and Education.* Cambridge: Cambridge University Press.

Noddings, Nel. 2007. *Philosophy of Education,* 2nd ed. Boulder, CO: Westview Press.

Noddings, Nel. 2010. *The Maternal Factor: Two Paths to Morality.* Berkeley, CA: University of California Press.

Pettersen, Tove. 2008. *Comprehending Care: Problems and Possibilities in the Ethics of Care.* Lanham, MD: Lexington Books.

Polaris Project. "Human Trafficking Statistics." <http://www.cicatelli.org/titlex/downloadable/human%20trafficking%20statistics.pdf> [accessed 7/25/14].

Robinson, Fiona. 1999. *Globalizing Care: Feminist Theory and International Relations.* Boulder, CO: Westview Press.

Robinson, Fiona. 2011. *The Ethics of Care: A Feminist Approach to Human Security.* Philadelphia, PA: Temple University Press.

Ruddick, Sara. 1989. *Maternal Thinking: Toward a Politics of Peace.* Boston, MA: Beacon Press.

Sevenhuijsen, Selma. 1998. *Citizenship and the Ethics of Care: Feminist Considerations on Justice, Morality and Politics.* London: Routledge.

Siddle Walker, Vanessa, and John R. Snarey. 2004. *Race-ing Moral Formation: African American Perspectives on Care and Justice.* New York: Teachers College Press.

Simola, Sheldene K. 2007. "The Pragmatics of Care in Sustainable Global Enterprise." *Journal of Business Ethics* (74)2: 179–88.

Slote, Michael. 2001. *Morals from Motives*. Oxford: Oxford University Press.

Slote, Michael. 2007. *The Ethics of Care and Empathy*. New York: Routledge.

Slote, Michael. 2010. *Moral Sentimentalism*. New York: Oxford University Press.

Stengel, Barbara S., and Alan R. Tom. 2006. *Moral Matters: Five Ways to Develop the Moral Life of Schools*. New York: Teachers College Press.

Tronto, Joan C. 1993. *Moral Boundaries: A Political Argument for an Ethic of Care*. New York: Routledge.

Tronto, Joan C. 2013. *Caring Democracy: Markets, Equality, and Justice*. New York: New York University Press.

Walker, Margaret Urban. 2003. *Moral Contexts*. Lanham, MD: Rowman and Littlefield.

Walker, Margaret Urban. 2006. *Moral Repair: Reconstructing Moral Relations after Wrongdoing*. Cambridge: Cambridge University Press.

Part I

Care and Justice

2

Care and justice, still

Virginia Held

How should we understand justice and care and the relation between them? I have been thinking about this question for over twenty years. I published an early paper called "The Meshing of Care and Justice" in 1995 trying to answer the question, but I am still trying to figure out what to think. However, unlike some questions on which I have given up—such as "what is a social relation?"—I have not given up on this one. I think it is becoming clearer. And so this chapter is an attempt to show how.[1]

From its beginnings, the ethics of care has been developed in contrast with the ethics of justice. I locate the beginnings of what I mean by the ethics of care in the early 1980s, with Sara Ruddick's exploration of mothering and the thinking it involves, Nel Noddings' phenomenological account of caring, and Carol Gilligan's psychological accounts of different and gender-related interpretations of moral problems. I mean by the ethics of care the new, feminist moral outlook and theory that have developed by paying attention to, and recognizing the moral relevance and importance of, previously discounted caring practices (Held 2006).

These practices were very different from the legal and political ones that the dominant normative moral theories of Kantian ethics and utilitarian consequentialism seemed designed to guide. Moral theory was concerned almost entirely with universal principles and rules, with impartial judgments, with rights and obligations, or with the interests of self versus the interests of all. Accompanying political theory focused on hypothetical contractual agreements, on universal rights, and on maximizing individual interests in a version of a marketplace. Questions about what we ought to do were to be answered by rational deduction from abstract rule to particular case, or rational calculation of costs and benefits. To motivate persons to act as they should, the dominant theories looked to rational recognition of the Categorical Imperative or the Principle of Utility.

Practices of Care

The practices of care we started to pay attention to called for very different approaches and values. A mother taking care of a small child for whom she is responsible does not pit her own interests against those of the child, aiming to maximize her interests in competition with the child's, or altruistically her child's at her own expense. Although taking care of children is full of conflict, parents aim at the relation between themselves and their children being loving, trusting, and considerate. They aim at the well-being of their children along with themselves, at what would be best for them *together*, at their mutual interests, rather than at individual gain. They attend closely and receptively to the particular child for whom they are caring, responding to his particular needs with sensitivity and effectiveness. To evaluate whether a parent is caring well for a child, an evaluation must be made as much from the point of view of the child as of the parent. Good care needs to be respectful, to avoid being domineering.

In deciding what to do when caring for a particular child, one relies rather little on universal rules and the rights and duties they imply. One focuses on the particular characteristics of the unique person in one's care, trying to understand her needs and responding to them. Empirical findings on beneficial and harmful effects are important but not morally decisive. One fosters the trust between parent and child so central to a good relation. Rather than relying on rational recognition of the validity of a universal principle to motivate one's actions, one does what is needed because one cares for the child. One's emotions of empathy, sympathy, benevolence, love, motivate the often very burdensome labor of care.

Sometimes, if caring emotions flag and one's actual emotions turn ugly, one may fall back on a sense of *duty* to keep going in a caring task, but one can recognize this as an inferior rather than a superior motive.

Understanding the values in caring work and practices, we can cultivate and promote these values, extending them to others beyond the family. The domain of friendship has many similarities and calls for many similar values. So does the wider social group, and as we explore these values we can see how they can be extended to very distant others. As Hume observed, "the happiness and misery of others are not spectacles entirely indifferent to us..." (Hume 1983/1751, 57) The values of care have vast implications for political and economic activities and institutions, and can be extended to a global context.

Care and Justice

Mothering, taking care of children, caring for the ill and elderly, had not been considered relevant to moral theory, but as feminists started attending to these caring practices they could see that they were extremely relevant. And soon after the philosophical beginnings of the ethics of care emerged, the psychological findings of Carol Gilligan and her colleagues solidified the contrast between the traditional moral theories and the values of care as a contrast between justice and care. Gilligan delineated the two "perspectives" of justice and care, and identified them with a tendency of men to adopt a justice perspective, and a tendency of some women to adopt a care perspective. Gilligan outlined these perspectives as alternative ways to interpret a moral problem (Gilligan 1982). And perhaps I contributed to the solidification of the contrast by publishing a collection of readings called *Justice and Care: Essential Readings in Feminist Ethics* (Held 1995). These readings illustrated the contrasting approaches.

As the perspectives have evolved, we can say that from the perspective of justice one looks for universal rules to apply impartially to particular cases, one considers fairness and the rights and obligations of all, one assumes each person involved to be a free and equal agent. From the perspective of care, in contrast, one attends with sensitivity to particular others in actual historical circumstances, one seeks a satisfactory relation between oneself and these others, one cultivates trust, one responds to needs, aiming at and bringing about as best one can the well-being of the others along with that of oneself. Although they can perhaps be understood most clearly in the personal contexts of family and friends, the values of care are not limited to these. They are values for fellow members of one's community, one's society, and for distant others around the globe.

The perspective of justice conceptualizes persons as autonomous individuals; that of care sees persons as relational. Where justice assumes persons to be independent, care understands that instead of being Hobbesian or Lockean or Kantian individuals, we all start out as helpless infants. Without the care that incorporates different values than those of the dominant moral theories, we would not have survived, and we continue to be interdependent for the rest of our lives, embedded in social relations.

As Grace Clement writes, "[P]rior to the care/justice debate, moral philosophers tended to focus on general principles rather than attention to contextual detail, on the self as an independent individual rather than the self in relation to others, and on varying commitments to equality rather than commitments to maintaining relationships." She concludes that "distortions tend to arise with the exclusive focus on justice considerations and neglect of care considerations." Among many other distortions, "[m]ost moral philosophers... have trivialized women's traditional role as moral educators" (Clement 1996, 110). And by understanding interests purely individualistically, justice can "motivate actions in the interests of others only by requiring that one sacrifice one's own self-interest," whereas care "allows us to understand the extent to which our interests are inseparable from those of others . . . " (111).

Although they have important differences, the dominant moral theories of Kantian ethics and utilitarianism are rationalistic moral theories of justice. The newly explored outlook of care can be developed as an alternative *moral* theory, the ethics of care. The dominant moral theories are based on rational foundations claimed to be universal. They are clearly more suited to widespread acceptance than the varied customs of different traditional social groups and cultures. But the ethics of care is based on experience, experience that really is universal, the experience of having been cared for, without which we would not exist, and the experience of caring.

Gender Bias in Moral Theorizing

I think it's clear we need both justice and care, as outlooks and perspectives, as values of practices and institutions. Unlike Michael Slote, who thinks care as benevolence or compassion can do all the work needed in a moral theory, I think we must call on the principles of justice to champion rights, demand equality, and clarify fairness (Slote 2007; Held 2011a). But unlike those who think traditional moral theories of justice can be revised to handle all our moral concerns, I think care and its related moral theory are essential. So, the question is still: how to integrate them?

Daniel Engster argues that an adequate theory of justice should include adequate attention to care. He thinks that care should be seen as within justice. The title of his book *The Heart of Justice* captures well the idea. Care, he thinks, is the most important part of justice. Without care, no one would even live, let alone live well. "There would be no individual liberty or equality, community values or good life," he writes, "without the caring practices necessary to sustain and foster human life and society" (Engster 2007). Justice should assure that everyone gets the necessary minimums of care. Engster argues that "caring should be placed at the center of a public conception of justice and applied to the basic institutions and policies of society so that more support and accommodation is provided for care work" (13).

Engster's aim is to construct a theory of *justice* that appropriately includes within it an adequate appreciation of care. Fiona Robinson, with more of a focus on international affairs, seems to have a similar view. She is not working to devise a new *moral* theory, an ethics of care, but to see that our existing theories, such as theories of justice and of security, appropriately understand the central importance of care. She shows how and why such theories should pay the kind of attention needed to such global problems as widespread poverty, the migration of care workers, the deficits of care in so many ways and places (Robinson 2011).

I agree that theories of justice for legal and political institutions, and conceptions of security for human beings, should show why we must provide necessary levels of care for all persons. These should be covered by principles of distributive justice and protected by rights to basic necessities, within societies and at the global level (Held 1984). Much of the labor involved in the care that is needed should be paid labor, and not left to families and voluntary organizations to struggle with alone. Societies should take responsibility for care as they should for justice.

I do not agree, however, that moral theories of justice can adequately cover the concerns of care. I do think we need an *alternative moral theory*, the ethics of care, and that this outlook must have priority over political theories of justice.

The approach of Engster and Robinson seems to me to be *applying* a theory of justice to the activities of care. Care is essential to us all. If we lack it, we cannot survive or flourish. Of course, principles of fairness should recognize this, and apply to it: everyone should be able to get the care to which they should be recognized as entitled by right. But thinking this doesn't overthrow the gender hierarchy entrenched in our *theorizing*.

I think we need to do the latter and recognize that we need a new *moral* theory, not just a new application of the dominant justice thinking. I think moral theory should have priority over political theory, and that paying attention to care and its activities and values requires new moral and thus political theorizing, not just a new application of a traditional theory of justice.

Normative moral theory is the most general theory, aspiring to provide guidance for what we should value and how we should act as human beings in any domain of activity from the personal to the political, from worker in healthcare to judge in a courtroom, from parent with a difficult child to friend in a dangerous situation. It aims to be comprehensive.

When we act in more limited roles as citizens or legislators or educators or spouses, we should often or also be guided by more restricted and specific recommendations.

Since we all, at least to some extent, inhabit these different domains simultaneously, it is difficult to sort out the normative recommendations and descriptions of reality appropriate for us and for them. But this has always been the case, and is perhaps less problematic from the perspective of care than from more traditional perspectives.

It was formerly imagined that conceptual order could be achieved by a radical separation of public and private. In public life, men were to be guided by abstract principles of justice for persons assumed to be free, equal, self-interested, and self-sufficient. They were to be governed by institutions to which they could consent from an imagined disinterested position. In the private sphere, in contrast, they were to head households in which their authority would be exercised benevolently without governmental interference.

Contradictions between regarding men as considerate of others in the household and motivated by self-interest beyond were ignored. Contradictions between valuing equality in the public sphere and not valuing it in the family were overlooked.

The gross deficiencies in the conceptualizations of and practices within the domains of public and private have been made clear by feminist critiques. There is by now widespread recognition that the personal is political, that what happens in political life deeply affects the lives of interdependent women and men in the family, and that the values and realities of "private life" have profound implications for public, political life.

Some care theorists accept existing moral theories, such as Kantian ethics, but revise them to include appropriate attention to care, concluding, for instance, that we have a duty to care. I think these too are not going far enough in overthrowing the gender hierarchy in theorizing.

Many, probably most, of those who write about care notice how different its ontological commitments need to be. Understanding care leads us to a relational view of the person, and away from the view of the person as liberal individual: free, equal, autonomous, self-sufficient, adult. The outlook of care understands us as dependent and interdependent. It emphasizes and values caring relations, not just the dispositions or actions of individuals. These views, among others, seem to require a kind of moral theory different from the dominant ones.

The dominant moral theories are closely aligned with the dominant political theories of the past few centuries. I am emphatically not a historian and will not venture a stand—though I wish others would—on whether the moral theories led to the political ones, or the political ones to the moral. I suspect that the dominant moral theories are reflections of the historical development of liberal political, economic, and social institutions and life. But what matters for us here is that they are compatible, they are reflections of each other.

Care theory may be a reflection of the growing influence of women in society, but as a moral theorist, I think moral theory ought to have priority, to guide us on how we ought to organize and conduct social and political and economic and personal life. I think care theory needs to be a new moral theory, not only a new area of application for previous moral and political theory. The ethics of care should have priority over its political theory the way the dominant moral theories of justice, if they were satisfactory, should have priority over their associated political theories. But which moral theory should we accept?

The Domains of Society

Whatever the direction of historical influence, existing political theories of justice reflect existing moral theories of justice. Consider how the existing theories of justice not only overlook care, but privilege various segments of society, the legal and political, and ignore others. Rawls asserted that "justice is the first virtue of social institutions" (Rawls 1971, 3). If you apply this claim to the legal institutions of society, it is highly persuasive. But social institutions include far more than the justice system of the law and its enactments and enforcements. Educational institutions are certainly social institutions, but their first virtue is hardly justice. Of course, they should treat persons fairly, but their priority is to promote the values of education. Opportunities for education should be distributed fairly, but first systems of education must be created.

Or consider the social institutions composing the healthcare system. Healthcare should be available to all in ways that are fair. But first the institutions must be developed. They should take justice into account in the ways they treat patients and the general public, but justice is not and should not be their first concern. They rightly aim first of all to promote the values of health, to treat the wounded, cure the ill, and prevent disease. (Actually, many healthcare institutions in the United States at the present time aim primarily at making money, and profit, but this is clearly not what their priority ought to be, so they pretend to aim primarily at health.) Similarly, social services, whether public agencies or private charitable institutions, are social institutions whose aims of providing for the poor and meeting the needs of the afflicted do not have justice as their first concern.

What about the economy? Although it ought to be vastly more just than it is at present, it may be questionable that it ought to have justice as its *first* virtue. Before a society can assure a just distribution of its wealth and income, it must have the wealth and income to distribute.

Finally, the family is a social institution monumentally left out of the conception of society that sees justice as the primary value of its institutions. Yes, there should be far more fairness in the family than there has traditionally been, but justice should not be the concern it puts above all others. The distinction between public and private, and the idea that the public has relevance for moral theory in a way that the private does not, accounts for much of this oversight of the experience of women in moral theorizing, but that distinction is now being dramatically overhauled by feminist rethinking.

We have to wonder whether our conceptions of society as they have come to us from the dominant moral and political theories are not affected by a gender bias that focuses on the activities associated with men and hardly notices those associated with women, such as taking care of children, educating them, and caring for the ill and infirm. Those domains of society associated with women have had little effect on moral theorizing and do not fit well with traditional moral theory.

When we do focus on these other segments of society, we can see that they are and ought to be guided far more by the values of care than of justice. And we can see as an empirical matter that if more resources were devoted to these undervalued segments of society, the need for the legal activities and enforcements of the segments that play so large a role in dominant theorizing would diminish.

For instance, if care is adequate when persons are young, they will have fewer problems with the law when they are older. To take just one example, there is a great deal of evidence that preschool programs more than pay for themselves later (Gayl 2008; Heckman and Masterov 2007; Schweinhart et al. 2005).

This is not to say that as the caring activities of a society would expand, government funding should shrink. Public funding is often the best way to carry out the care we all should provide for each other. But the share of that funding devoted to law enforcement within society, and military force globally, could diminish.

Arguments that care needs to be socialized rather than to remain entirely the responsibility of families and private charitable or religious institutions are thoroughly persuasive (Hamington and Miller 2006; Tronto 2013). They become then, to some extent, parts of political systems. But care institutions do not then become simply yet another part of legal or political systems. To an important extent they remain, though previously neglected in moral theorizing, in separate domains of society.

A Comprehensive Morality?

If we try to correct for the past neglect of caring practices and values, should we then take care and justice as somehow of equal importance, as women and men should be regarded as equal? This would seem to leave us with Carol Gilligan's unsatisfactory conception of alternative perspectives: we encounter a moral problem, and see how it looks from the different perspectives of justice or care. But then what? Which should we choose to act on? If it is a moral problem, we do not just want to see how it looks from the different points of view. We want to figure out what to do about it. So, should we do what a care perspective would recommend, or what a justice perspective would demand? Thinking of them as equally valid and as applicable to whatever the problem is helps us to clarify alternatives, but does not guide our answers. Grace

Clement's suggestion, that for any moral problem we should use the approaches of both justice and care, suffers from the same indeterminacy (Clement 1996).

What I propose is to see the ethics of care as a comprehensive morality within which it can be appropriate to see various ethics of justice as applicable to the limited domains of the legal and political. I take the network of caring relations as the wider domain of society as a whole. Within it are subsystems with their own priorities. This wider domain of society as a whole includes the weaker caring relations of civil society that enable legal and political and other institutions to function. The wider domain includes also the strongest bonds of care, in families and among friends. It is composed of relations that are primarily informal, in contrast to the formal relations of legal and to a lesser extent political systems. While legal and political institutions ought themselves to be more caring than they have been, they should still, I think, give priority to justice. But while legal and political institutions should look for moral guidance primarily to moral theories of justice, institutions and persons in the wider domain should look primarily, I think, to the ethics of care.

We can think of all this, I suggest, in terms of larger and smaller and overlapping yet distinct circles or domains. I definitely recognize the difficulties with the metaphors with which we try to conceptualize these matters. There are problems, for instance, with the architectural metaphors of foundations and structures or superstructures built on them. There are problems with the biological metaphors of organisms and ecosystems emerging and diminishing. I have come to think that the best approach (an approach is itself a metaphor) is to be aware that any metaphor we use is only that, and necessarily unsatisfactory, but arguably the best we can do. So I argue for the metaphor of circles, overlapping but distinct, if we think of a cross-section of society. But of course they are also embedded in history, changing over time, growing larger or smaller, dimmer or brighter.

Given persons are in relations in and belong to multiple systems. In some senses they belong to many systems at any one time and over time. In other senses they act in different roles at different times and attend to the different relations differently. Persons navigate back and forth and around their positions as, say, parents and workers and citizens and plaintiffs and volunteers. In their different roles they can appropriately give priority to different moral values.

Of given issues, we need to decide in which domain to primarily place them. And in saying that in a given domain, a given value should have priority is not to say that other values then become irrelevant. For instance, within the caring relations of the family, though the values of care should have priority, we often need to make room for the values of fairness. Within the family, although the relations are primarily caring relations, sometimes they are highly competitive or legal and should look first to justice for guidance. For instance, if siblings engage in a competitive game, say of tennis, for that limited interaction, fairness should prevail. Or, if one sibling buys out the share of another in some jointly inherited property, for that limited issue, their relation is a primarily legal one and should put justice first, although the more general considerations between them, even in these cases, should remain those of care.

Many institutions providing care, such as welfare assistance, healthcare, daycare, or education, are and should be in some sense part of the political system because public financing is the best way to meet the needs they serve. Insofar as the political system includes supporting and directing them, it should especially emphasize the values of justice and the general welfare in providing fairly for the needs of all, along with the values of care that may motivate doing so at adequate levels. But in the practices themselves of meeting the needs of patients, clients, children, and students, these sectors of society should foster especially the values of care and understand how care requires empathy, sensitivity, trust, and the effective meeting of needs. It requires listening to others as well as acting.

If all this seems unduly vague and confusing, consider that we do have a somewhat clear idea of what we mean by a legal system. And yet, it is very unclear how it should be distinguished from a political system. Liberal theories of justice characteristically treat them as if they were somehow the same. But they are definitely different. Consider social movements. These are very important to, and recognized in, political systems. Perhaps, as some claim, there cannot be significant change without them. And yet, social movements barely register in legal systems and how they are conceptualized. In a half dozen books on legal theory by writers I admire—Dworkin, Hart, Fuller, some collections—none had anything to say about social movements. But social movements are certainly important to political systems. So even though the ways of distinguishing legal and political systems are in doubt, we can speak meaningfully of them as different.

Or consider economic systems. We have a somewhat useful idea of what we mean by the economy of a society, but there are good reasons to reject the view that it includes and determines everything else. Laws, for instance concerning property, and political policies of many kinds have enormous effects on economic systems, yet there are good reasons to understand the economy of a society as distinct from its legal and political systems.

I see legal and political systems as overlapping but distinct. And both are distinct from economic systems, though again there is large overlap. And these are distinct from the healthcare or education systems of a society. Social policies determined by political processes shape the economy, healthcare, education, the family and much else. Politics and the law can have a large effect on how healthcare or education is handled in a society, as we can often be acutely aware. Nevertheless, politics and the law do not deliver healthcare, the actual work of treating patients or preventing illness. They do not themselves educate children. Law and political institutions greatly affect the economy but do not themselves produce most goods and services. And all these segments of society are different from the social bonds of families and the informal groupings of friends and voluntary associations. The institution of the family has been changing greatly in recent years, and families can be very different from traditional notions of nuclear and even extended families. Groupings of friends can amount to families. Yet we can still recognize the family as a fundamental social institution, and acknowledge the great importance of families (Noddings 2002).

We can also recognize culture as a domain of societies, segments of societies, regions composed of several societies, and potentially of global society. Culture reflects and produces images, emotions, ideas, attitudes. It can contribute greatly to social change, to sensitivity toward and understanding of and willingness to take account of unfamiliar others and distant persons. If culture would be produced and guided increasingly by the values of care, prospects would improve for global understanding, non-violent resolution of conflicts, improved meeting of needs.

It is useful and not impossible, then, to discern these different domains of society. And we can well understand how these different domains should give priority to different values and be guided by moral approaches with different emphases. And all these different domains exist somehow within that of a society as a whole, usually a national one but potentially a global one, within which social relations must be at least minimally caring or the society will disintegrate.

There is huge overlap between various domains. The model here should be that between the legal and the political, which are not easy to distinguish and yet are not the same. Somewhat similarly, the provision of social services is an important function of government, but the welfare system and even more clearly the healthcare system can be distinguished from the political system despite their overlap. The system of education in a society is usually largely funded by government, but again, it is not simply part of the political system. And culture is certainly affected by other domains but is not the same as any of them.

These different domains of social activity can, then, be distinguished, and we can consider which values ought to have priority in guiding them. There is a misleading way in which the law can be thought to cover everything because whatever is not prohibited is permitted. In a similarly misleading way, it may be thought that since power is involved in all that people do, everything that happens is somehow political.

However, in trying to understand society and what we as conscientious members of it ought to do, it is more helpful to recognize distinctions between kinds of contexts.

Sociological Views and Normative Recommendations

When sociologists look at society, they discern such major institutions as the family, the political system, the economic system, the legal system, sport, education, science, the medical system, the military, and so on (e.g. Robertson 1981; Smelser 1994). These different components of society serve different needs and are guided by different values and norms.

Sociologists describe these values and norms, such as the value of a fair trial and the norm of informing suspects of their rights for the legal system, and the value of unbiased search for truth and the norm to conduct research for the institution of science (Robertson 1981, 84). The intent of sociology is merely to describe the dominant values and norms. The task of moral philosophy, in contrast, is to provide the arguments with which to improve them. My arguments aim at recommending which values and norms ought to have priority for persons in their different roles. It is entirely appropriate that persons in different roles in different institutions should be guided by different moral norms and values, and should give precedence to different moral approaches. It is these issues to which my arguments are addressed, my recommendations directed.

Legal and political institutions should be guided by moral theories. I have characterized both Kantian ethics and utilitarianism as moral theories of justice, but there are significant differences between them, of course. I think a deontological Kantian moral approach is most appropriate for legal systems, but a consequentialist pursuit of the general welfare or the public interest most appropriate for political systems. I've developed this argument at some length in my book *Rights and Goods* (Held 1984).

It may be confusing to think of a twofold division of moral approaches, those of justice and care, and then a three- or fourfold division of moral theories, those of Kantian ethics, utilitarianism, sometimes virtue theory, and the ethics of care, and then still another division between the values to which to give priority in the legal and political spheres, justice, and the general welfare. But once one is familiar with the arguments, I think the positions can be clear enough. I have tried to show why Kantian ethics and utilitarianism should both be considered rationalistic moral theories characteristic of the justice approach in ethics. I've argued that legal systems ought to be guided by Kantian moral values, political systems by utilitarian ones. And then I've argued that the ethics of care rather than either of these ethics of justice should guide much of what goes on in society and should have priority in much of how persons live their lives beyond the legal and political systems. I have said little here about virtue theory, and the way care ethics is not, in my view, a kind of virtue theory. Elsewhere I have tried to indicate how the ethics of care is a vast improvement over virtue theory in its guidelines, its ontological assumptions, its appeal to experience across cultures, and its ability to include other moral theories (Held 2006).

In the widest circle of society as a whole are the contexts of families and friends with their strongest and most lasting caring relations, and also the institutions of civil society with their weak, sometimes transient, yet necessary relations of at least minimal care. For a national state to exist there must be at least sufficient caring among its members to support state identity. Governmental institutions can in turn support the caring relations of civil society by their programs, for instance by subsidizing educational and cultural ventures. For legal and political institutions to function, people must care sufficiently that the rights of fellow citizens are respected, that obligations to them are met. They must care enough for the political interests of fellow citizens to accept majority decisions for elections, the policies of winning parties, and the like.

Society as a whole contains the strongest caring relations of families and groups, and the weakest yet important relations of civil society. Both of these sorts of relations are largely informal. Located somewhere between these are the formal relations of legal and political systems.

In the domain of law, justice should be granted priority. It includes the legal institutions that structure the society and shape its politics and other major institutions. When what we are justified in enforcing with the use of violence is at issue, we can say that our most important consideration should be justice. And those rights and obligations of justice that ought to be reflected in the law should be assured through deontological arguments, regardless of whether they meet with popular approval or serve the interests of majorities.

In political decisions, in contrast, the public interest, or common good, or general welfare—some version of what would be in the interest of the public as a whole, or of all or most in society—should prevail (Held 1972). Utilitarian and consequentialist calculations can be best for deciding on budget priorities and policies concerning, for instance, support of economic and social endeavors.

The might of the state, however, does not make right, and political decisions are not always good decisions. From the perspective of morality, we can argue that although, on grounds of care, justice and the public interest should be accorded priority in these limited domains of the legal and the political, care should retain its overall priority. Many of the social institutions the law allows and influences and that political processes support should have values much closer to those of care than of justice as their highest priorities; the values, for instance, of education, of health, of sustainable growth, of responding to particular needs. And as these are given greater support and attention, the need for the enforcements of law and coercions of political decision diminish.

In this intermediate region is also the economy. As it would be guided—both voluntarily and by governmental requirement—increasingly by the values of care, it would do more to provide what members of society actually need, and would be structured less to bring further advantage to the already advantaged. Its relations would more often be caring and cooperative rather than competitive and conflictual. Its markets would be limited rather than ever expanding (Held 2006).

The ethics of care should guide the widest circle of society and the relations between the domains within. It should allow and recognize that although the law should be far more caring than it is, encouraging more mediation and conciliation and less confrontation, justice should still be accorded priority within its legal system. But it should understand how this system should itself be limited, and in most circumstances shrinking, as society overall would become more caring and employ better institutions than the law for dealing with many of its concerns. It should allow pursuit of the general welfare, impartially ascertained, to have priority in its political system over the welfare of particular persons in caring relations. This domain of the political should also be understood as a limited one in society, not the way all persons should be guided morally in the whole of their lives.

In a comparable way, the ethics of care might allow and recognize the pursuit of individual gain as legitimate in many of society's economic pursuits, but might promote a vast expansion of caring, cooperative economic activity. And it would surely promote an expansion of culture guided by moral and aesthetic values rather than by mere economic gain.

In the family, justice certainly has a place. We ought to be fair to one another. Advice to squabbling siblings can often be some version of: whoever cuts the cake gets the last piece. And yet, considerations of care should trump those of justice (and if the reader recognizes here a reference to Dworkin, it is intended). If a member of the family urgently needs exceptional medical attention, no one gets cake. When siblings resort to the courts to settle an inheritance, or spouses engage in legal battles in a divorce, we regard it as unfortunate. One hopes such legal battles can be avoided as the individuals involved consider what would be best for the larger family or for the next generation.

Care and Society

Within the family, as beyond, better the law than the gun, but better consensus than the law, the cooperative solution than the legal battle. A caring approach would recognize the good grounds for one solution or another in innumerable situations, making the invocation of law less necessary.

Also at the level of a society, justice should not always have priority. An institution responding to a disaster or dealing with a threatened famine should not necessarily put justice first. If one is trying to prevent massive starvation, one's highest priority is not a fair trial for the person who steals a bag of grain. When looting is forcibly prevented, it is more to ensure that more people will get what they need than to punish the looters.

As Hume understood, justice (which he interpreted too narrowly as having to do with property) applies to conditions of moderate scarcity. In conditions of extreme scarcity, justice breaks down, and when there is no scarcity, justice is not needed. Hobbes and many others have assumed that in conditions of extreme scarcity, or absence of law and enforcement, men would descend into brutal, every-man-for-himself conflict. This is not all that should be considered. Care often can and does endure.

When writing about moral theory, Engster argues that we need a theory of obligation to show why we ought to care and ought to promote and cultivate caring practices in society. Here he suggests that rational defenses of obligation can strengthen care. I can agree that, though care theory is different from Kantian theory, it can welcome any support provided by rational arguments in addition to its bases in caring emotions. Unlike Kantian theory that rejects the moral value of emotional inclinations, the ethics of care need not reject any rational support it can receive, even though it can recognize, with Hume, that *mere* rational recognition can be weak motivation.

Similarly, in considering the debate between Kantians and consequentialists, the ethics of care can accept the best arguments of both. No, the moral worth of an action is not only a matter of consequences. Motives matter, and intending to do the caring thing even if the consequences turn out less than well can have moral value. But consequences matter a great deal also, and caring should bring about what really does meet in an effective way the needs of those being cared for.

The ethics of care would clearly recommend societies and a world in which the values of care would be far more strongly developed and emphasized, and the institutions of law and enforcement and coercive political power decreasingly needed. The ethics of care appreciates the values incorporated into practices of care and understands how they should be extended to the wider society and the globe.

Sara Ruddick focused her attention on the values discernible in practices of parenting, and showed how they were highly relevant to promoting peace between societies. "Many mothers know," she wrote in a characteristic passage, "what many military enthusiasts forget—the ability to destroy can shock and awe but compelling the will is subtle, ultimately cooperative work"

(Ruddick 2009, 307). Nel Noddings, in her book *Starting at Home*, examines the values of caring in the family and shows how they should be extended to social policies. I, and others, have tried elsewhere to indicate some of the implications of the ethics of care for social institutions and global arrangements (Held 2011b; 2015).

In the domains of law and politics, it may be acceptable to adopt, for their purposes, conceptions of persons as independent liberal individuals. But elsewhere persons should be recognized as the relational beings they more fundamentally are. What I have been suggesting in using the metaphor of overlapping circles, and the values that ought to have priority in the various domains, is something like society and morality seen from the outside by a moral observer. But the most important point of view for morality is that from the inside: the point of view of the conscious agent looking out on the world and deciding how to live and what to do. From this perspective, those close to me probably matter most, the legal system and its political counterpart are well beyond, and society as a whole with its different domains are rather far in the distance. The metaphors now have to be different. But we live with this enormous incompatibility—between the world we try to see from the outside as an observer and the world we try to understand from the inside as a conscious agent—across the board in everything we think about everything. It is not more of a problem when we consider care and its morality.

Let us not forget that the ethics of care is only a few decades old, almost nothing in comparison with the long history of the dominant moral theories. It is still very much in the process of development. I have come to think that the ethics of care is potentially a comprehensive moral theory constructed from an understanding of care *and* the justice already so theorized and thought about for centuries. Possibly this new ethics should be just thought of as ethics or moral theory, not the ethics of care or the ethics of justice. But that would be for the future. Ethics *tout court* now, as a matter of usage, designates the ethics of justice, or occasionally a virtue ethics missing the insights of care. So at least for the foreseeable future the ethics of care needs to be the focus of those of us who recognize the shortcomings of the dominant moral theories. And we can show how the ethics of care can and should include the concerns of justice, the general welfare, and the virtues.

Where does this leave other values, such as artistic/aesthetic ones? Care permits and encourages the pursuit of other values. Often they need to be argued for on their own merits, not because they promote peace or better care, but because they enrich life and experience. I have briefly tried elsewhere to explore the kinds of social and cultural institutions that would contribute appropriately to this aim, but those arguments are for another day.

Note

1. Earlier and related versions of this chapter were presented at the University of Oxford, England, in a lecture series on the ethics of care, 22 October 2014; at the US Military Academy, West Point, NY, 26 April 2014; at the New York Society for Women in Philosophy's Weinberg Lecture, 22 November 2013; at the University of Verona, Italy, Conference on Caring, 10 October 2013; at the University of North Carolina, Chapel Hill, 3 October 2013; and at Goethe University, Frankfurt, Germany, 15 May 2013. Several related papers have been published elsewhere. I am deeply grateful to the many persons who gave me their thoughts on these occasions and after them, and whose comments on related papers influenced this chapter. I wish to thank especially Andries Baart, Susan Brison, Gina Campelia, Rowan Cruft, Eva Kittay, Serene Khader, Diana Meyers, Cara O'Connor, Graham Parsons, Petr Urban, Iakovos Vasiliou, Susan Wolf, and the editors of this volume.

References

Clement, Grace. 1996. *Care, Autonomy, and Justice*. Boulder, CO: Westview Press.

Engster, Daniel. 2007. *The Heart of Justice: Care Ethics and Political Theory*. Oxford: Oxford University Press.

Gayl, Chrisanne. 2008. "The Research on Pre-K." <http://www.centerforpubliceducation.org/Main-Menu/Pre-kindergarten/Pre-Kindergarten#sthash.aw3mSxwg.dpuf>. Alexandria, VA: Center for Public Education.

Gilligan, Carol. 1982. *In a Different Voice: Psychological Theory and Women's Development*. Cambridge, MA: Harvard University Press.

Hamington, Maurice, and Dorothy C. Miller (eds.). 2006. *Socializing Care: Feminist Ethics and Public Issues*. Lanham, MD: Rowman and Littlefield.

Heckman, James, and Dimitriy Masterov. 2007. "The Productivity Argument for Investing in Young Children." *Review of Agricultural Economics* 29(3): 446–93.

Held, Virginia. 1972. *The Public Interest and Individual Interests*. New York: Basic Books.

Held, Virginia. 1984. *Rights and Goods: Justifying Social Action*. New York: Free Press/Macmillan.

Held, Virginia (ed.). 1995. *Justice and Care: Essential Readings in Feminist Ethics*. Boulder, CO: Westview Press.

Held, Virginia. 2006. *The Ethics of Care: Personal, Political, and Global*. New York: Oxford University Press.

Held, Virginia. 2011a. "Care, Empathy, and Justice: Comment on Michael Slote's Moral Sentimentalism." *Analytic Philosophy* 52(4): 312–18.

Held, Virginia. 2011b. "Morality, Care, and International Law." *Ethics and Global Politics* 4(3): 173–94. Open access journal.

Held, Virginia. 2015. "Gender, Care, and Global Values." In *The Routledge Handbook of Global Ethics*, edited by Darrel Moellenndorf and Heather Widdows, 49–60. New York: Routledge.

Hume, David. 1983 [1751]. *An Enquiry Concerning the Principles of Morals*, edited by J. B. Schneewind. Indianapolis, IN: Hackett.

Noddings, Nel. 2002. *Starting at Home: Caring and Social Policy*. Berkeley, CA: University of California Press.

Rawls, John. 1971. *A Theory of Justice*. Cambridge, MA: Harvard University Press.

Robertson, Ian. 1981. *Sociology*, 2nd ed. New York: Worth.

Robinson, Fiona. 2011. *The Ethics of Care: A Feminist Approach to Human Security*. Philadelphia, PA: Temple University Press.

Ruddick, Sara. 2009. "On Maternal Thinking." *Women's Studies Quarterly* 37(3 and 4): 305–8.

Schweinhart, L. J., et al. 2005. *Lifetime Effects: The High/Scope Perry Preschool Study through Age 40*. Ypsilanti, MI: High/Scope Press.

Slote, Michael. 2007. *The Ethics of Care and Empathy*. London: Routledge.

Smelser, Neil J. 1994. *Sociology*, copyright UNESCO. Cambridge, MA: Blackwell.

Tronto, Joan C. 2013. *Caring Democracy: Markets, Equality, and Justice*. New York: New York University Press.

3

Care ethics and liberalism

Michael Slote

If care ethics is to represent a systematic alternative to rationalist/traditionalist approaches to morality, it has to speak and speak persuasively about political issues. Yet in that area it seems to have a marked disadvantage vis-à-vis liberal Kantian or Rawlsian views about rights (and justice to the extent that it involves the honoring of rights), because of the way or ways we typically think and speak about political or human rights. Not just rationalist/liberal philosophers but ordinary Americans too think we have a fundamental and/or self-evident right to various civil liberties: for example, to freedom of speech and freedom of religious worship. And because this intuitive or at least familiar way of conceiving political morality seems far from anything care ethics would want or be able to say, care ethics has a problem. One way out of the problem would be and in effect has been simply to grant that liberalism is right and says all the right things about political/legal issues, thus treating care ethics as mainly an approach to the ethics of personal or private relationships. That has—with certain important qualifications—been the approach taken by Virginia Held and certain other care ethicists (Held 2006).[1] But this way of pursuing care ethics is problematic on a number of theoretical grounds.

First, it concedes that the original impulse or motivation behind care ethics—the idea of connection with and caring about others as ethically basic—can't adequately deal with political issues, and since Kantian ethics and various other forms of rationalism can and do claim to cover the whole of ethics, both private and political morality, care ethics will seem less comprehensive and less adequate if it has to borrow from other views to fill out what it says otherwise about morality or ethics. Care ethics will then be a kind of hybrid, and it will be understandable in ordinary philosophical terms if more uniform and systematic approaches like Kantianism and consequentialism are preferred to what is merely partial and in need of supplementation *by one of those other approaches.*

But there is another problem too with the proposal to limit the ethics of care to the private sphere. Even if we grant the personal isn't *entirely* the political, it is obvious nowadays that these two spheres or aspects of morality intersect and interact in very important ways. So how can care ethics keep its approach to individual/personal morality clear of implications for political morality, rights, and justice? And there is more to be said. I have argued in *The Ethics of Care and Empathy* (Slote 2007) that the basic philosophical/moral ideas behind care ethics are actually inconsistent with liberal political/legal views (that was my main purpose in writing this book). Care ethics from its inception in the 1980s has put great stress on connection with others, and the kind of liberalism we are focusing on here emphasizes autonomy (rights) in a way that insists on the moral separateness of individuals. It is difficult to believe that this difference, this *opposition*, wouldn't lead to different moral judgments about specific ranges of political/legal cases, and that is just what we in effect do find. In what follows, I shall mention some important areas where there is a normative conflict between what liberalism says and what care ethics, if at all true to its founding theoretical/moral motivations, will want to say, and I think two things follow. The first is that we had better not try to harness care ethics to or with political liberalism because that leads to forms of inconsistency we should surely wish to avoid. But, second, it follows that if care ethics wants to speak about political issues, it needs to speak with its own distinctive voice and thus to cover the full range of issues and cases—both personal and political or mixed between them—that Kantianism, etc., seek to deal with. And this, as I mentioned above, creates problems for care ethics because it deals with political questions in terms of empathy, caring, and connection rather than speaking of basic and independently intuited political rights in the way that comes so naturally or easily to thoughtful Americans and American political thinkers.

So the question then arises whether there is any way for the care ethicist to persuade people that we shouldn't think of political rights and justice in traditional terms, but should reformulate or reconceptualize our thinking about rights in the less familiar coinage of empathic concern and sensitivity. I think there is, and the present chapter is going to be my attempt to make a persuasive or strong case for making the change-over, for reconceiving our political ideals along care-ethical lines. Certain other care ethicists have already made efforts to theorize about political values in basically care-ethical terms, but they haven't, I believe, taken on the task I shall be undertaking here. Even if they have been critical of liberalism, they haven't reckoned with how easy it is for Americans to conceive political morality along liberal philosophical lines. They have not tried to show the familiarity and naturalness, at least for Americans, of thinking of political rights as having a rational and/or intuitive status that doesn't intersect with or depend on empathy, emotion, and caring—they have not specifically attempted to show how and why this familiar and traditional approach is normatively inadequate and simply cannot work.[2] And that is what I will be seeking to do here.

I am going to begin by focusing on issues from political life where care ethics and liberalism needn't disagree. However, in order to see how and why this can be so, it will be helpful to clarify some terms or concepts that care ethics needs to rely on not only in dealing with political examples but in its "home territory" of personal moral issues. And then we will proceed to the types of cases where care ethics and liberalism disagree, again making use of concepts that care ethics distinctively needs, but now attempting to show how and why this allows care ethics to frame political issues in ways that are superior to anything liberalism can provide. And the most important concept for us to start talking about is empathy.

The word "empathy" didn't exist till the twentieth century, and in fact Hume used the term "sympathy" to refer both to what we would now call sympathy and to what we nowadays think of as empathy. And just to make sure we are all on the same page, let me say, briefly, that the difference between empathy and sympathy is approximately the difference between Bill Clinton's feeling someone's pain and someone's feeling bad that someone else is in pain and wanting to help them or see them helped. "Empathy" has a broader use than this suggests—for example, one can take in or absorb another's attitudes or opinions via a kind of empathic osmosis that Hume talks a great deal about. But in any event, empathy is important for our purposes here because it is natural to suppose and there is a lot of psychological evidence in favor of the view that caring about others depends on the development of empathy in individuals. (There is some controversy about this idea, too, but I propose to put the controversy to one side for purposes of the present chapter.)[3]

Now it is true that we tend to feel more empathy for suffering we witness than for suffering we merely know about at a distance, and more empathy for the suffering of those we know and care about than for the suffering of strangers or people we know less well. And these facts of partiality can make us wonder how or whether we can derive plausible views about rights and justice from considerations concerning empathy and empathic concern for others. However, as the literature on empathy and moral development makes fairly clear, it is possible for mature individuals and even adolescents to feel substantial empathy with and concern for large groups of individuals they don't know personally, and this gives care ethics an entry point for talking about issues of social (or international) justice in terms of empathy and without having to bring in rationalist/liberal notions (or utilitarian or libertarian views) to supplement what it has to say about individual moral obligations and actions. Moreover, even if empathy is inevitably and irrecusably partial, empathy can be cultivated and widened via processes of moral education that the literature on moral development has described in some detail. So let's not too quickly assume that empathy and caring based in empathy are incapable of the task I am setting for them and that, if I am correct, care ethics itself sets for them.

But can a care ethics grounded in empathy really deal plausibly with all the different aspects of social or international or legal justice? Some have argued that it cannot and have mentioned the issue of tolerance as a good example of why we need something other than sheer feeling and motivation based in feeling in order to deal with people's rights to religious freedom. It is often held, for example, that religious liberties need to be rationally grounded in autonomy rights because sheer feeling will sometimes lead people not to tolerate religious practices that they find abhorrent or disgusting. And a typical liberal conclusion, then, is that we should fully respect the emotion-independent rights of free worship of those whose religion we strongly dislike and that we show such respect if we tolerate views and practices we dislike out of a conviction or intuition that people have a basic right to have those views and participate in those practices.

But this whole picture is morally distorted. Someone who allows others to worship freely even though they have nothing but disdain for those others or their views *doesn't* show full, genuine respect toward or for those others. It would be much more respectful if one tried, in an open-minded fashion, to see things from their perspective, if one could muster some empathy for that perspective, and didn't allow oneself simply to hate or contemn what the others think or do. (This needn't lead one to ultimately agree with those one initially disagrees with.) Liberals and ethical rationalists believe that justice and rights are tied to respect, but as we have just seen, that assumption, far from supporting rationalism and liberalism, actually works against their political ideals/vision and in favor of the care-ethical emphasis on empathy and emotion. A care ethics that stresses empathy will say that there is something wrong with or limited about the liberal/rationalist notion of respect because what the liberal conceives as full respect isn't the fullest kind of respect: liberalism doesn't recognize the importance of trying to empathize with those one disagrees with as a basis for the fullest kind of respect.

I am not, however, saying that everyone has a moral obligation to try to empathize, in open-minded fashion, with those they disagree with. That seems over-demanding. But it isn't too demanding to morally require that one not persecute people for their religious beliefs and not force them to give up their rituals and observances if one hasn't made a genuine effort to see things from their perspective. And this is precisely what historically hasn't happened. All the persecutions that have occurred throughout history appear to have occurred in the absence of any attempt to see things from the point of view of those being persecuted. However, somewhat apart from the issue of empathy, there is also the issue of sheer caring. Could persecution and torture in the name of one's religion count as a form of caring and thus pass the moral muster of any plausible care ethics?

Consider the Spanish Inquisition, for example. Apologists for the Inquisition both then and since have sometimes said that heretics and non-believers were tortured out of a (caring) concern for the welfare of those being tortured (the good of their immortal souls). But as John Locke wisely and wittily pointed out in his *Second Treatise of Government* (Locke 1960), the "dry eyes" of those who tortured heretics give the lie to the claim that the inquisitors were concerned with the welfare of those they tortured. But then, you say, couldn't someone with tearful eyes be genuinely seeking the well-being or happiness of those to whom they were denying religious freedom and possibly even torturing? Dan Engster has suggested to me that St Augustine might have been such a person, someone who would have been genuinely upset about the use of force on unbelievers, but who would have counted as genuinely caring in doing what he did or advocated doing. But I am not so sure.

Someone doesn't demonstrate caring motivation in a given instance if they say they want to help a given person, but don't do the relevant homework about how best to help that person. One has to want to learn how to help someone if one is to count as genuinely caring about them. But then consider Augustine. He was no doubt a great mind, a great philosopher, but (though we don't often say this) he was also a fanatic. He favored persecuting or excommunicating the Pelagians (whose supposed doctrinal sin was that they thought human beings could become morally better through their own unaided efforts), and more generally he wasn't open-minded vis-à-vis those who religiously disagreed with him. But if you are genuinely trying to help someone, you have to be open-minded about issues that are relevant to the question of how to help that person. And, by contrast, St Augustine was in effect saying to those who disagreed with him: I know the truth and you don't and so I know what is best for you without having to consult with you about what would in fact be good for you. If this is supposed to justify forcing people to worship differently for the sake of their immortal souls, such a justification simply doesn't work in care-ethical terms. St Augustine's lack of open-mindedness, his unwillingness to see things from the point of view of those he disagreed with and was willing to use force on, counts as a form of egotism; and to pursue another's well-being in an egotistical closed-minded manner is to be less than fully concerned about their welfare.

Indeed, Augustine's lack of religious toleration greatly resembles what we deplore about many stage mothers or fathers. The stage mother who, for example, tells their child they have to practice ballet six hours a day and who, despite all the protests of their child, tells the child that they are forcing them to do this for the child's own good is closed-minded and egotistical vis-à-vis their child, and neither such a parent nor Augustine in his mode of intolerance and persecution can really constitute a good instance of caring. So just as carelessness or laziness about obtaining relevant information can undercut someone's claim to have acted in a caring manner, so too does acting at the behest of egotistical (non-open-minded) fanaticism count as less than fully or genuinely caring; and I believe, therefore, that an ethics of care can tell us why religious intolerance/persecution is unjustified in moral terms. But liberalism can tell its own story of why these things aren't allowed, so my main point here is that (perhaps surprisingly) an ethics of care that emphasizes empathy (and empathic open-mindedness) can rule out religious intolerance and persecution just as definitively as liberalism can. But then one should also add that (as I mentioned earlier) there are aspects of (the fullest) respect for other people's religious or other views that care ethics can capture through the idea of empathy and that liberalism has totally ignored. However, as we shall see, this isn't the strongest argument care ethics can mount against liberalism, and before we get to the stronger or strongest case against liberalism, I think it would help the case of political care ethics if I pointed out some other areas where it can account for our received or intuitive moral/political opinions just as easily as liberalism can.

Consider, for example, issues of justice and rights that concern the welfare or wealth of members of society. Liberalism assumes (as libertarianism does not) that justice needs to be connected with some degree of welfarist equality or at least with improving the lot of those who are worst-off in society. But care ethics has similar things to say about this issue because of the emphasis it places on empathy. I mentioned earlier that empathy is partial to what is perceived as opposed to what is merely known about, but empathy is also partial to sheer badness. Someone's awful lot in life engages our empathy much more strongly than someone's being in a fairly good or mediocre position that allows for substantial improvement. And this is another way of saying that empathy favors *compassion* over *sheer benevolence*. So a care ethics of justice can say that justice requires greater help or aid for those whose welfare condition is bad than for (groups of) those whose condition is simply not wonderful, and this leveling implication sits well with what liberals say and most of us feel about social (and international) justice.

Finally, care ethics also favors democracy over other forms of government for reasons having to do with empathy and the kind of full respect that requires a willingness and ability to empathize with others. Rulers/leaders in the Far East often say that there is no reason for their states/societies to be governed democratically. Westerners may place a great value on democracy and self-government, but, they say, there are different "Asian values" that actuate people in their own countries. There is, they claim, a natural Asian deference to authority that makes democracy much less relevant in the East than it is thought to be by those Westerners who seek to impose their values throughout the world (see Bell 2000).

Doesn't this remind you of what used to be said about women? It used to be said that women are naturally deferent to men and that that is why it is inappropriate to give them the vote. And this kind of argument works no better for or with Asians than it does for or with women. It is true that after being beaten down by patriarchal/sexist social mores or their own parents over a period of years ("you don't really want to be a doctor, dear, or to go to university; you'd be much happier as a nurse or full-time homemaker"), a girl or woman may end up not thinking for herself and mainly deferring to others. But if their aspirations and ideas are actually listened to, little girls don't become the deferential "angels in the house" that some of them were praised for being during the Victorian era. And there really is no reason to think things are or would be any different with East Asians. (Think about what has been happening in recent years in rural Thailand.) Once again, empathic respect for what the other wants is the key to justice, and if people know about the possibility of democracy and aren't browbeaten into denying or devaluing their own desires and aspirations, they will want democracy. And a full empathic concern for them will seek to gratify or fulfill that very understandable human desire. So here, as with various other areas of justice and political thinking, a care-ethical approach is or can easily be consistent with what liberals think and what most of us antecedently believe about what is required by justice and/or our rights as human beings.

But of course in the United States at least, issues of justice are typically framed in terms of rights in a way that seems to have no reference to empathy or caring and that seems to reach out for some kind of rationalistic justification. The American "Declaration of Independence" declares that various truths about human rights are self-evident, and this is or is normally seen as an appeal to sheer rational intuition. (Can anything be self-evident to empathy?) So a care-ethical approach to justice has to say that this normal (American) understanding of justice gets things wrong, puts things on the wrong basis. It has to say that the real source of what is just or unjust (and of corresponding rights) lies in a relation to human empathy. It has to say that such empathy picks out what is appealing about justice in more humane terms than any understanding of rights and justice that relies on (abstract considerations of) reason and is entirely independent of all feeling can allow.

Part of the argument for this conclusion we have already given: we have seen that ideal or complete respect, far from being a matter of honoring abstract rights independently of how we feel, depends on our genuinely empathizing with how others see and feel about things. But there is another reason too for thinking that justice cannot be as ethical rationalists/liberals conceive it. If the rationalists and liberals actually come to mistaken views about particular ranges of practical cases, then the considerations on which they base what they say about those cases cannot be the basic foundational considerations that underlie properly conceived justice (or rights). And I shall now argue, therefore, that care ethics gives us a better practical/normative answer than liberalism does to certain important political issues and, for that reason, a better account of the foundations of justice, as well.

Most liberals who have recently spoken of the right of free speech have invoked the roughly Kantian notion of autonomy (e.g. autonomous self-expression) as the basis of that right. And for most cases this seems plausible enough. But liberals use the same notion of autonomy to defend hate speech as a form of free speech, and this leads to controversial results. An example that often comes up in the literature concerns the march and subsequent speech making that neo-Nazis sought permission for in the 1970s in the town of Skokie, Illinois. Important academic liberals like Ronald Dworkin, Thomas Nagel, and T. M. Scanlon have argued that the autonomy rights that underlie and justify freedom of speech also justify allowing the neo-Nazis to march and speechify in Skokie (something they never in fact did).[4] But the neo-Nazis chose Skokie for a reason: it was a town with a large population of Jewish Holocaust survivors, and empathy with those survivors might make us hesitate and more than hesitate to allow the neo-Nazis to march, demonstrate, speechify, etc., in such close and immediate proximity to the survivors.

But the academic liberals, knowing about the Holocaust survivors, nonetheless favored allowing the march, etc., on grounds of (the importance of) rational autonomy. However, these same liberals also tended to see the situation in Skokie in a way that downplays or ignores the effects of the march, etc., on the survivors. Many of us—including care ethicists—would defend free speech that is merely offensive or frustrating to those who hear it; but what the neo-Nazis were proposing to do was likely to do more than offend and frustrate. The sheer knowledge that something like this was going on at such close quarters in their country of supposed refuge from the Holocaust (and the survivors were likely not just to know about the nearby march but to hear some of what was going on with their own ears) would very probably have had a (re)traumatizing effect on some or many of the Holocaust survivors, and this amounts to psychological damage, not mere frustration and offended feelings. But the liberals never mentioned this possibility, and I think this showed a certain lack of empathic sensitivity in their intellectual position. Sure, if the effects would just be offense and frustration, then autonomy considerations would have sufficient force to justify allowing the march. But when actual harm is at issue—and it is important to realize that not all harm is physical—then the weight of empathic and humane considerations seems to me—and has seemed to many feminists and care ethicists—to favor a refusal to let the neo-Nazis march in Skokie rather than somewhere else.[5] The frustration of the neo-Nazis is nothing as compared with the retraumatization of Holocaust survivors. And in that case the liberal/rationalist "autonomy defense" of free hate speech in the Skokie case seems misguided.

Moreover, the wrong answer about the Skokie case seems to come from putting too much emphasis on rational autonomy and not enough on (sensitivity to) human feeling, its causes and effects. So this case (and it really is a range of cases) suggests that justice is better grounded in such feeling than in purely rationalist considerations. And let me now mention another case (or range of cases) that points toward the same conclusion.

In the past and in many jurisdictions even today, judges are reluctant (and the law doesn't readily allow them) to issue restraining orders against husbands or boyfriends who their wives or girlfriends say have threatened them with violence or have already done violent things to them. Often further judicial/legal process is or has been required, and this has often meant that women are (further) injured or even killed before the further process has taken its course. But why has there been so much reluctance to issue the restraining orders (or to have the women guarded through additional police patrols, etc.)? In large part it is out of a sense of the importance of autonomy rights of freedom of movement (and assembly). But this means that until very recently (and only in certain jurisdictions at that), the legal/judicial emphasis has been on autonomy rights rather than the welfare (rights) of women, and I think most of us nowadays—and not just feminists and women—would say that the law has erred in placing so much emphasis on autonomy rights and so little on dangers to women (and children).

But the liberal has precious little room to renavigate these waters. To do so is to place more emphasis on welfare than on civil liberties and the committed liberal (e.g. Rawls, as we shall see in just a moment) is likely to be very uncomfortable with doing so. However, if one thinks the basis of morality and justice doesn't lie in abstractly, rationally considered or intuited rights like autonomy, and sees these things, rather, in relation to our own human empathic sensitivities to issues and realities of human welfare, one will once again favor welfare over autonomy. And this is what we nowadays feel is appropriate. We feel that restraining orders and police patrols or bodyguards can be justified much earlier or much more broadly than traditional political thinking allows, and in the light of its ability to deliver a morally more plausible view of what is called for in cases of threatened or actual abuse, the care-ethical way of grounding its view of such cases and all others is further supported.[6] So even if most Americans think in terms of rationalistic bases for their own intuitions about justice and rights, a care-ethical account of what is foundationally involved in justice and rights delivers more plausible and acceptable normative judgments about various ranges of practical legal cases.

I know of no comparable advantages of the rationalistic approach over the care-ethical in regard to other cases, and all this, therefore, constitutes a reason to accept a generalized empathy-emphasizing care-ethical theory of rights and justice—and to abandon the traditional liberal way of conceiving these matters.

And let's be clear about the difference here. Rawls's liberal theory of justice, as applied to developed societies, gives basic civil liberties a lexical priority in relation to (what can be seen as proxies for) considerations of welfare, and on any plausible reading of what he says, this means that the neo-Nazis should have been allowed to march and give speeches, even if that would have brought a cost in human welfare to the Holocaust survivors in Skokie. It also means that the law and the courts should hesitate or more than hesitate to interfere with the autonomy rights of free movement of accused husbands who have not yet been allowed or subjected to any legal proceeding or trial.[7] Liberalism in some important contemporary instances really does seem to yield the wrong answers to the sorts of questions we have been discussing, and that in itself gives us reason to question its rationalistic emphasis on autonomy (as traditionally conceived) and its whole way of seeing political issues of morality. Our whole country may buy into that way of seeing things, but if that yields normatively unacceptable results, we have to start theorizing about things differently, and I am arguing that care ethics gives us a way of doing so that yields the right normative answers across a wide range of political issues.[8]

Of course, the defender of liberalism might at this point try to find cases that care ethics can't handle and that liberalism can. But that is something I myself have been unable to do, and if the liberal can't do any better, then they should at the very least start worrying about their own views and pay some serious attention to what care ethics can and does say about political morality. And there is another, possibly deeper reason why rationalist/Kantian liberals should worry about their own views, a reason based on what Carol Gilligan (1982), following psychoanalyst Nancy Chodorow (1978), has said about the differing childhood experiences of girls and boys.

Both girls and boys have traditionally been raised by their mothers much more than by their fathers, and this has an asymmetric impact on their development. To meet social or family expectations, boys have had to distance themselves from their mothers in a way that girls traditionally have not, and boys have therefore typically ended up emphasizing and valuing autonomy and separateness and systems of rules of the kind that exist outside the home much more or much more frequently than girls have. But liberalism à la Rawls and Scanlon places great emphasis on autonomy and systems of rules or principles, and to that extent it reflects or at least corresponds to a typical male, rather than a typical female, upbringing.

This ought to give the Kantian/rationalist liberal pause, but never has. There is no sign in the literature of ethics and political philosophy that liberal philosophers like Rawls and Scanlon (or ethicists like Derek Parfit who also place great emphasis on public systems of rules) have taken notice of what Gilligan and Chodorow say about the difference between typical male and typical female upbringings, and if they did, the fact that their philosophical views correspond so closely to what happens in typical male (but not female) development should make them wonder (but would it?) whether their views are more determined by their upbringing(s) as males than by cogent arguments.[9] Of course, even after wondering about this, they might still try to offer good philosophical arguments for liberalism and against care ethics and other normative views. But to proceed, as these philosophers have, as if the issue of the influence of upbringing (raised by Chodorow and Gilligan) didn't exist seems to me to be wrongheaded or else oblivious in a way that one might describe as academically/intellectually negligent. Alternatively, and using Gilligan's terminology, one could describe this lack of reaction from liberal philosophers as a rather new and distinctively academic instance of men not listening to the voice of women. Now care ethicists may face a similar problem, given what Chodorow and Gilligan say about the relation of care thinking to typical traditional female upbringing. But the care ethicists have all at least read Gilligan, and so they know about the statistical relation between different kinds of upbringing and different moral orientations; whereas the male philosophers I have just mentioned haven't even got that far with the perplexing issue of how upbringing affects or should affect theoretical moral views.[10] So as I see it, and primarily on the basis of the arguments I offered earlier, there is reason to favor care ethics over liberalism as an approach to political issues of morality.

Notes

1. Held holds that even if valid (liberal) political morality is in important ways independent of caring, it has to be situated within a larger context that embodies the values of caring. But that doesn't, I think, affect the points I am making in the main text. Also, I hope it is clear that the political liberalism I am speaking of here is the Kantian/Rawlsian variety of liberalism, not Millian (or more generally utilitarian) liberalism.
2. Here I am most specifically thinking about what Nel Noddings says about and against liberalism in her *Starting at Home: Caring and Social Policy* (Noddings 2002).
3. See, e.g., C. D. Batson's *Altruism in Humans* (Batson 2011). In my *A Sentimentalist Theory of the Mind* (Slote 2014, chapter 4), I argue that the doubts that have been

raised recently about the role of empathy in producing or sustaining altruism are largely misconceived.

4. For references to the work of Dworkin et al. and a much more extensive discussion of this case, see my *The Ethics of Care and Empathy* (Slote 2007, chapter 5).
5. But couldn't a homophobe claim they were injured by having a gay rights parade go near their house, and couldn't a racist make a similar claim about civil rights activism occurring near their home? Well, they could make such claims, but we have to judge for ourselves whether such claims are plausible, and I think most of the readers of this chapter would agree that the claims are rationalizations and pretexts rather than reality-based. Of course, a racist judge might buy such claims and it is sometimes difficult to know when psychological irritation ends and genuine psychological damage begins. So there are certainly slippery slope issues that arise in principle (and without anyone being prejudiced and rationalizing their prejudice), and this certainly bears practically on how courts can and should function regarding these kinds of cases. But the main point here is that it in fact would be just not to allow the neo-Nazis to march and speechify in circumstances like those that obtained in Skokie, something that care ethics claims for but liberalism does not. Finally, even if a racist is psychologically damaged by the accumulation of the events of black progress, that damage, supposing it really to exist, reflects their immoral (in both liberal and care-ethical terms) moral beliefs and dispositions, and the damage that would have been sustained by the Holocaust survivors doesn't reflect any immorality on their part (only on Hitler's). That is also morally relevant to distinguishing these cases.
6. But what if the wife is lying about her husband's having abused or even threatened her? Won't it then be unfair to the husband if the restraining order is issued on her say-so? In that particular instance an injustice will, I agree, have been done, but the issue is one of just administrative or judicial *policy*, and if the lying wife has no previous record of lying to or misleading officials, then the just policy—for reasons having to do with generally ensuring women's safety—will dictate taking her at her word and issuing the (temporary) restraining order. In certain jurisdictions the law allows dogs "one free bite": even if they bark and growl menacingly, they can't be legally sent to the pound, etc., until and unless they have actually bitten someone. And surely we can and should accord this much scope or leeway to complaining women: one free lie, as it were. In the kinds of cases I am talking about, the interests at stake for wives are more serious than those at risk for husbands, and the care-ethical approach would therefore argue that in all fairness they should trump the (full exercise of the) liberty rights of husbands. The possibility that a wife may be lying for the first time in a judicial proceeding doesn't alter that basic non-equation. However, I am also assuming that any temporary restraining order against the husband won't go on his permanent public record. To make the point I want to make, our case has to be one in which the well-being of the woman is just pitted against the husband's temporary freedom of movement.
7. On the lexical priority of liberty, see *A Theory of Justice* (Rawls 1971, sections 11, 26, 39, and 82). Rawls never dealt with the Skokie case directly or, as far as I know, with issues of spousal abuse. But what he says about freedom of speech in *Political*

Liberalism (Rawls 1993, 295f.) supports the present interpretation of his views. Note too that, although American liberals (unlike libertarians) typically favor strict or stricter gun control, it seems difficult to reconcile such a view with belief in the priority of the basic liberties (in what Rawls [1993, 297] calls "reasonably favorable conditions"). If liberals are inconsistent on this point and could come to recognize this, then perhaps the sheer moral weight of what favors gun control could lead them away from liberalism and in the care-ethical direction I have been arguing for here.

8. If we Americans think of our political morality as based in rationally intuited rights of autonomy that trump other ethical considerations, but at the same time are moving or have moved to normative views about hate speech and violence against women that are inconsistent with such a basis for morality, that shows us not to understand or to have understood ourselves very well. What we have taken to be paramount (for us) turns out not to be morally paramount (for us) in ways that can only by and large be quite surprising. So the implications of care ethics are eye-opening, but that is only because we have misapprehended, misunderstood what morality, our own morality, is all about. And, if I may say, I think this ignorance is partly of our own doing. Emotion and thinking about emotion makes many or most of us uneasy and even anxious, so the idea that morality is based in an empathy-rooted emotion like caring is a deeply unsettling and uncomfortable one. But it is time, I think, for us to face these realities, and all the recent focus on both empathy and caring in our culture and our society (HMOs advertise themselves as, for example, "the caring folks") makes it somewhat more likely that we will do so.
9. See, e.g., John Rawls (1971); T. M. Scanlon, *What We Owe to Each Other* (1998); and Derek Parfit, *Reasons and Persons* (1984) and *On What Matters* (2011). All these philosophers (even Parfit in *On What Matters*) are influenced by Kant, but it is worth noting that recent female neo-Kantians (e.g. Onora O'Neill, Barbara Herman, Marcia Baron, and Christine Korsgaard) don't place the same emphasis on systems of rules that male neo-Kantians do. Again, this is something that seems fairly predictable, so I think we all should pay more attention to and worry about issues of psychological origin.
10. The idea that a view's origins can be relevant to assessing our reasons for believing it is a familiar theme in the work of Bernard Williams and has also been advocated by Alison Jaggar, by me, and by other feminists.

References

Batson, C. D. 2011. *Altruism in Humans*. New York: Oxford University Press.

Bell, Daniel. 2000. *East Meets West*. Princeton, NJ: Princeton University Press.

Chodorow, Nancy. 1978. *The Reproduction of Mothering*. Berkeley, CA: University of California Press.

Gilligan, Carol. 1982. *In a Different Voice: Psychological Theory and Women's Development*. Cambridge, MA: Harvard University Press.

Held, Virginia. 2006. *The Ethics of Care: Personal, Political, and Global*. New York: Oxford University Press.

Locke, John. 1960. *Second Treatise of Government*. In *Two Treatises of Government*, edited by P. Laslett. Cambridge: Cambridge University Press.

Noddings, Nel. 2002. *Starting at Home: Caring and Social Policy*. Berkeley, CA: University of California Press.

Parfit, Derek. 1984. *Reasons and Persons*. Oxford: Oxford University Press.

Parfit, Derek. 2011. *On What Matters*, 2 volumes. Oxford: Oxford University Press.

Rawls, John. 1971. *A Theory of Justice*. Cambridge, MA: Harvard University Press.

Rawls, John. 1993. *Political Liberalism*. New York: Columbia University Press.

Scanlon, T. M. 1998. *What We Owe to Each Other*. Cambridge, MA: Harvard University Press.

Slote, Michael. 2007. *The Ethics of Care and Empathy*. London: Routledge.

Slote, Michael. 2014. *A Sentimentalist Theory of the Mind*. New York: Oxford University Press.

4

A theory of justice as fair terms of social life given our inevitable dependency and our inextricable interdependency

Eva Feder Kittay

Introduction: Defining the Problem

Carol Gilligan (1982) famously counterpoised an ethic of care to an ethic of justice. Reconciling the two ethics has occupied much of the literature by care ethicists. The two ethics have sometimes been thought to be aligned with a public/domestic divide, but many of the theorists of care have made the case that care ethics is pertinent to the more than intimate relationships among individuals. Fifteen years after Gilligan's publication, Virginia Held wrote:

> Feminist understandings of justice and care have by now made clear . . . that these are different values, reflecting different ways of interpreting moral problems and of expressing moral concern . . . that neither can be dispensed with: both are highly important for morality. . . . What remains to be worked out . . . is how justice and care and their related concerns fit together. (Held 1995, 128)

Sarah Ruddick, one of the first to argue that the practices and values of maternal care have a broader canvas than mothering, has also insisted that justice, conceived of as non-domination, has a place in family life (Ruddick 1995). Okin too insisted that whatever might be said for the values of care, we need a concept of justice within the family no less than care (Okin 1989). Yet while Held has stayed with her original position that these are two different moral perspectives, she has increasingly shrunk the areas of life governed by principles of justice to a small handful, mostly those that involve the adjudication of legal matters (Held 2006).

Arguably, not all have believed that justice and care are different values that reflect different moral orientations. Michael Slote, for example, argues that we should understand both as motivated by empathetic concern for others (Slote 2007). He shows how a theory of justice may be developed by analogy with an ethic of care in intimate realms. The position I wish to develop is not far from Slote's, although analogy and empathy play a lesser role, and some of the values of justice which are not accommodated in an ethic of care continue to play a role.[1] Nel Noddings (2002) argues that the same values that guide care practices, such as mothering, and especially those developed by Sarah Ruddick (1989), can be used to deal with many injustices in society. She sees the distinction between justice and caring *for* others (which requires that we be in actual contact with the cared-for) as mediated by the notion of "caring about." Noddings now says that "caring supplies the basic good in which the sense of justice is grounded" (Noddings 2002, 22). Once again, this does not sound as if care and justice reflect "different ways of interpreting moral problems and of expressing moral concern," even if they are still distinct concepts.

Joan Tronto (2013) and Daniel Engster (2007) offer us two well-developed political notions that are imbued with the ethic, practice, and value of care. Tronto speaks of one particular political form of a just social arrangement, namely democracy, which she claims is both indispensible to good care and cannot be fully realized without care. When Engster places care at "the heart of justice," he does so in a closely related sense. Since the work of society is to provide for needs that can only be satisfied through public goods and services, and since such needs to be cared for and to do caring should be available and accessible to all, a society that doesn't attend to matters of care will not be a just society. Engster builds on some of my own work in which I conceptualize society as a set of nested dependencies. Unless the core of that nested set is well maintained, we do not have an orderly, just, and (with Tronto) democratic society.

There is an interesting ambiguity in many of the works that confront the relationship between justice and care. Care is sometimes treated as a moral value; the term used in this way has a normative content. Care in this sense is the ideal at the ethical core of an ethic of care. In its purely normative sense, care means what we mean when we speak of "good care."[2] It is the virtues, obligations, and consequences of good care that are delineated by an ethic of care and which derive from practices in which care is done well. Care at other times is used as a descriptive term that may be broadly applied and found in a large variety of practices (Tronto 1993; Tronto 2013; Bowden 1997). Care in its descriptive sense is akin to a commodity, something people need and desire that can be of varying quality, distributed fairly or unfairly, and in adequate or inadequate doses. The work of care can itself be a desired and desirable labor or a burden. As a burden of social cooperation (or a condition of living together on fair terms), it too is subject to principles of distributive justice (Kittay 1999; Engster 2007; Abel and Nelson 1990).

Feminist theorists have generally held that distributing both the receiving and giving of care can be done fairly or unfairly, and have generally agreed that this is a matter of justice. In this regard, there is no inherent problem about meshing the values of care and justice—although how to fit care, even as a commodified good, in among the other goods that distributive justice concerns itself with continues to be a question worth pursuing. The problem of meshing care and justice is more problematic when care is viewed as an inherently ethical practice: that is, care in the normative sense it has within an ethic of care.[3] Here an ethic of care still appears as a rival ethic to an ethic of justice—at least with regard to some areas of life.

In this chapter, I want to make a recommendation about how to speak of care both in its fully normative and its descriptive sense with respect to justice. We hold fixed the distinction between an ethic and a political theory, wherein political theories are applicable to social institutions, while ethical theories govern relationships between individuals, and say that justice is a virtue of political institutions. Yet, political theories of just societies are based on an ethic: that is, on an understanding of what constitutes moral relationships among the members of a community. The question of justice can be said to be the question of how we arrange our social institutions so that citizens can realize an ethical life.

Rawls's theory of justice, for example, is primarily built on a Kantian ethics (Rawls 1971). The ideal just society that Rawls envisions has Kantian moral subjects who strive to always act toward one another as ends in themselves. The political structure is meant to foster and support this ethical ideal. But if political theories reflect an ethical ideal, then we can propose alternate theories of how we want to govern ourselves that are based on a different ethical ideal. I (along with other care theorists) want to contend that social institutions are just if the ethical ideal includes care in the fully normative sense. Care ethics here is not a rival of *justice* but a rival of some of the other ethical theories that have served as the ground of justice theory.

The task for care theorists who want to take the guiding values, virtues, modes of ethical deliberation, and so on, into the public domain is to build a theory of justice for political institutions. My proposals in this chapter complement the work of others in envisioning a society in which good-quality care is available to all and viewed as a responsibility shared by all, as well as one in which people act toward one in accord with an ethic of care. In such a society, care, in the descriptive sense, is most importantly focused on the question of our inevitable dependency and our inextricable interdependency.

The chapter is essentially programmatic. It is not an argument for such a theory of justice, nor a systematic account. It tries to identify elements of such a theory rather than to build it, since that is a project for a much longer work.

Changing the Focus of Social Justice

The point of a theory of social justice, John Rawls (1971) tells us, is to provide the "fair terms of social cooperation." Although this proposition seems at first to be uncontroversial, it is, I suggest, tied to a picture that has held political philosophy in its thrall since at least the modern period. It begins with a view of the person that David Gauthier (1986) sets down with great perspicuity: "A person is conceived as an independent centre of activity, endeavouring to direct his capacities and resources to the fulfillment of his interests. He considers what he can do, but initially draws no distinction between what he may and may not do" (1986, 9).

The assumption, which Rawls makes explicit, is that these "independent center[s] of activity" have the capacities required to fulfill those interests. They are drawn to cooperate because these cooperative endeavors better allow them the fulfillment of their interests.

From the perspective of our unfettered subjectivity, we clearly appear to ourselves to be an independent center of activity. But fulfilling our interests almost inevitably involves other people and institutions and even those very interests are shaped by and drawn from others. The problem for political philosophy as it has mostly been thought of can be gleaned from the another claim that Gauthier makes: "[T]he contractarian sees sociability as enriching human life; for him, it becomes a source of exploitation if it induces persons to acquiesce in institutions and practices that but for their fellow-feelings would be costly to them" (1986, 9).

The latter portion of this sentence is doubtless true. Some persons can and do exploit the sociability of others to take on labor and responsibilities that ought to be more fairly shared. But Gauthier and other contractarians (and contractualists) go astray when they presume that sociability is only an *enhancement* to a form of life that could possibly go on without it. In fact, the exploitation of which Gauthier speaks arises precisely because human life *cannot* go on without sociability and the work and responsibilities it imposes.

The view that sociability is a mere enhancement has led philosophers to go to great lengths to explain why independent and free beings, who have their own view of their own good, should give up so much freedom and independence to unite with others in mutually constraining arrangements. Philosophers have resorted to explanations such as the innate sociality of humans, our vulnerability to the harm others can visit upon them, the idea that we can do better materially when united, and the belief that human life can realize its particular dignity only when in concert with others: in short, that we form societies because doing so is mutually advantageous, and doing so justly is the rational and reasonable course.

All these explanations have some merit. But they seem to skirt what is most obvious: that we are born dependent and stay dependent for a long period, and that the care and protection of dependent beings is a shared enterprise most successfully carried out when responsibility is shared between the individuals closely connected to the dependent and the community at large. Humans as a species have little choice about the need for collective action insofar as they have evolved in such a way that their very survival depends not on them alone. That is, the idea that we can begin by thinking of persons as "independent centers of activity" involves more than the normal distortion of an idealization. There is an incoherence at its heart. It may be logically possible for there to be such beings, but such "persons" cannot be human persons who have inherited the social capabilities and needs that make human life possible and that make human life, in all its variety, what it is.

Yet in the picture that begins with Gauthier's characterization of persons, the political significance of the demands and consequences of our inevitable human dependency (that is, the dependency of the very young, the very old and frail, many forms of disability and illness) and our inextricable interdependencies, which are often unbidden but inescapable, are all excluded by fiat.[4] In our inevitable dependency we are, by definition, not independent, equally situated or even roughly equally empowered. Given the inextricability of our interdependence, we are never fully independent. Nor are we able to engage in cooperative ventures around production on the same terms as those freed from dependency concerns. Our sociability, which has enabled us to survive our early dependency and our ability to live past childbearing age, and which has been harnessed to care for us when illness and disability occur, has meant that we can develop the emotional and cognitive abilities that give rise to complex social organization and cooperation.

The very demanding nature of that care has meant not only that human mothers/fathers individually care for their young, but that they can do so only through arrangements of shared caregiving.[5] While many of our primate relatives have capacities of empathy needed for the care of their own offspring, humans, alone among the great apes, have the capacity for empathy that has given rise to forms of trust, cooperation, and sociability sufficiently extensive that we allow others, even non-kin, to watch over our vulnerable infants. These are the capacities and needs for sociability that we call upon when we ask ourselves and others to act with justice toward others. All human life, and most especially life in the complex societies for which we seek adequate conceptions of justice, is highly interdependent, and all this interdependence begins with the fact of our inevitable dependency.

Inevitable human dependency differs from socially induced dependency, such as when one person or group robs others of the power to enable their survival and flourishing. Slaves are forced to be dependent on masters for their most basic needs by laws and cruel treatment. Under patriarchal regimes, women are compelled to be dependent on men for the well-being of both their dependents and themselves as they are denied other means by which to take care of their own and their family's needs. Mobility-impaired people who can propel themselves with a wheelchair are made dependent when public spaces are inaccessible with a wheelchair. These and similar forms of dependency are removed by giving people rights, opportunities, or entitlements and by the creation of public spaces that enhance people's "freedom of functioning," to use Amartya Sen's (1995) notion.

Inevitable human dependencies can sometimes be conflated with socially constructed dependencies. Inevitable human dependencies take different shapes in distinct historical periods, cultures, and societies. And sometimes, a form of dependency that seems inevitable in some circumstances can be seen as constructed in another. In highly patriarchal societies, where women are not permitted to engage in gainful employment and are expected to fulfill gender roles purportedly dictated by nature, their dependency on men appears inevitable. In more gender-egalitarian societies, women's economic dependence on men is the paradigm of a constructed dependency. In a not dissimilar manner, the seemingly inevitable inability of people with significant sensory or motor disabilities to be gainfully employed is a constructed dependency borne of prejudice and lack of accommodation. With ramps, appropriate technologies, and open attitudes, this inevitability vanishes. But for the most part, it is important to understand that some dependencies are not constructs and are inevitable in the sense that they are rooted in our biology and not constructed by social arrangements, even if the form they take will be culturally shaped. A person with paraplegia may be dependent on a personal assistant, but not dependent financially if employment opportunities are truly open to people with disabilities. Still, the need for an assistant to help with certain activities of daily living is not constructed. The need of my daughter Sesha, who cannot feed, toilet, or do anything for herself, is not socially constructed.

There are also dependencies that are *derived*: that is, they are dependencies that one person has because of the relationship they bear to someone who is inevitably dependent.[6] Persons who are responsible for the care and well-being of an inevitably dependent person may themselves be more or less dependent according to the extent of the other's dependence on them. For example, a person with the full responsibility of caring for an entirely dependent infant is herself dependent on others to supply what a caregiver requires to meet both her needs and those of her dependent. As the infant grows into a child and then an adult, the dependency becomes less marked.

While at any given time, a certain portion of the population will be inevitably dependent, we are all vulnerable to different degrees and sorts of inevitable dependency; and we are all vulnerable to becoming more or less derivatively dependent. While some of us may be able to opt out of caring for a dependent (and in this way opt out of becoming derivatively dependent), inevitable dependency and derivative dependence are frequently conditions we find ourselves in, not conditions we seek or choose.

At best, our independence is relative, but at heart it is really a fiction, a construct that has more or less value to various actors in different situations. When battling imposed dependences, the cry for "Independence!" can be crucial in the struggle against oppression. A woman who asks for the right to enter the workplace so she can be economically independent is asking for the right to be recognized as a particular sort of efficacious self-determining agent. A disabled person who demands workplace accommodation so that she can be independent is similarly asserting the right to such recognition. But workers are nonetheless dependent on their bosses; entrepreneurs are dependent on their investors and their customers, etc. Entering the workforce and being able to earn a living is not independence as such but independence from certain oppressive conditions, and a dependence on other conditions that are hopefully more respectful of our desire to be efficacious agents.

We are inextricably interdependent. The notion of social cooperation captures elements of this interdependence, but retains some of the fiction that as self-determining and self-sufficient agents we can take or leave this cooperative arrangement if we do not agree to the terms. To insist on our inextricable interdependence is to say that, regardless of the social arrangements we *chose* to enter into, what is not a matter of voluntarism is the fact that we must be engaged in *some* social arrangements, some forms of dependency, and interdependence.

This is because a social structure needs to be in place to meet the needs of dependents and dependency workers and those who provision dependency workers. The most ubiquitous of dependency relations, that of infant and caregiver, requires more than a dyadic relationship. Because human infants are as needy and helpless as they are, a single person alone can rarely succeed without social supports to care for that infant. For this reason, argues Sara Hrdy (2009), humans could evolve into the sorts of creatures we are only because we (and we alone among apes) had to engage in shared caregiving, a sharing of responsibilities and resources that both depend upon and help develop social capacities such as trust and cooperation. The complex social and political structures that characterize human societies, the liberal democratic structures that appear to many as requirements for a just society, would be impossible, perhaps even inconceivable, without the capacities that arise out of the necessity of dependency relationships, and the trust that they require and engender.

If a theory of justice is to provide principles that, as Joshua Cohen (2001) has put it, leave "no one less well-off than anyone needs to be" and each one's "life matters as much as anyone's," then surely, we still want fair terms for the forms of social cooperation for production in which we engage. But we will require more than this: for to view social arrangements from the perspective of dependency means that just social arrangements require attention to our dependency needs and the relationships that sustain us in our dependency. Starting from this perspective, it is impossible to see how a theory of justice can be adequate if it leaves out the needs of care in all their variety. Caring for each other with our different needs and capacities are the first order concerns of social arrangements. It is these social arrangements that in turn make possible the many other forms of intercourse that fulfill human desires and aspirations. But social arrangements need a political conception of justice if they are to fulfill care needs for each person and do so in an equitable fashion.

Hence the need for a conception of justice that incorporates the facts of inevitable human dependency and inextricable interdependency and so folds in the concerns of those who give and receive care into the vision of a just society. If we are to respect the critical nature of social arrangements for actual human beings, human beings "as they truly are," we want a theory of justice that provides principles not for the fair terms of social cooperation, but for the fair terms of social life given our inevitable dependency and our inextricable interdependency. Both sets of "fair terms" affirm the importance of fairness in ordering social arrangements; the second eschews idealized normal fully cooperating agents in favor of actual human beings in the dependency and vulnerability, including the very young, the disabled, the frail elderly, the caregivers, and the assistants.

An important thing to notice is that when we consider our mutual dependency and interdependency, we see that fair terms are needed to govern social arrangements, whether or not we are in a condition of moderate scarcity. Even under conditions of no scarcity, human beings are still in need of care, and care is itself a relatively scarce resource insofar as care, when properly performed, requires a great deal of attention, energy, and even sacrifice on the part of the caregiver. Such dependency needs—while not independent of considerations of scarcity—are inevitable even in conditions of affluence. An infant living in the midst of plenty still needs someone to procure those goods if she is to survive. A person with significant impairments may still be disabled even in the midst of plenty if she cannot access those goods she requires for her well-being.

Concepts and Principles of Justice Based on an Ethics of Care

When based on these considerations of care, the question of justice is transformed. We ask: "Given our interdependence and our mutual dependence, what are the fair terms that should govern the basic social and political institutions if we are to live together, work together and care about each other?"[7] Another way to put this is to say that what we require is a theory of just social arrangements that will allow us to flourish, regardless of our relationship to dependency. That is to say, no matter where we may be situated in a continuum of inevitable dependency and no matter what sorts of dependency relationships we may find ourselves in, we will have the opportunity to flourish to the same extent that those without such constraints have.[8] Such a theory asks: "What institutions do we require to support each other and to enable each one to flourish, given our different capacities and our different relationships to dependency and care? What are the governing principles for establishing and maintaining such institutions?"

At best, Rawlsian principles that govern fair terms of social cooperation are a subset of such fair terms when they are sufficiently broadened to include everyone, not only the "normal and the fully cooperators." Such a theory of justice does not merely fairly distribute care as one commodity among others, but forms a social order in which participants act toward one another in accordance with an *ethic* of care.

A theory of justice that is guided by an ethic of care will need to include concepts, conceptualizations, and values derived from an ethics of care.[9] Among these are the following:

1. *Self.* This theory of justice will need to recognize that the primary constituents of a society are not simply individuals with their own interests, but individuals who exist in varying relationships of inevitable dependency and inextricable interdependency. At the same time, as it recognizes individuals as connected, it must also preserve the integrity of each individual. Such a theory is neither communitarian nor individualist, but balances commitments to individuals and to their relationships.
2. *Equality.* While the liberal and democratic value of equality should be preserved in a commitment to moral parity for all, the idea of equality should not presume an equality of situation or power, even in an idealized conception. In my previous work, I have suggested a relational understanding of equality in which we recognize each other as "some mother's child": that is, as someone in whom care has been invested, as none of us could survive, much less thrive, without such care.[10] Whether we use this aphorism or some other formulation, the point is that our equality resides in the relational nature of self and self-formation.

3. *Rights and responsibilities*. The importance of understanding the relational nature of the self pervades all the concepts that figure in a theory of justice based on an ethic of care. In a theory of justice based on a deontological theory or a liberal ethics, the right is prior to the good. Responsibilities are usually understood to derive from conceptions of the good, while duties are derived from a concept of the right. Instead, in a theory of justice guided by an ethics of care, responsibilities are based not only on individual conceptions of the good, but also on the legitimate (i.e., non-coercive)—even if not fully chosen—connections that we bear to one another. (Illegitimate connections, such as a slave may bear to a master, do not result in responsibilities on the part of the slave, for whom the connection is a coerced one. The non-chosen, but legitimate connection a child has to a parent does issue in responsibilities on the part of the child as well as the parent.) Responsibilities also issue from imbalances in power among people who are in connection, so that the more powerful have responsibilities to those dependent on them. An ethic of care, as Gilligan (1982) presented it in her early work, and as people such as Card (1991), Walker (1998), and Joan Tronto (2013) have insisted, is at once an ethic of responsibility and any theory of justice based on an ethic of care has to have the idea of responsibility as a central political concept. With a justice based on a deontological theory such as Kant's, rights can only be constrained by other rights. But in a justice based on a care ethic, responsibilities and rights (with their correlate duties) are mutually constraining. That is, rights do not always trump responsibilities, nor do responsibilities always trump rights. Consider, for instance, a caregiver who finds herself needing to stay beyond her scheduled time because a medical appointment of her charge goes on longer than expected. As a worker, she has a right to leave at her appointed hour. Here, however, her responsibilities trump her right. But she also has a right to demand that such overtime be well compensated—this right might trump responsibilities that an agency has to use its funds primarily for the benefit of its clients. A resolution to a conflict between a right and a responsibility must be settled in a contextual way that also respects other principles in the theory of justice.
4. *The realm of care*. A concept of justice guided by an ethic of care has to take the realm of care as a natural and central focus of political life, not an add-on. That strategy has persistently been shown to give short shrift to the needs of care (see Kittay 1999; 2012; Nussbaum 2006; Fineman 2000).
5. *Freedom and needs*. Such a theory understands freedom as the freedom to engage in desired and desirable relationships as well as the freedom to be left alone. But just as important, such a theory understands that freedom

is impossible if our needs are not met. We are no freer if we are hungry because we are unable to feed ourselves when left to our own devices than if our hunger results from someone preventing us from eating. Therefore legitimate needs issue not only in rights, but in a social responsibility to meet such needs.

6. *Asymmetry of power and the problem of domination.* A theory of justice based on an ethics of care will need a way to legitimate power differences that are due to asymmetries in inevitable dependency and inextricable interdependency. That is, given the recognition that constituents of a political order go through periods of inevitable dependencies, and that dependency and care of dependents creates inextricable interdependencies, which also involve asymmetrical power relationships, we need a theory of justice that will recognize that some power inequalities are inevitable and will establish means by which to protect the vulnerable from both domination and neglect. Such protection from domination and neglect is as primary a responsibility of a just social order as is protecting constituents from the infringement of their rights.
7. *Covenant v. contract.* Such a theory cannot be thought of as a contract. This is because those whose interests most need protection are those least able to come to the table. Contract theory does important work in political theory. It provides a framework for what constitutes legitimate coercive state power. It gives equal dignity to each contracting party. Is there a political concept that can serve the same end, when the constituents are understood not to be equally situated, not equally empowered and not necessarily capable of autonomous action? Is there a political concept that can express the mutual constraint of rights and responsibilities? There is a notion closely related to contract that may be helpful, namely that of a *covenant.* The term has many meanings and is sometimes used as just a particular form of contract. But the way in which I wish to understand it is as an acknowledgment of a relationship or agreement that already exists, wherein we accept the responsibilities or submit to the conditions entailed in being in that relationship. For example, when we purchase land that is covered by a covenant, we accept the responsibilities and constraints that come with the land. And while it is true that the purchase is a contract between buyer and seller, it is the land, not the seller, that is violated if the covenant is not respected. Or consider the duties a parent owes to a child. These are not the consequence of a contract between parent and child. The relationship of a parent to a child is instead bound by a covenant that parenthood entails and which raises

legitimate expectations on the part of society at large as well as the child in particular.

8. *Allocation and distribution.* Justice based on an ethic of care has as its aim the possibility of a flourishing life regardless of one's condition of dependency or relation to dependency. This aspiration can be thought of as a shared conception of a central good: that people care about each other. It leads not necessarily to a distributive principle but to a principle of allocation that attends, first, to matters of dependency. The principle would require that institutions be so arranged that conditions of dependency are not simultaneously conditions of deprivation—or at least not greater deprivation than the economic circumstances of one's society necessitates. The guiding conception of the good yields both responsibilities on the part of social institutions to assure that conditions of dependency do not become conditions of deprivation—as they do in societies where the poorest 25 percent of a population are children and where the disabled are consistently poorer and more poorly represented in employment, and in valued positions in public life—and the right of people to be able to access what they require to have flourishing lives, no matter what their relationship to dependency may be.

The above paint a picture of society that contrasts significantly with ones found in theories of justice based on more traditional ethical theories. The next question we ask is: what sorts of principles govern a society so reconceived?

Principles of a Care-Based Conception of Justice

Material deprivation is only one way that conditions of dependency can impede the possibility of a flourishing life. Abuse, neglect, and exclusion are wrongs that a person in a condition of dependency is often powerless against. Without adequate care and assistance that has institutional support and protection, the possibilities of having a flourishing life under conditions of dependency are greatly diminished. Principles of justice that begin with an ethic of care and with inevitable human dependency will be ones that form around non-exploitation, non-deprivation or neglect, non-abuse, and sustaining bonds of care and assistance.

First Principle: Non-deprivation and Non-discrimination

This principle would demand that public resources and opportunities be distributed in such a way that meeting dependency needs receive prima facie priority over other concerns; and that opportunity not be denied because of dependency needs. In one sense, all so-called basic needs, food, water, shelter, etc., are dependency needs. Yet, I generally hesitate to endorse a pre-given set of needs as I agree with Fraser that needs contestation is a part of political life (Fraser 1989). What I have in mind instead are questions of public policy, such as whether a state should provide universal childcare even if it needs to increase taxes; whether a state should insist that all buildings be accessible even if this proves costly and means that other concerns receive lesser funding, and so forth. (This principle is based primarily on conception 4 above, that taking care of dependency needs is a, if not the, central aim of social organization, and also on 8, that allocation as well as distribution is a concern of justice.)

Second Principle: Non-exploitation for Dependency Workers (Caregivers and Assistants)

The second principle is needed to protect those who tend to others in a condition of inevitable dependency from exploitation and deprivation of resources and opportunities. This principle maintains that the labor of caring for dependents must be never coerced, must be fully compensated, and must not close off other opportunities to those who assume such responsibilities (see conception 5 above). The problem of exploitation is rampant in dependency work, in part because the conditions of such labor often involve affective attachments that form to vulnerable persons and especially those who are vulnerable to our actions. The other's vulnerability, our own attachments, and the fact that we feel ourselves indispensable to that person's well-being mean that we accept conditions of our labor that undercut our own interests, conditions we would not accept given a set of viable alternatives (see Bubeck 1995; Kittay 1999). This principle leans on conception 1 above, the recognition of the relationality of the self; 3 above, the need to balance rights and responsibilities; and 6 above, the asymmetry of power.

Third Principle: Non-exploitation for Dependents

Furthermore, the vulnerability of dependency leaves the dependent open to exploitation as well. If someone hands us a lifeline in the form of care, and especially if we develop a bond of affection toward that person, then we are at risk of being exploited in order to have our needs and wants met. A third principle is needed to protect against such abuse. This principle provides for the institutional protections and recourse to opportunities that can help assure that people in states of dependency are not left exposed to abuse and exploitation, and can have the greatest amount of freedom commensurate with their capabilities and without impeding the freedom of others. (This principle engages conception 5 above, the conception of freedom as requiring the meeting of dependency needs, and again the asymmetry of power in dependency relations, 6 above.)

Fourth Principle: Support for Sustaining (Effective and Non-exploitative) Caring Bonds

Fair terms of social life given our inevitable dependency must recognize the importance of *bonds* that form between a dependent and those who assist and care. This principle is to support and protect bonds formed through care. This fourth principle must assure protections and resources that enable the caring bonds to be sustained without becoming exploitative or abusive. The invocation of a covenant rather than a contract (see conception 7 above), along with a relational conception of the self (1 above) and of equality (2 above), are ways of recognizing the inherent importance of the bonds themselves.

Inextricable Interdependencies: the Terms of Reciprocity

What about our inextricable interdependency? Sarah Hrdy has argued that we were emotionally human before we became cognitively human. Our ability to cooperate around caregiving co-evolved with our large brains, our need for high-quality food, and our extended dependency in our early years. We simply would not have evolved into the beings we are, along with our extensive social competencies as well as intellectual capabilities, had we not been able to trust one another enough with our infants to procure the necessities of human life. And we would not have been able to trust others in this way if our infants did not form connections with people other than mothers. Today, even given the ideology of intensive mothering, no one raises a child alone. There are schools, babysitters, physicians and nurses, grandparents and other relatives, siblings, and of course people who provide the material resources needed to sustain life, sociality, and culture. Furthermore, if only to a very minimal extent, everyone who lives beyond infancy has benefitted from such care. We are all, all of us, in debt.

The notion around the idea of fair terms of social cooperation that is intuitively vivid and compelling is reciprocity. When we receive, to the extent that we can, we need to give. Alasdair MacIntyre (1997) speaks of the virtues of acknowledged dependency as revolving around an ethic of giving and receiving. Of course, we are indebted to those who have cared for us, but our way of reciprocating does not necessarily depend on our returning our favors to them. When we are in debt, another form of reciprocity has us not pay back but pay forward. "What goes round comes round." In my other work, I have called this a principle of doulia, a notion that Engster (2007) especially has expanded upon and carried into the political domain.

I want to give a refined version of that principle here.

Refined Principle of Doulia

We are obligated to give care to those who need it to the extent that we are able and in a position to do so; and when we are in need of care, we are owed that care by someone who is well positioned to give it and who will be appropriately compensated and cared for when they need care. I now add an obligation on the part of the one receiving care: one is obliged to respond to care graciously, to the extent that one is able, when the care is offered thoughtfully, in good faith, and with requisite competence. Fischer and Tronto (1990) have called the response to care the fourth stage of care. But it is one that care ethicists, with the notable exception of Tronto (1993) and Noddings (1984), have by and large ignored. By *the gracious reception of care* I mean being willing to acknowledge the care and not to demand more than the one giving the care can give without depleting herself. Such caregiving is respectful of carer and cared-for alike. This added obligation of the cared-for is needed to complete another's act of care. Without the cared-for's uptake, the caregiver's actions are not yet care in a fully normative sense. The insistence that "care needs to be completed in the other," as Noddings puts it, is what distinguishes care from paternalism because paternalism requires only the imposition of what the pater regards as being in the interest of the other, while care, in its fully normative sense, requires that what the caregiver provides is recognized, or comes to be affirmed at some later time, as in fact being in the cared-for's interest by the one receiving the care. Furthermore, understanding that care has to be completed in the other shows us that care (in its fully normative sense), and in particular being cared for, is an active uptaking and not a passive submission.

How does the obligation to receive care graciously when offered in good faith, competently, and thoughtfully enter into a political conception of justice? First, that care requires uptake becomes an adequacy criterion for laws and policies, thereby protecting against pernicious paternalistic policies. Because receiving care *graciously* requires that the care receiver be attentive to being *overdemanding*, the boundaries between care-giver and care-taker must be acknowledged to add validation to the non-exploitation principle for dependency workers and all forms of caregiving.

What the principle of doulia, the principles of non-exploitation, non-deprivation or neglect, and the support for caregiving bonds, amounts to is this: fair terms of social life, given our inevitable dependency and our inextricable interdependency, are meant to insure (first) that when one is in a condition of dependency, whether as dependent or dependency worker, the dependency does not blight our prospects for a good life, and (second) that the condition of dependency when fairly dealt with will "leave no one less well-off than anyone needs to be." The social arrangements of the institutions of society are not to leave those in conditions of inevitable dependency to think that they fail to be "treated with respect as an equal, one whose life matters as much as anyone's," to employ the ideals that Cohen (2001) sets out.

This may seem like an outrageous demand to some, not because it may be costly, but because, the objectors will say, it seems obvious that our life goes better if we are not in a condition of dependency (leaving infancy and early childhood aside—though my ten-year old grandson might not agree to this exception!). That dependency impedes flourishing is fate, not injustice. Here the insights and the activism of the disability movement should set us straight. People with disabilities consistently report at least as good if not a better sense of well-being than those without disabilities—once, that is, one adjusts to the disabling condition and if the situation one lives in offers needed supports. Yes, the skeptic may say, but what about those with severe disabilities, highly limited cognitive function, unimaginable disfigurement, not to mention persistent pain? Here too biographies and autobiographies do not bear out the sorrowful conceptions of these lives that many abled people envision. People complain of not having what they need to make their lives go well, not the inherent impossibility of it going well.

Without social institutions which are based on principles that provide fair terms for attending to human dependency and inextricable interdependency, many are unable to enter into the relationships that Rawls refers to as social cooperation. *With* such fair terms, even those who are not situated to enter into Rawlsian relationships at all are still counted among those whose lives should be no "less well-off than anyone needs to be."

Rawls claimed that the conception behind the original position allows people to revise their conception of the good even radically and nonetheless not lose their public persona. He writes of the "profound and pervasive shift[s], or reversal[s], in [our] final ends and commitments . . . On the road to Damascus Saul of Tarsus becomes Paul the Apostle." Yet, he continues, "such a conversion implies no change in [their] public or institutional identity" (Rawls 1971, 85). For many that road to Damascus is the introduction of disability into one's life, either when that disability affects them directly or when it affects them indirectly as a carer. One parent I know remarked, "when I had Tommy [his son who was born with a chromosomal anomaly], I finally understood that my life had a point to it." Living with my daughter has compelled me to question many of the philosophical verities that had previously directed my life. Before I had Sesha, I had believed that all the problems of the world were caused by injustice. Now I have come to believe that injustice itself only arises because of a failure to care. It is something I could have learned independently, yet my experiences with Sesha have made this more vital. Living not in an ideal state, as Sesha's mother, my public persona has also changed. I am still a citizen, but my standing as an equal is compromised because I am not assured that Sesha has equal standing; to the extent that her dignity is slighted, my dignity is slighted; to the extent that her needs are not met, my own languish; and to the extent that she lacks full protection, I lack full protection.

The contract has the advantage that it incorporates the idea of political association formed in freedom. Centering social life on a covenant that respects dependency may appear relatively inglorious. But although dependency in its neediness and necessity seems an inherently undesirable condition, there are many conditions to which we are subject that are not necessarily viewed as unfortunate. The fact that we require food does not make food loathsome. On the contrary, we turn our need for food into occasions for sociality and artisanship—even artistry, cultural identification, and so forth. We are compelled to breathe air, a fact we rarely rue and simply accept as a condition of being alive. By removing the political, social, and economic disadvantages that attach to dependency, we can look again at the fact of human dependency and see it not as an impediment to living well, but as a source of value: a source of connection, an occasion for developing our capacities for thought, empathy, sensitivity, trust, ingenuity, and creativity; in short, as providing for us the conditions of our distinctive human dignity. Dependency (which is always set up against independence), when properly managed and fairly dealt with, is paradoxically not the enemy of freedom but the very condition of the possibility of our freedom.

Am I offering up the principle of doulia and its lemmas, insofar as they form the basis of a theory of justice based on an ethic of care, as an alternative to justice as the fair terms of social cooperation? Might there a different interpretation of the initial choice condition, say, where we imagine that under a veil of ignorance no one knows their particular relationship to dependency, but does know that we each have such a relationship and vulnerability under which we would choose these principles over Rawls's two principles? Might we be offered a menu of options that we can consider, along with Rawlsian principles and Nussbaum's (2006) capabilities, each in a pure form and in a mixed form? And might we then speak of contracting to affirm such principles?

I have claimed that properly managed dependency is the condition for the possibility of our freedom.[11] That surely suggests that there is more that we want out of our social arrangements than to have dependency needs fairly managed or our care needs adequately addressed. So what principles would we choose to govern the remainder of social life? To the extent that care considerations and our dependency and our relations to dependency do not leave us exploited or deprived, to the extent that we understand that dependency needs do not diminish our dignity, or at least need not, to that extent we are freed to explore all the human possibilities of a good life that are predicated on our dependency on one another, and plausibly our dependency on non-human animals and our environments as well. We will worry less about work–family balance, and talk less about the burdens of care, because social institutions will be geared to allow us our time caring for those we love without depreciating our income or social standing. Institutions of our society will be geared to meet needs that derive from inevitable dependency and inextricable interdependency. Joan Tronto, Bowden (1997), and others have shown that many social institutions are already engaged in care even though they might not be viewed as such because of gendered considerations. These will be subject to a conception of justice that is better suited to those institutions than the rights-based ethics that currently constrain and distort their functioning. People with disabilities will not have to fight for inclusion, as it will be a given that, without the presence of diverse bodies and minds, our lives are all poorer and that as a society we need to do all we can to be sure that every institution is fully inclusive. All are covered under the terms of the covenant.

If we valued the connectedness of the dependency relationship as much as we value productive labor in a society based on "fair terms of social cooperation" (where cooperation means participation in productive labor) then we would do all we could to insure that dependency relationships with dependent adults as well as dependent children were protected and each adult capable of productive labor would have the ability to engage in dependency work along with or instead of other labor. Our industries would be more geared to fashioning equipment that reduced unnecessary dependencies, and our heroes would include those who were valiant in their care of others, as well as those who showed us the dignity of all lives, no matter the extent of the dependency. What I mean to say is that dependency, as much as other needs that become sources of innovation, connection, and creativity (think about hunger and food), would so transform our world that what would be left of contracts specifying the fair terms of social cooperation is simply unknown.[12]

Notes

1. They do so for Slote as well insofar as they can be shown to develop directly from our empathetic concern for others. For example, he argues that notions such as rights, respect for autonomy, and others associated with a distinct justice ethics can be shown to derive their moral character from an extended empathetic concern for

others. My view is not so morally monistic—that is, I do not want to try to derive all moral values from a singular human capacity.

2. The sense of care in the phrase "good care" is essentially descriptive—otherwise the goodness of the care would already be part of the meaning of care itself, just as we do not speak of "good justice." If what we refer to is not good, it is not "justice." Justice, unlike care, does not have a set of practices that it descriptively refers to, although there are practices of justice, e.g., the legal system.
3. As I have indicated above, the tack that I wish to take is already being pursued by several other theorists without being elucidated as clearly as it might be.
4. A fuller discussion of the concepts of inevitable dependency and inextricable interdependency is given later in this chapter.
5. Here my account echoes the theme of Tronto (2013), which argues that a democracy can only be fully democratic when it includes shared responsibility for care.
6. See Kittay (1999) and Fineman (1995).
7. I take it that this is akin to what Joan Tronto (2013) has recently spoken of as "caring with."
8. We should add that flourishing here is not necessarily understood in the Aristotelian sense. There are different ways of conceiving what flourishing may be, but in my view of care ethics, flourishing demands at the very least that the person cared for assents to and desires the good(s) required for their flourishing. It includes the notion that engaging in care activities is an important aspect of a flourishing life for most people. It also allows for many different capacities to be cultivated, depending on the talents and dispositions of the individual involved. A person with capacities as limited as those of my daughter Sesha, and as dependent, has no less an ability to flourish than do I, although what that means for her is quite different from what that means for me.
9. Tronto (2013), Held (2006), Slote (2007), Engster (2007), Sevenhuysen (1998), Noddings (1984), Fineman (1995), and myself, among others, have attempted to bring an ethics of care into the political arena. My proposal draws in substance and spirit from all these efforts.
10. Tronto (2013) has proposed that we are equal in that we are equally in need of care. But I prefer my original formulation—Tronto's formulation is problematic as care needs are vastly different, between individuals, and at different points in an individual's life. My own formulation has often been misunderstood, and people object that some children are not cared for by their biological mother. But I mean by "mother" some mothering person or persons. And furthermore, I mean that we all are beings whose welfare, at least at some point, is or was significant to someone. Perhaps one might say that our equality consists in the fact that all of us have needed someone's care and all are equally vulnerable to being in need of care. But that is just what I mean by the aphorism.
11. I speak at greater length about managed dependency in Kittay (forthcoming).
12. Here I echo the claims of Virginia Held, who argues that if we allowed the ethics of care its full scope, the domains in which the rule of justice was necessary would be fewer than we can currently imagine. The difference between us is only that I would say that the ethics of care is operative through a justice based on care, although I grant (at least on some days) that there may still be domains where a justice based on more traditional ethics could still be needed (Held 2006).

References

Abel, Emily K., and Margaret K. Nelson. 1990. *Circles of Care: Work and Identity in Women's Lives*. Albany, NY: State University of New York Press.

Bowden, Peta. 1997. *Caring: Gender-Sensitive Ethics*. London/New York: Routledge.

Bubeck, Diemut. 1995. *Care, Gender, and Justice*. Oxford: Clarendon Press.

Card, Claudia. 1991. "The Feistiness of Feminism." In *Feminist Ethics: Problems, Projects, Prospects*, edited by Claudia Card, 3–35. Lawrence, KS: Kansas University Press.

Cohen, Joshua. 2001. "Taking People as They Are?" *Philosophy and Public Affairs* 30(4): 363–86.

Engster, Daniel. 2007. *The Heart of Justice*. Oxford: Oxford University Press.

Fineman, Martha Albertson. 1995. *The Neutered Mother*. New York/London: Routledge.

Fineman, Martha Albertson. 2000. "Cracking the Foundational Myths: Independence, Autonomy, and Self-Sufficiency." *American University Journal of Gender, Social Policy and Law* 8(13): 13–29.

Fischer, Bernice, and Joan Tronto. 1990. "Towards a Feminist Theory of Caring." In *Circles of Care*, edited by Emily K. Abel and Margaret K. Nelson, 35–62. Albany, NY: State University of New York Press.

Fraser, Nancy. 1989. *Unruly Practices: Power, Discourse, and Gender in Contemporary Social Theory*. Minneapolis, MN: University of Minnesota Press.

Gauthier, David. 1986. *Morals by Agreement*. Oxford: Clarendon Press.

Gilligan, Carol. 1982. *In A Different Voice*. Cambridge, MA: Harvard University Press.

Held, Virginia. 1995. "The Meshing of Care and Justice." *Hypatia* 10(2): 128–32.

Held, Virginia. 2006. *The Ethics of Care: Personal, Political, and* Global. Oxford/New York: Oxford University Press.

Hrdy, Sarah Blaffer. 2009. *Mothers and Others: The Evolutionary Origins of Mutual Understanding*. Cambridge, MA: Belknap Press.

Kittay, Eva. 1999. *Love's Labor: Essays in Women, Equality and Dependency*. New York: Routledge.

Kittay, Eva Feder. 2012. "Getting from Here to There: Claiming Justice for People with Severe Cognitive Disabilities." In *Medicine and Social Justice: Essays on the Distribution of Health Care*, edited by Rosamund Rhodes, Margaret P. Battin and Anita Silvers, 313–24. Oxford/New York: Oxford University Press.

Kittay, Eva. forthcoming. "Dependency." In *Keywords in Disability Studies*, edited by Rachael Adams and Benjamin Reiss. New York: New York University Press.

MacIntyre, Alasdair. 1997. *Dependent Rational Animals: The Virtue of Dependence and the Virtue of Acknowledging Dependence*. Berkeley, CA: University of California Press.

Noddings, Nel. 1984. *Caring: A Feminine Approach to Ethics and Moral Education*. Berkeley, CA: University of California Press.

Noddings, Nel. 2002. *Starting at Home: Caring and Social Policy*. Berkeley, CA: University of California Press.

Nussbaum, Martha. 2006. *Frontiers of Justice: Disability, Nationality, Species Membership (The Tanner Lectures on Human Values)*. Cambridge, MA: Belknap Press.

Okin, Susan Moller. 1989. *Justice, Gender, and the Family*. New York: Basic Books.

Rawls, John. 1971. *A Theory of Justice*. Cambridge, MA: Belknap Press.

Ruddick, Sara. 1989. *Maternal Thinking*. New York: Beacon Press.

Ruddick, Sara. 1995. "Assault and Domination." In *Care and Justice: Essential Readings*, edited by Virginia Held, 204–24. Boulder, CO: Westview Press.

Sen, Amartya. 1995. *Inequality Reexamined*. Oxford: Oxford University Press.

Sevenhuysen, Selma L. 1998. *Citizenship and the Ethics of Care: Feminist Considerations on Justice, Morality and Politics*. Amsterdam: Taylor and Francis.

Slote, Michael. 2007. *The Ethics of Care and Empathy*. New York: Routledge.

Tronto, Joan C. 1993. *Moral Boundaries: A Political Argument for an Ethic of Care*. New York: Routledge.

Tronto, Joan C. 2013. *Caring Democracy: Markets, Equality, and Justice*. New York: New York University Press.

Walker, Margaret Urban. 1998. *Moral Understandings: A Feminist Study in Ethics*. New York: Routledge.

5

Care ethics and "caring" organizations

Nel Noddings

Over the past three decades, the relation between ethics of care and ethics of justice has been much discussed (Gilligan 1982; Engster 2007; Held 2005; Noddings 1984). Early on, the two approaches to ethics were contrasted; a bit later, attempts were made to absorb one into the other and/or to show that neither is complete without the other. Drawing on theories of justice, writers have often used the adjective *just* to describe societies, institutions, practices, and even schools that establish and maintain justice. Only recently have we seen the adjective *caring* applied to organizations such as large employers, nations, and schools. I will argue here that we should apply such labels cautiously. Organizations can certainly address some particular needs, but they cannot *care* in the sense required by care ethics. Assuming that they can do so may lead to a corruption of the concept of care. Before launching that argument, however, it is necessary to identify and analyze some important distinctions that arise in discussion of justice and care.

Justice and Care

It is generally recognized that justice is a rights-based ethic and care is needs-based. The concept of needs is enormously complex (Braybrooke 1987; Tronto 1993), and we'll have to say much more about it, particularly distinguishing needs from wants and desires. However, it seems clear that the concept of needs is more basic than that of rights. Indeed, it seems that rights begin as expressed needs (or wants) and become rights when claimants finally can exercise the power to satisfy their needs. Then it requires care—attentiveness and responsiveness—to extend those rights to others. It also requires care to perceive and understand that others may not evaluate a "right" as we do.

Another important difference between the two types of ethics is that care ethics is a relational ethic, whereas the justice approach is anchored in the individual, in his/her rights, duties, and liberty. In part, this distinction arises from the roots of care ethics in women's experience, the long history of responsibility for the welfare of children and the maintenance of caring relations. This history is clearly important, but overemphasis on it sometimes causes confusion between *caring* and *caregiving*. Caregiving as an activity—paid or unpaid—can be engaged in with or without the care described in care ethics. While it is true that experience in caregiving, women's traditional experience, seems to engender the attitudes defined in care ethics, it is important to distinguish the activities from the overall ethical approach. It is also worth mentioning that the relational approach has been described by Martin Buber (1970), who advised us to start political and social theorizing with neither the individual nor the collective. "In the beginning," he wrote, "is the relation" (1970, 69). Thus, although care ethics is widely (and rightly) considered to be closely related to women's experience, it is broader and deeper than "feminist ethics." As Virginia Held has pointed out:

> Care is probably the most deeply fundamental value. There can be care without justice: There has historically been little justice in the family, but care and life have gone on without it. There can be no justice without care, however, for without care no child would survive and there would be no persons to respect. (2005, 17)

As a relational ethic, care ethics recognizes the roles of both carer and cared-for in establishing and maintaining the caring relation. The carer is attentive, open to the possibility of being affectively moved and experiencing motivational displacement, and responds in a way to meet the needs of the cared-for or, at least, to maintain the caring relation. The cared-for completes the relation by acknowledging the efforts of the carer. It is important to note here that the response of the carer may or may not be efficacious in the long run. As carers, we occasionally make mistakes. This is another reason why care theorists put such emphasis on the relation. By maintaining the caring relation, we keep open the possibility of correcting our responses. An infant may smile and cuddle closer to the parent, a patient may sigh with relief as the nurse relieves her pain, a student may offer a comment or question that promotes further exploration of a point made by the teacher. The response of the cared-for need not be gratitude; it is merely (and significantly) an expression acknowledging that the caring has been received. The role of the cared-for is essential, and its recognition is central to care ethics. In traditional, rationalist ethics, a moral agent's act is judged by its conformity to the appropriate principle. In virtue ethics, it is judged by conformity with the requirements of character laid down by the finest model. In care ethics, a carer's act must be evaluated with respect to its effects on the relevant web of care, but there is no caring *relation*—no matter how hard the carer works—if there is no acknowledging response from the cared-for. This requirement is especially important when we consider the possibility of "caring" organizations.

Let's return briefly now to the topic of needs. In addition to the difficulty of distinguishing needs and wants, there is also confusion over assumed (or inferred) needs and expressed needs. Some human needs can obviously be assumed; we all need food, shelter, and clothing. It is still possible, however, to make mistakes even with these needs when we fail to communicate with those thought to be in need. Organizations have been known to flood survivors of natural disasters with clothing when they really need food or with food when they need building materials. But a deeper confusion arises in some theoretical descriptions of needs. When theorists such as Abraham Maslow suggest a hierarchy of needs, we are led to believe that people can address only one level of need at a time: that is, that one cannot aspire to a higher need until a lower one has been met (Braybrooke 1987). However, even if people cannot work actively on a higher level of need (and this is by no means certain), they may still feel such a need strongly. People may very well feel—or express in some way—simultaneous needs for food, safety, respect, even self-actualization. It is important to remember this as we move to globalize care. The message, once again, is to care—to attend, listen, and observe, and to maintain relations of care and trust.

In education, most of what is done in schools is based on assumed needs, and there is some justification for this. After all, adults do have some knowledge about what children need to achieve satisfactory and satisfying lives. However, the best teachers listen not only for expressed needs but for expressed wants and interests. To have one's interests recognized and encouraged is itself a basic need, whether or not it is directly expressed. Understanding this, teachers offer far more in the way of information, stories, and informal histories than will appear on tests. Not every story or account will appeal to every student, but the plenitude of such offerings should ensure that most students will find their interests encouraged. To teach only that which all students *must* learn is to reduce teaching to mere instruction, and teachers are more than instructors. Good teachers are models of intellectual, aesthetic, and moral life. This ideal is recognized in care ethics when we respect the difference between assumed and expressed needs. To address expressed needs, teachers work to establish relations of care and trust with their students. Within such relations, intellectual dialogue can become meaningful.

It is also necessary to distinguish between caring-for and caring-about. It is not possible to care-for everyone in the world; caring-for requires the attention and response cultivated in relation. It is possible, however, to care-about—to be concerned for—multitudes at a distance. The question arises how this caring-about is to be translated into caring-for. A natural disaster such as an earthquake or flood usually brings an outpouring of caring-about, but the response is often short-lived, and sometimes the transition from caring-about (concern) to caring-for is disrupted by inefficiency or even corruption.

But, again, there is a deeper theoretical problem. If we suppose that those about whom we are concerned want (or need) exactly what we would want in their situation, or that we can assume knowledge of their situation from a few salient facts, we are likely to make serious mistakes and evoke distrust and resentment rather than gratitude. As we discuss global and organizational caring, it should become clear that organizations (such as schools) cannot care-for directly. They must concentrate on establishing conditions under which caring-for can take place, under which relations of care and trust are established and maintained. We—as individuals or organizations—cannot do for every child what we wish for our own. In caring-about all children, we can work intelligently to support the conditions under which good people can supply the direct caring-for needed by every child.

Caring-about may be thought of as the foundation of justice in care theory. We can and should care about everyone and work from that basic attitude to establish policies that will facilitate the caring-for that must occur on-site. Both forms of caring are essential. Clearly, we can care-about and then fail to move on to caring-for, and I'll say much more about this common failure. But it is also possible to care-for those closest to us and ignore or even allow others to mistreat people who need care.

Care ethics recognizes the centrality of *emotion* or *feeling* in moral life. In this, we might trace our philosophical roots to David Hume and the moral philosophers who emphasized the role of feeling in moral motivation (Noddings 2010; Slote 2010). Reason is required in analyzing situations and evaluating our resources, but we may achieve understanding and yet remain bystanders. Hume put it this way:

> What is honourable, what is fair, what is becoming, what is noble, what is generous, takes possession of the heart, and animates us to embrace and maintain it. What is intelligible, what is probable, what is true, procures only the cool assent of the understanding. (1983/1751, 15)

To be motivated to act, we must *feel* something. When a large group of people react to the suffering of others at a distance, they care-about the sufferers and may act by contributing funds for their relief. This laudable caring-about, however, may or may not be realized in caring-for. As we explore ways in which to translate caring-about into caring-for, we will again encounter a complex of problems involving the concept of needs. Needs, whether assumed or expressed, must be interpreted, and that task must be undertaken at both the level of caring-about and that of caring-for.

Can Large Organizations Care?

In a recent article in the *New York Times*, Nicholas Kristof (2013) drew attention to the debate over whether foreign aid helps or hurts those meant to receive it, and he has provided some evidence on both sides of the debate. Sometimes the aid publicly announced for relief is actually directed toward political purposes and little reaches the purported recipients. Other times, the whole campaign is simply mishandled and inefficient. And too often, aid encourages corruption in both caregivers and receivers. What is missing in all of these cases is the activation of genuine caring-for, the person-to-person relationship characterized by attention, dialogue, recognition of expressed needs, and immediate response moved by the feeling aroused when people are in direct contact with those in need. Kristof documents the difference revealed in the work of Rea Dol in Haiti. Whereas much of the aid money meant for Haiti after the earthquake seems to have disappeared without a constructive result, "Dol soldiers on and works closely with a network of other Haitians also trying to build a better Haiti" (Kristof 2013, 11). She has established a school and a library, and she works directly with both donors and recipients. In this case, the caring-about of students in Los Altos, California, has been translated into caring-for by Dol and a working group in Haiti. The success of Dol's project and that of so many on-site NGOs underscores the importance of relationships in caring-for.

Fiona Robinson notes that reaction to the world's growing interdependence has been "to return to the universalism of Kant" (1999, 45). Robinson comments that this turn is ironic because a genuine understanding of globalization should lead us to appreciate differences not only between individuals but between groups, nations, and cultures. Care ethics is not aimed at removing all of these differences but, rather, at developing relationships that will disclose which should be removed by cooperative action and which should be sustained and appreciated. A common mistake under the Kantian return is to assume that we all share a common conception of justice and place the same value on individual rights. Robinson points out, rightly, that such a faulty conception of universality often leads to paternalism or even domination in an effort to correct others and shape their societies in our image.

It may be the paternalism felt by recipients of care that causes the passivity decried by some critics of both foreign and domestic aid. When people feel that they are recipients of aid because they are both needy and somehow deficient, they may sullenly accept their inferior status and simply give up. In some cases, acceptance may be accompanied by resentment, and then the possibility of corruption is increased. The ungrateful recipients of "care" feel justified in taking all they can get. This result underscores the importance of recognizing the simultaneity of needs. Those in economic need may at the same time need respect and the assurance that they are capable of helping themselves. Meeting this need should not excuse laziness or cheating. On the contrary, it should be part of building relations of care and trust through which competence will grow on both sides. As Joan Tronto has argued, "an adequate account of needs, and of capacities, should be embedded in an understanding of care as an ongoing and multifaceted process" (1993, 139). I would add that, as the relationship develops, both parties—initial caregivers and recipients—should enter each encounter as potential carers and cared-fors. This is a mark, generally, of adult, equal relations. Realistically, we must admit that some recipients of care will not become more individually responsible; some may indeed become more lax and dependent. In such cases, a paternalistic program may be justified, but when should that possibility enter the interpretive discussion?

Nancy Fraser raises a host of questions concerning the interpretation of needs. Focusing on the homeless, she asks: "Do homeless people need forbearance, so that they may sleep undisturbed next to a hot-air vent on a street corner? A space in a subway tunnel or a bus terminal? A bed in a temporary shelter? A permanent home?" (1989, 163). Now, of course, she is right to point out that, at the level of political discourse, there are multiple participants in the conversation and many competing interests. But all of this, important as it is, takes place in the "caring-about" mode. In that mode, Fraser admits, the needs of the homeless are assumed (or inferred) by various groups, and the right of the contesting groups who are making the assumptions to speak authoritatively is also assumed. The people in need are not usually included in these conversations.

Too often, it is supposed that what has been decided at the caring-about stage is definitive. On-site carers, then—those charged with providing care—simply have to follow the directives, albeit, one would hope, with compassion and respect. Care ethics advises caution here. In attempting to establish a caring relation, a carer asks the question suggested by Simone Weil: "What are you going through?" Weil insists on meeting the other "not only as a unit in a collection, or a specimen from the social category labeled 'unfortunate,' but as a man, exactly like us" (1977, 51). One can disagree with the last phrase, "exactly like us," and yet endorse her basic advice that we must start with attention to the individual cared-for. In listening, we may move away from assumed needs toward expressed needs. Maintaining the caring relation makes it possible for both parties to suggest revisions in the mutual understanding of needs.

Weil's emphasis, one central to care ethics, is on attention. The carer listens to and observes the cared-for. Weil writes, "This way of looking is first of all attentive. The soul empties itself of all its own contents in order to receive the being it is looking at, just as he is, in all his truth" (1977, 51). Now again, one may argue against Weil that it is simply not possible for the soul to empty itself of all its own contents, but care ethics argues that it *is* possible for the carer to put aside his or her own projects for the moment and allow the expressed needs of the cared-for to take precedence. When this occurs, the carer often feels with or for the cared-for and experiences motivational displacement; his or her motivational energy flows toward the needs of the cared-for.

At this point, another important feature of care ethics should be mentioned. When the carer is attentive, she is in a *receptive* mode. This is very different from the mode described in the original definition of empathy as projection into a work of art or another's mind in order to understand it. On that definition, empathy is projective and cognitive. In contrast, care ethics postulates the carer as receptive and feeling; she receives the other into her own mind and center of feeling; she does not project herself into the other. It is for this reason that I have been reluctant to use the word *empathy*. Today, *empathy* is notoriously ambiguous. It is sometimes used as a synonym for sympathy. In some interpretations, the cognitive aspect—empathic accuracy—is dominant; in other approaches, the affective dimension is emphasized; often, there is confusion between empathy as a process and empathy as a feeling that results from a process. The term badly needs further analysis (Noddings, 2013a).

In the projective mode, at the level of caring-about, we often ask how we would feel, what we would need, if we were in the other's situation. This is not a useless move. Indeed, it readies us to conform to the biblical injunction to do unto others as we would have done unto us. It prepares us to invoke justice. When we move to caring-for, however, we recognize that the other is an *other*, not necessarily exactly like us, and we must enter a receptive mode in order to find out what the other is going through, what he or she needs. We listen for expressed needs and do not assume what the other needs by reference to our own experience. Notice that both questions are useful, but one is better used at the level of caring-about, the other at the level of caring-for.

The brief answer to the question whether large organizations can care is that, in their policies and public statements, they can express their concern; they can care-about. To translate that form of caring into genuine caring-for, they must provide the conditions under which on-site workers can engage in caring-for.

Moving from Caring-about to Caring-for

In the policy discussions of large organizations, we are necessarily at the level of caring-about. I mentioned earlier Nancy Fraser's formidable list of questions on the problem of homelessness. There have been arguments made in favor of respecting the rights of the homeless to *be* homeless—to sleep under bridges or on the sidewalks, to beg outside restaurants, to disrupt traffic on city streets. When such arguments are made, one response is to consider others in the web of care. Will granting a particular right to the homeless cause distress to or violate the rights of others in the community? Will schoolchildren feel unsafe as they must walk past homeless men lying in corners or doorways for shelter? Will the aesthetic sense of the community be offended and business hurt by the decision of consumers to avoid areas inhabited by the homeless? Should we be ashamed even to raise such questions? Care theory insists that we listen when we are addressed. These questions must be discussed; both questioners and potential recipients of care may be enriched by the dialogue. To squelch questions that suggest insensitive class differences simply pushes their objections beneath the surface. When a woman says, "I don't like walking past dirty, drunken old men lying in doorways," it doesn't improve matters to remind her that the "dirty old men" are suffering more than she is and that she should be more compassionate. The focus has to be concentrated on the question: what shall we do about it?

Fraser (1989) and Tronto (1993) both emphasize the difference in power inherent in discussions of social policy. Those making policy are in positions of some authority; those in need of care typically have little power to change their situation. Often, even the vocabulary and grammar of the two groups are markedly different. To be sure, this power difference often works to satisfy the needs of those in power, but in trying to develop an appropriate vocabulary at the level of caring-about, we must exercise our receptivity and keep the conversation open. We can act to improve the condition of dirty old men without scorning the aesthetic interests of fussy old women. This is an important point at which to remind readers that care theory is not just about caregiving, important as that is. More basically, it is about how we should meet and treat each other. Weil's question—what are you going through?—is relevant in every human encounter.

At the policy level, power differences exist between caregivers and care recipients, but the ideological differences mentioned above sometimes lead to conditions under which the needs of care recipients are actually neglected. The policy-makers throw their energy into fighting each other. For example, one group may describe itself as liberal and generous, the other as conservative and compassionate. Both present moral arguments, one inclined more toward equality and rights, the other toward paternalism. The contest over who are the "good guys" displaces the real problem. It would seem sensible to pull the debate away from a purely theoretical argument to one more clearly directed to the problems at hand. The policy making of caring-about will still occur at some distance from the real-life recipients of care, but it need not concentrate on condoning or condemning paternalism or on general, theoretical positions concerning the role of government in welfare. The goal is not to separate policy-makers into two (or more) warring camps, each claiming to be right. The goal is to work together to improve the lives of those needing care and to support the on-site caregivers.

Well-conducted discussions on the problems of homelessness will recognize the expressed needs of policy-makers, community members, caregivers, and recipients of care. It should become clear that acts of paternalism are sometimes necessary, as are acts that allow freedom to do what many of us deem unwise. How should we choose? In *Starting at Home*, I wrote:

> A responsible society needs an attitude that will allow it to exercise sensitive control. I argue, for example, that people should not be allowed to sleep on the street (even if they claim this as a right), but that the relevant public must respond to complaints that shelters are not safe, hygienic, or consonant with the promotion of human dignity. We ought not to be deterred by charges of "paternalism" unless we are indeed guilty of exercising control without attentive love... In contrast to self-righteous love, attentive love listens, it is moved, it responds, and it monitors its own action in light of the response of the cared-for. (Noddings 2002, 136–7)

Thus it is necessary to establish regular communication between those discussing care at the policy (or caring-about) level and those working directly with the recipients of care. How does the conversation change at the level of caring-for? The carer must listen and watch for expressed needs among those requiring care. These will vary from one recipient to another. In the case of homelessness, for example, some will express a need only for shelter; some will emphasize safety; some will hope for privacy; and some (families, usually) will express a need for a *home*, a living space uniquely their own. In a recent series in the *New York Times* (Elliott 2013), it was revealed that one family—mother, stepfather, and eight young children—were housed in one room, no kitchen, a bathroom shared by other residents. The Auburn Family Residency, where they lived for three years, is described in the first article in the series as "a decrepit city-run shelter for the homeless" (1). Even the shortest conversation between care worker and recipient would reveal desperate needs that are not being met.

We see here a failure at all levels. Cramming a large family into one room (without privacy partitions) should be forbidden at the policy level. Caregivers at the level that should be caring-for should press for more options. The needs of one man under treatment for alcohol addiction are surely very different from the needs of a large family. The caregivers are negligent in another way. Part of their job, as carers, should be to establish relations of care and trust not only with their clients but *among* their clients. The carers could recruit residents to clean the filthy bathrooms, watch for the safety of women and children in the halls, and work together to make the serving of meals more efficient and pleasant. As things are now, the residents trust neither the care workers nor each other.

The adults in the family described here are also at fault. The father rarely works, and he spends money foolishly. The mother admits to stealing and has spent occasional nights in jail. She is always ready for a fight and encourages her children to engage in physical combat to protect their interests. Perhaps the children should be placed in foster care, but . . . they love one another and derive their only sense of permanency from clinging to each other. It is this love for each other that should be built upon. It could provide a powerful motivating force.

In the earlier mention of Rea Dol in Haiti (Kristof 2013), it was noted that she works closely with members of the group needing help. It would certainly make sense to do this—at least, try to do it—at the Auburn residence. Are there residents willing to help themselves and others? Are care workers willing to help in securing more financial support for cleaning supplies, paint, and the like? Is there regular, reciprocal communication between those charged with caring-for and those at the caring-about level? Do policy-makers invite suggestions from on-site workers, or do they simply insist on "accountability"? If the latter is the case, then there is an absence of caring at the level of transition from caring-about to caring-for. At every stage, we must remember that there is no caring relation if the cared-for does not acknowledge the effort to care. When neither the homeless nor the social workers charged with their care feel cared-for, there is clearly something wrong with the system.

When we read about situations such as those in the Auburn Family Residency, we not only deplore the lack of attention to expressed needs at every level, but also think more tolerantly of paternalism. After all, there are good fathers and bad fathers. A government agency must sometimes exercise control of those citizens who seem, on sound evidence, unable to take responsibility for their own lives. We allow this reluctantly because we regret the loss of freedom it involves. The alternative, however, may be worse. To allow people to live in squalor, to permit their children to skip school often, to steal when they want to provide a birthday cake, to continue their lives in addiction, and to insist that they are not responsible for all of these misfortunes cannot be defended in the name of freedom. Isaiah Berlin put it well when he said, "to admit that some of our ideals may in principle make the fulfillment of others impossible is to say that the notion of total human fulfillment is a formal contradiction, or metaphysical chimaera" (1969, 167–8). Commenting on this assessment in an earlier work, I said:

> If by coercion of the mentally ill [or socially irresponsible], we produce for them a better life than they might have had, the loss of freedom is to that degree justified. If their lives are not improved—and here we have to listen to their evaluation of their own experience—then, as Berlin would put it, the loss of freedom is absolute. (Noddings 2002, 258)

Caring Schools

In our discussion of caring in social services, we saw that failures to provide care can occur at the level of caring-about (policy making), at the level of caring-for, or in the transition from one level to the other. It was granted in that discussion that a system of care must provide for both assumed and expressed needs, and that it is sometimes necessary to exercise paternalism. In this brief exploration of caring schools, I will argue that today's schools have gone too far in the direction of paternalism: that is, we are exercising too much control and too little attentive love.

The tendency, ostensibly driven by a sense of justice, is to force all students into a college preparatory program, regardless of their talents and interests. As a result, courses in music, the arts, and vocational pursuits have been drastically cut. Policies established at the caring-about level concentrate on providing the same education for all students, thereby depriving many students of opportunities to develop their own special abilities. Indeed, it has become almost heresy to suggest that some students, perhaps many, are better suited to programs other than the conventional academic preparation. I agree that all students should have an opportunity *to choose* (not be assigned to) an academic program, but they should also have the opportunity to choose, under careful guidance, a really fine vocational program, and at present we are unwilling to spend the money required to develop and sustain such programs (Noddings 2013b). This is a failure at the caring-about level.

A second example of failure at the policy level is the establishment of zero-tolerance rules. Fortunately, school people are beginning to speak out against these rules. To punish each forbidden act in exactly the same way—whether the offense was committed by accident, by a first-offender, with or without an apology—cripples the efforts of teacher-carers to relate to their students as individuals. Policies of this kind undermine efforts to care-for.

At bottom, today's policy making is too narrowly concentrated on standardized teaching and testing. When smaller class-size is recommended, for example, policy-makers ask whether the result will be higher test scores. They seem to forget that there other, more important, outcomes to seek. Smaller classes provide greater opportunities for teachers and students to develop relationships of care and trust. Schools would almost certainly do better on the issues addressed under zero-tolerance rules if they encouraged teachers to spend more time in developing these relationships instead of trying to control behavior through threats of punishment. Teachers and students should be encouraged to work together to build a safe, cooperative, and creative learning environment.

Possibly the worst failure in translating caring-about into caring-for is the overemphasis on instruction at the cost of relationships. Teachers are not just instructors. If that were their only job, we might do well to turn the job over to computers and online courses. Students are influenced by their teachers not only as instructors but far more deeply by them as persons. Doris Kearns Goodwin, in her account of the journalists working for *McClures*, notes, "Each of the four journalists [Ray Stannard Baker, Lincoln Steffens, Ida Tarbell, and William Allen White] was deeply influenced by a teacher" (2013, 201). We hear stories like this again and again, and yet the current insistence is on strictly planned lessons involving a learning objective, direct instruction, practice (often rote), and assessment. Sometimes, the lesson is even scripted.

Sound educational policies would encourage the creation of relationships of care and trust between teachers and teachers, teachers and students, students and students. Relationships of care and trust are developed person-to-person through attention and dialogue. Mark Edmundson writes:

> Why does the encounter need to take place face-to-face, rather than online? Because the student and the teacher need to create a bond of good feeling, where they are free to speak openly with each other. They need to connect not just through cold print but through gestures, intonations, jokes. The student needs to discover what the teacher knows and what she exemplifies about how to live; the teacher needs contact with the student's energy and hopes. (2013, 46)

Conclusion

Large organizations such as social services, schools, and nations cannot care directly: that is, they cannot care-for in the sense prescribed by care theory. Caring-for requires a person-to-person relationship in which both carer and cared-for play essential roles. No institution can do this. What it can do is to provide and support the conditions under which caring relations can prosper. If these conditions are met, the population involved—again, both carers and recipients of care—should report positively on the efforts to care.

With advocates of justice, care theorists agree that organizations, nations, and societies should care-about the welfare of everyone. But the policies promulgated at the caring-about level must support the work of those doing the person-to-person on-site, the real work of caring-for.

References

Berlin, Isaiah. 1969. *Four Essays on Liberty*. Oxford: Oxford University Press.

Braybrooke, David. 1987. *Meeting Needs*. Princeton, NJ: Princeton University Press.

Buber, Martin. 1970. *I and Thou*, translated by Walter Kaufmann. New York: Scribner's Sons.

Edmundson, Mark. 2013. *Why Teach? In Defense of a Real Education.* New York: Bloomsbury USA.

Elliott, Andrea. 2013. "Invisible Child." *New York Times*, 9–13 December.

Engster, Daniel. 2007. *The Heart of Justice: Care Ethics and Political Theory.* Oxford: Oxford University Press.

Fraser, Nancy. 1989. *Unruly Practices: Power, Discourse and Gender in Contemporary Social Theory.* Minneapolis, MN: University of Minnesota Press.

Gilligan, Carol J. 1982. *In a Different Voice.* Cambridge, MA: Harvard University Press.

Goodwin, Doris Kearns. 2013. *The Bully Pulpit: Theodore Roosevelt, William Howard Taft, and the Golden Age of Journalism.* New York: Simon and Schuster.

Held, Virginia. 2005. *The Ethics of Care: Personal, Political, and Global.* Oxford: Oxford University Press.

Hume, David. 1983 [1751]. *An Enquiry Concerning the Principles of Morals.* Indianapolis, IN: Hackett.

Kristof, Nicholas D. 2013. "Can Foreign Aid Help This Girl?" *New York Times (Sunday Review)*, 8 December.

Noddings, Nel. 1984. *Caring: A Feminine Approach to Ethics and Moral Education.* Berkeley, CA: University of California Press.

Noddings, Nel. 2002. *Starting at Home: Caring and Social Policy.* Berkeley, CA: University of California Press.

Noddings, Nel. 2010. *The Maternal Factor.* Berkeley, CA: University of California Press.

Noddings, Nel. 2013a. *Caring: A Relational Approach to Ethics and Moral Education.* Berkeley, CA: University of California Press.

Noddings, Nel. 2013b. *Education and Democracy in the 21st Century.* New York: Teachers College Press.

Robinson, Fiona. 1999. *Globalizing Care.* Boulder, CO: Westview Press.

Slote, Michael. 2010. *Moral Sentimentalism.* Oxford: Oxford University Press.

Tronto, Joan. 1993. *Moral Boundaries: A Political Argument for an Ethic of Care.* New York: Routledge.

Weil, Simon. 1977. *Simone Weil Reader*, edited by George A. Panichas. New York: Moyer Bell.

Part II

Applications

6

The supportive state

Government, dependency, and responsibility for caretaking

Maxine Eichner

Until recently, the liberal political theory that has animated American political thought and public policy has had little to say about the inevitability of dependency in human lives and the important role that families play in dealing with dependency.[1] Liberalism, particularly in its American incarnations, has largely conceived of citizens as able, autonomous adults, and has focused on them as individuals rather than as members of families. Conceptualizing citizens in this manner has helped to ground the important moral ideal that all citizens should be treated as free and equal, which in turn has justified the state's role in safeguarding freedom and equality. Yet while the liberal conception of humans as autonomous adults may be an important moral ideal, as care theorists have pointed out, it does not reflect the reality of the human condition. In reality, citizens spend most of their lives dependent on one another to some greater or lesser degree. Citizens are born completely dependent and live in near-total dependence on others for roughly the first decade of their lives, and in considerable dependence during their second decade. During these first two decades, they require large amounts of caretaking and human development to become healthy, flourishing adults and contributing members of the polity.

A small but significant number of citizens will never achieve a substantial degree of independence from the caretaking of others because of physical or mental disabilities. Most others will enter an adulthood in which they are largely, although never completely, independent. All adults have some periods in which they require significant caretaking because of physical or mental illness. Further, a considerable portion of adults will experience serious disabling conditions that will leave them dependent for long periods of time, if not permanently. And as they age and approach the end of life, most adults will become increasingly dependent on others for care.

Recognizing this dependency makes the picture of what citizens need from society more complex than conventional versions of liberal political thought would have it. If adults are conceived as capable and autonomous, the respect for human dignity that grounds liberalism requires, above all, ensuring their freedom and equality. To ensure these, central liberal institutions provide for sovereignty of the people; a limited state; and the security of its citizens. Once we adjust the image of citizens to account for the dependency in the human life cycle, however, respect for human dignity entails more than just protecting citizens' individual rights: caretaking and human development come to the fore as every bit as important to human dignity as safeguarding citizens' liberty and security. The importance of caretaking and human development, in turn, calls attention to the role of the family, which, as our society is currently structured, has been the institution largely responsible for performing these functions.

To the scant extent that liberal theory has attended to families, it has generally conceived of them as if, like the adults who head them, they properly are and should be autonomous. The goal of public policy, in this view, is to keep the family as free as possible from state intervention. Moreover, insofar as dependency needs of children arise, this theory contends that the autonomous adults who head families should properly deal with them, without action by the state.

This view of family autonomy, however, like the view of individual autonomy, is a gross oversimplification. In truth, the ways in which families function are always deeply and inextricably intertwined with government policy. To mention just a few examples, child-labor laws keep children financially dependent on their parents; equal employment legislation has encouraged women's movement into the labor market and out of the home; and Social Security survivors' benefits influence some recipients not to marry. Most importantly, for the purposes of this chapter, law and public policy affect families' ability to deal with dependency needs. Because of this, and the critical role that sound families play in the lives of flourishing citizens and a flourishing society, the family–state relationship must occupy a central position in liberal democratic theory. The centrality of dependency also means that questions asked of political theory must be amended: no longer is it sufficient simply to ask what a just distribution of societal goods among citizens would be, or how we should best organize society to protect citizens' rights. We must also ask how we can bring into being, care for, and develop the faculties and virtues of sound citizens. Putting these issues center stage, however, requires revising fundamental tenets of liberal theory. In this chapter, I begin that revision.[2]

Expanding the List of Important Liberal Goods: Supplementing Freedom and Equality with Caretaking and Human Development

To begin with, the marquee of important liberal values must be expanded so that freedom and equality share top billing with the added goods of caretaking and human development. Yet the two newcomers cannot simply be added to the existing list while leaving the other goods unchanged. Instead, adding caretaking and human development to the pantheon of liberal goods necessarily reorients how both of the heretofore dominant liberal values of liberty and equality should be conceived. The recognition of dependency requires discarding the idea of complete freedom, conceived in terms of independence from others, as an impossible and unpalatable goal; dependency will always be a part of life to be managed in any human society committed to the dignity of its citizens (Fineman 2004, 36). Yet we should still hold tight to the portion of freedom that embodies the ideal of autonomy—the notion that humans should be able to plan and pursue their own course in life (Spragens 1999, 122).[3] Recognition of the fact of dependency in human lives, and a focus on the human life cycle, however, make it clear that autonomy of this sort is not a condition that simply appears at birth, and which the state may adequately respect through ensuring individuals' freedom to be left alone to enact their life plans. Instead, this sort of autonomy is an achievement that takes time and requires certain circumstances. Without caretaking and adequate development of their capabilities, individuals could not become the (largely) autonomous citizens whose choices are worthy of respect.

The recognition of dependency in the human condition also has significant consequences for equality, the good generally given second billing behind liberty in our tradition of liberal thought. The copious amount of care work that dependency necessitates has profound implications for gender, economic, and racial equality. The great extent of the care work required means that many citizens—disproportionately women and minorities—spend a good part of their adult lives engaged in caretaking for children or ill or aging adults (AARP 2009, fig. 7, fig. 2).[4] The failure to recognize dependency as an integral issue for political theory has led to the exploitation and inequality of those who perform dependency work (Kittay 1999, x, 40). Putting dependency in proper theoretical perspective therefore requires thinking through how a society can fairly distribute its care work, and the benefits and burdens that accompany it.

Adding caretaking and human development to the aspirations of a liberal democracy not only transforms liberal theory; it also, necessarily but unfortunately, complicates it. Contemporary liberalism already embodies an unsettled internal tension between liberty and equality, which is responsible for the conflict between libertarians and progressives. Resolving what a just government would do to balance considerations of freedom and equality is difficult enough; adding in supporting caretaking and human development as well, complicates this situation further. Does the state have a responsibility to provide universal childcare, which would require higher taxes, therefore restricting citizens' freedom to use their money as they would? Questions like this make for more complicated political theory.

Yet an adequate liberal democratic theory has no alternative but to embrace this larger list of goods, given that caretaking and human development are fundamental to a healthy polity. A theory that eliminates these other goods in order to produce determinative results, such as that attempted by John Rawls in his hugely influential work, *A Theory of Justice*, which defines the state's role only in terms of pursuing freedom and equality, attains its determinacy at the cost of ignoring goods of critical importance (Rawls 1971). Rather than artificially restricting the important goods at stake, what is called for is a more nuanced theory and more nuanced public policies that carefully calibrate this mix of goods and, as far as possible, ameliorate the tension among them (Spragens 1999, xv). Where this tension cannot be resolved through carefully-crafted policies, hard choices must be made among this expanded list of goods. At least a revised vision of liberal theory can do so explicitly and thoughtfully, rather than by ignoring the existence of important goods.

In the rest of this chapter, I begin to sketch out what such a revised vision of liberal theory that incorporates caretaking and human development would look like. Incorporating these goods, I argue, requires transforming the role of the state from a neutral protector of individual rights to a state that supports the development of its citizens' capacities. It also requires recognizing the centrality of families to a healthy polity, and considering the ways that they can best be supported in their caretaking and human development responsibilities. Finally, it necessitates transforming the dominant notion of family privacy, conceptualized in terms of the state leaving families to succeed or fail on their own lights, to one in which the state supports families in their caretaking and human development activities but enables them to make important decisions for themselves.

Rethinking the Role of the State: from Neutrality to the Support for Caretaking and Human Development

Incorporating the goods of caretaking and human development as a central concern of liberal theory requires revising the conception of the role of the state.[5] The dominant view of the role of the state in liberal theory, most famously put forth by John Rawls in *A Theory of Justice*, is that it should be neutral with respect to different ways of life (Rawls 1971). As Ronald Dworkin expressed this view: The state "must be neutral on . . . the question of the good life [and] political decisions must be, so far as is possible, independent of any particular conception of the good life, or of what gives value to life" (Dworkin 1985, 191). William Galston aptly summarized this view of the liberal state as "presid[ing] benignly over [different ways of life], intervening only to adjudicate conflict, to prevent any particular way of life from tyrannizing over others, and to ensure that all adhere to the principles that constitute society's basic structure" (Galston 1991, 80).

Both communitarians and feminists have demonstrated that what was taken by Rawlsian liberal theorists to be neutral actually embodies a particular conception of the good life premised on autonomy and individual choice.[6] Adapting liberal theory to recognize citizens' dependency needs points out further difficulties with the Rawlsian view of the state's role. If we conceive of citizens as able, autonomous adults, the state best respects their dignity by constructing a private realm that is off-limits for state action, and by limiting the role of the state to protecting individuals' rights to be left alone. Incorporating dependency into our understanding of human relations, however, transforms the focus of the liberal project: respect for human dignity now demands more than the protection of individual rights and freedoms. It also requires that the state actively support individuals in receiving the caretaking and conditions for human development necessary for them to become responsible, self-directing citizens. This responsibility of the state to support caretaking and human development becomes every bit as fundamental as its responsibility to establish an adequate police force and military in order to safeguard citizens' individual rights.

Transforming the conception of the state's role from neutral protector of individual rights to active supporter of caretaking and human development does not mean the state should abandon its commitment to neutrality entirely, but it must transform this commitment. As Rawls recognized in his later work, his earlier commitment to keep the state neutral with respect to citizens' visions of the good life was too constraining to foster a healthy policy: certainly a liberal state must be able to distinguish between good citizens and psychopaths. Rawls therefore eased his earlier requirement, asserting that the liberal state need be neutral only in the less restrictive sense that it may not impose any particular vision on its citizens based only on some citizens' personal philosophies of right and wrong, which Rawls referred to as "comprehensive" views of the world. In Rawls's later, more permissive view of the state's proper role, state action must be neutral in the sense that it can be justified in a manner that citizens with a broad range of world views can accept—what Rawls called "public reason" (Rawls 1993). The requirement of public reason posits that state action is supportable only insofar as it is grounded on a set of public ideals and principles—a sort of public morality.[7] The state's support for caretaking and human development is eminently defensible under standards of public reason. Recognizing the fact of dependency as an inevitable feature in human life, and the interplay of this dependency with the respect for human dignity that is central to liberalism, give the state strong public reasons to act to support these goods.

In sum, focusing on dependency complicates the state's role in a liberal polity. No longer can the state be seen as simply safeguarding individuals' rights to be left alone. Instead, the state has a responsibility actively to support specific goods, including caretaking and human development. Focusing on how to support these goods leads ineluctably to consideration of the family–state relationship.

The Family as a Central Political Institution

Mainstream contemporary liberal theory pays little attention to the institution of the family because citizens are taken as autonomous and able. Families, in its view, exist in the private realm, and are only relevant to the public discussion in the limited ways that they affect freedom and equality. Once we take into account the fact of dependency, and we focus on citizens during the course of the human life cycle, however, the role of families in caretaking and human development becomes a central subject for political theory. To begin with, the issue of what groupings of people will be recognized as families becomes an important subject for consideration. While the issue of what constituted a family was long thought to be resolved by nature, as feminist theorists more recently observed (Minow 1997, 250; Nussbaum 2000a; 2000b), it is in fact an issue heavily freighted with legal and political considerations. Indeed, the legal and political nature of this issue has been placed front and center in the battles over same-sex marriage. And as an issue that sounds in law and policy rather than nature, the question of whether particular groupings should be recognized as families should be answerable to principles of justice.

Just as there is no natural, pre-political family, so there are no natural, pre-political ways in which families function. In today's complex society, as I discussed earlier, the ways in which families function are always deeply and inextricably intertwined with government policy (Olsen 1985). The state is not only involved in determining what constitutes a family and when family relationships are dissolved, it is also involved directly and indirectly in a multitude of other ways. For example, the state reinforces parents' authority over children by subjecting the children to court supervision should they disobey their parents; by preventing other adults from caring for them;

and by allowing parents to have considerable power over whether children are institutionalized for mental-health reasons. As Frances Olsen points out, these policies generally go unrecognized as intervention by family privacy advocates only because they are so accepted that they are taken as inevitable (Olsen 1985).

And there are many other ways that state regulation and public policy affect family life. Some of these ways are more obvious: for example, the relaxation of divorce laws affects whether and which families stay together. Others are less obvious: for example, the state's regulation of other institutions outside the family deeply and profoundly affects the lives of families. The provision and mandating of education has shaped and continues to shape the lives of children and affect their parents' control over them. Equal employment laws likely contributed to the increase in divorces, as women in unhappy marriages began to have more financial wherewithal to divorce their husbands (DeWitt 1992). Laws governing the availability of health insurance influence which family members work (Lee 2007, 34; Gruber and Madrian 2002). And US welfare policy was, as Alice Kessler-Harris has demonstrated, constructed deliberately on a model that pitted work and family in mortal conflict, having considerable implications for the ways in which families function (Kessler-Harris 2001).

By the same token, the care that children receive from parents is inextricably intertwined with state policies. Parental care takes place in a matrix of constraints and entitlements that affect a parent's ability and opportunity to parent. The existence or non-existence of minimum wage laws, union rights to bargain, and overtime provisions affect parents' ability to meet the financial needs of their children (Mincy 1990). Welfare-reform laws in the United States that require recipients to work in order to receive welfare subsidies influence parents' ability to care for their children (Gennetian et al. 2002). The scope of family-leave laws affects parents' opportunities to stay home with their children (Lovell et al. 2007). The stability and security of a parent's job affects stress levels in the household, which also affect the quality of parenting. State support for and subsidizing of drug-treatment programs makes it easier or harder for parents to deal with drug addictions that can impair their ability to care for their children.

Along these same lines, the ways in which families function are intricately interlinked with economic and social conditions, which are also influenced by public policy. This tenet is dramatically illustrated by Friedrich Engels' description of working-class families in his account of factory life in Manchester, England in 1844. In that account, the grueling demands of the workplace drained families of their nurturing function, as men, women, and children worked from early morning to late at night. In this society, infants were left alone all day in their parents' unheated flats. The children they became were never properly socialized. In short, the pressure of economics suffocated feelings of love and affection, eviscerated caretaking, and led to the breakdown of the family (Engels 1975/1844, 424–5).[8] A more modern, if somewhat less dramatic, example is illustrated by the "Barriers to Marriage among Fragile Families" study in the United States. The Fragile Families study found that the poor job prospects of unmarried fathers reduced the chances of marriage between unmarried parents. Both partners, the study observed, thought that marriage should be an act that improves the economic status of the family; they were therefore reluctant to marry when the fathers lacked a steady job (Bendheim-Thoman 2003). The point is also made by contemporary studies that demonstrate the link between domestic violence in families and the surrounding economic and social circumstances.[9] These examples suggest that families' ability to produce and sustain sound, healthy citizens can be supported or retarded by their social environments, which, in turn, are influenced by public policy.

In these circumstances, the family has no "natural" baseline of functioning that it can be left to "apart from" the state and public policy, and that would be adulterated if the state were to intercede. Nor does the modern administrative state have a neutral, isolated position it can assume while leaving families autonomously to deal with their own affairs. Instead, the state is always and continually influencing how families conduct their affairs. The issue is not whether state policy will influence families, but whether it will be formulated with this inevitable influence in mind. When it comes to the ways in which families function, no family is an island.

Rethinking the State's Relationship with Families: the Supportive State

We come, then, to the issue of how to theorize the relationship between families and the state. I have argued already that the state has a responsibility to support caretaking and human development. To what extent should this affect the way it constructs its relationship with families? In a liberal democracy, we generally expect citizens to do things they reasonably can do for themselves. Does this mean, then, that the responsibility for dealing with dependency should fall in the first instance to family members, and only to the state if families fail? Rawlsian liberal theory and a good deal of public policy presume this. In this view, families are properly autonomous, providing for the needs of their members without state support.[10] As I have already suggested, however, in our world, the situation is more complicated than this version of family autonomy would have it.

Certainly when it comes to ensuring that family members receive caretaking, there are good reasons to expect that family members will shoulder much of the responsibility to provide or coordinate this care. Where children and spouses are concerned, doing so holds citizens accountable for obligations they have assumed. Citizens who have children should be responsible for their decision to do so, and should be expected to plan carefully and budget wisely for them, as well as to care for them.

Yet the view that family members should bear responsibility for the dependency needs of other family members does not necessarily exempt the state from responsibility for its citizens' dependency needs as well. In fact, there is little controversy over the proposition that the state bears at least some responsibility for dependent citizens. For example, few would argue that the state has no duty to remove children who are the victims of serious abuse from their homes. Instead, the controversy is not about *whether* the state has a duty, but about *when* that duty of the state is triggered. Opponents of state support argue that the state's duty is "residual" in the sense that it should be triggered only *after* families fail in some serious way (Case 2001, 1785).[11] The abuse example is, therefore, uncontroversial in terms of state action because the parents have failed to keep their children safe. The theoretical tenets embedded in current child-welfare law and in a broad array of public policies adopt this residual view of the state's responsibility.

Residual responsibility involves a type of apportionment of responsibility that Robert Goodin, in his schematization of the division of moral responsibility for vulnerable persons, refers to as "disjunctive." The defining feature of disjunctive responsibility is that, if *A* is vulnerable to *B* or to *C* or to *D*, then "any one of them could provide the needed assistance; and if any one of them does, none of the others need to" (Goodin 1985, 134). "The paradigm case... [of this type of responsibility] is that of the drowning child at the crowded (but unguarded) beach: any one of the bystanders could effect the rescue and, if any one does, the others need not" (Goodin 1985, 134). In the case of disjunctive responsibility, a particular person (for example, the nearest adult) may have a moral obligation to aid the vulnerable person before others attempt a rescue; this primary responsibility does not let all others off the hook, however. Once it becomes clear that the person with primary responsibility is not going to act, responsibility devolves to others (Goodin 1985, 134). This, in essence, is the theory proposed by those who advocate only a residual role for the state: parents are supposed to have primary responsibility for children's welfare; this duty devolves to the state only if parents fail in their responsibility.

But a disjunctive division of responsibility is not the only possible division of responsibility. As Goodin counsels, responsibility can also be divided in a "conjunctive" way, so that several persons—or, in this case, family members and the state—have a responsibility to ensure caretaking for societal dependents jointly (Goodin 1985, 136). The paradigm case for a conjunctive division of responsibility is a person trapped in a burning house. Not only does the firefighter who helps her out of the window have an obligation to do so; so do the firefighters who hold the trampoline below; and so does the emergency medical technician who provides medical aid. To spin this out still further, the firefighter also requires training, as well as sufficient equipment, from others to be able to do her job well. The fact that one actor bears responsibility to act, therefore, does not preclude concurrent responsibility on the part of others.

So which type of responsibility, disjunctive or conjunctive, should the state bear for meeting citizens' dependency needs vis-à-vis families? The intricate interconnections between families and the state make it conceptually inaccurate to conceive of a family acting *before* the state steps in. Instead, state action always and already affects families' capacity to deal with dependency issues. In addition, families and the state are not similarly situated when it comes to dealing with dependency needs. Families, given that they know their members' needs well and are generally the people who care about them the most, are better suited to performing the hands-on care and arranging other care for those with such needs. Yet they are less well suited to arranging institutions to support care. In contrast, the state is uniquely suited to ensuring that dependency needs are accommodated at an institutional level by establishing relevant laws and regulations. In this situation, it makes far more sense to conceive of the state's and families' responsibilities as conjunctive.

Returning to the example of the child drowning near multiple adult bystanders makes it clear why the model of disjunctive responsibility is a poor fit to the situation of responsibility for dependency. First, the actors at issue—families and the state—do not act independently of one another, as do the bystanders in the drowning example. Instead, institutions structured directly and indirectly by the state profoundly affect families' ability to care for their members. The child's best chance for achieving well-being is, therefore, not for the nearest adult to rescue the child single-handedly while the state acts just as another bystander. Instead, the child is best served by families and the state acting in conjunction with each other. To analogize to the drowning example, the state's position when it comes to care for dependents could be likened to a pilot in a nearby helicopter, who could drop a life preserver near the struggling child that would assist the adult in towing the child back to shore. Seen in this light, the positions of the relevant actors are considerably closer to the situation of conjunctive responsibility that Goodin describes, in which the actors should work together to protect the vulnerable person.

The beach rescue example, however, omits some of the strongest reasons in favor of conjunctive state responsibility for children and other dependents. Raising children, caring for dependents, and developing human capabilities are all activities that cannot be wrapped up in seconds or minutes like an ocean rescue. Instead, they are complex tasks that are part of a process that generally takes years. No family can reasonably accomplish all these tasks without some forms of help. During that time, moreover, dependents interact with a number of institutions aside from the family that profoundly influence their development, including schools, daycare centers, the labor market, and the healthcare system. By the same token, caretakers interact with a number of institutions, most prominently the labor market, that profoundly influence their ability to meet family members' dependency needs. Given the limits of families in controlling and navigating these other institutions, as well as the unique ability that the state has to exercise influence over these other institutions, there are strong reasons to assign the state responsibility along with parents and other family members.

When it comes to adults who are able to order their own affairs, the state does not have the broad ethical responsibility to protect their welfare that it does for vulnerable dependents. With that said, it is not just children and those with disabilities who need caretaking: all humans need care, even generally healthy adults. And as our society is organized, some large portion of the care that adults need will come, if it comes at all, from other adults with whom we share family relationships. The liberal state's commitment to human dignity, therefore, also makes it responsible for supporting stable caretaking relationships among adults.

Determining that the state and families are both conjunctively responsible for meeting dependency needs does not mean that the state's role should be identical to the role of families. Rather, each should bear responsibility for the area in which it has greater competence. This means that families should bear responsibility for the day-to-day caring for (or arranging the care for) children and others with dependency needs. Meanwhile, the state should bear the responsibility for structuring institutions in ways that help families meet their caretaking needs, and that support human development. This includes ensuring that families have safe and affordable caretaking options, as well as structuring other societal institutions, such as schools and communities, in ways that foster children's and other dependents' development and well-being. This division of responsibility recognizes the malleability and contingency of institutional structures. It does not artificially separate state action from the realm of families or presume that completely clear boundaries can even be drawn between them, but it does assume that certain spheres of authority will exist between the two. I call this vision of the state's role "the supportive state."

In dividing responsibility in this way, the supportive-state model respects citizens' autonomy by treating them as responsible citizens who are accountable for their choices and relationships with others. The liberal state, in this view, provides a scaffold on which citizens can construct their lives, but it does not plan their lives for them, or absolve them of the responsibility to plan carefully and budget wisely to achieve their goals. Yet it maintains that the meeting of dependency needs that these family members perform should be accomplished within institutional structures that facilitate caretaking and human development, and that it is the state's responsibility to secure such institutional structures. This approach recognizes the fact of dependency, and that the ability of families to nurture their members does not simply exist as a matter of nature, or spring up as a matter of spontaneous generation; instead, it is an achievement to be pursued jointly by both citizens and the state.

Determining the Parameters of the State's and Families' Responsibility for Dependency

Determining that the state and families have conjunctive responsibility for dependency does not mean that the state should scrap the ideal of familial autonomy as a goal; as with individual autonomy, however, the conception of family autonomy must be significantly revised. This revision would recognize that families have responsibility for meeting members' dependency needs, but it would also recognize that contemporary families' capacity to meet those needs is intimately related to the way that societal institutions are structured. Just as I argued that individuals sometimes require government action to become as autonomous as possible, the same is true for families. In this view, capable families that can meet their members' dependency needs are an achievement to be jointly pursued by families and the state, rather than an inevitability. State support should therefore be seen not as inimical to autonomy, but rather as an aid to it when it fosters families' capabilities.

But why can't families deal with dependency issues on their own since, in a liberal democracy, we expect citizens to do the things they can do for themselves? Residual views of the state's responsibility for dependency, of the kind reflected in this question, dominate public policy in the United States. Their basic premise—that parents are properly the ones who are responsible for children, and that the state should step in only as a last resort if and when parents have exhausted themselves and their resources—draws from classical liberal theory: liberalism's respect for individual autonomy and its emphasis on a limited state are premised on the view that, to the extent possible, citizens can and should plan and bear responsibility for their own actions and their own lives.

There are a number of problems with the notion of residual state responsibility when applied to the issue of dependency and families, however. As I suggested earlier, the conception that the state should step in only after families fail inadequately conceptualizes the complex interconnections that exist between the family and the state. There is no neutral position in which the state can locate itself until "after" families fail; state policies inevitably affect how, and how well, families will accomplish their caretaking and human development tasks. Moreover, the argument that families should bear sole responsibility for dependency overlooks the structural obstacles that families face. The fact of the matter is that there are critical institutional issues related to childcare and other forms of caretaking that are beyond the ability of most families to negotiate privately. For example, many jobs in the United States are organized in a manner that prevents workers from engaging in significant care work for children.[12] Until these job structures change, many of those parents who seek to shoulder caretaking responsibilities will be stymied from doing so.

Accordingly, the answer to the question of why families who deal with dependency issues should not have to do so on their own begins with the recognition that there is no "on their own" option available. Families and the state are sufficiently interconnected in contemporary society that state policies, regardless of whether they are explicitly formulated with families in mind, profoundly affect families' caretaking abilities. In addition, families and the state are not similarly equipped to deal with the same facets of dependency issues. Families are generally better suited to performing the hands-on care and the arranging of care for dependents. Parents, for example, generally know their children better than the state does, are better at discerning what is in their best interests, and are generally more motivated to promote their children's welfare because of the emotional bond between them. In contrast, the state is singularly placed to ensure that societal institutions are structured in ways that allow families to meet their caretaking responsibilities. Finally, raising children and caring for dependents are complicated, long-term projects. No family can perform these tasks completely on their own.

How far does the supportive state's obligation to support caretaking and human development extend? And how should the state weigh these goods against other goods and purposes of a liberal democracy? Clearly the answer to these questions cannot be determined through a kind of "moral geometry," in which a single, correct answer can be absolutely and firmly calculated once and for all. Nevertheless, some guideposts can at least mark out the parameters of this duty. At a minimum, the supportive state should arrange institutions in such a way that family members can, through exercising diligent but not Herculean efforts, meet the basic physical, mental, and emotional needs of children and other dependents and promote human development while avoiding impoverishment or immiseration. Translated into concrete government policies, this means that the welfare system must be structured in a way that those at the bottom of the economic ladder with dependents receive enough financial assistance so that they can provide them with decent environments that promote basic capabilities.

Insofar as they are required by the state's welfare policies to work outside the home, citizens with caretaking responsibilities must also have realistic access to good-quality, affordable daycare. Further, the state must regulate the workplace to ensure parents enough time with their children so that their children are well parented and supervised, and parents are not so pressed for time or frazzled by time pressures that it interferes with adequate caretaking. In this view, the state shirks its responsibility when it forces parents to choose between working to put food in their children's mouths and ensuring that their children receive adequate caretaking.

The state's threshold level of responsibility for structuring institutions to support caretaking and human development, it should be noted, is not a high one. It simply requires that children and other dependents be afforded decent conditions and sufficient caretaking to meet their basic dependency needs and to promote a minimally-adequate level of human development. A relatively wealthy polity should be able to do far better than simply clear this minimum threshold. With that said, millions of children in the United States are now being raised in conditions that do not meet this standard.[13] Above the state's threshold level of responsibility, state support is no longer an absolute obligation, but rather needs to be balanced against achieving other important goods. Although caretaking is not normally regarded as a distributive good, in many cases it functions in this way because expenditures to support caretaking require trade-offs with other goods. In weighing these trade-offs, the state should consider the importance of sound citizens to the polity's future, as well as its responsibility to avoid exploitation of those who perform significant caregiving—both important reasons for the state to prioritize care work above other uses of the state's resources.

In assessing whether to subsidize over and above this threshold level, a liberal polity can find a common-sense midpoint between, on the one hand, those who argue only for the most minimal state support for dependency and, on the other, those who argue the state should devote virtually unlimited funding to supporting caretaking and human development. One such sensible midpoint can be found by recalling the words of John Stuart Mill, who argued that the existing generation, even though it cannot make the next generation "perfectly wise and good, . . . is perfectly well able to make the rising generation, as a whole, as good as, and a little better than, itself" (Mill 1991/1859, 91). Seeking to do a little better for the next generation is a realistic but still ambitious goal that recognizes the considerable importance of caring for dependents, while also recognizing that there are other goods that a liberal democracy should pursue as well.

Finally, at some point toward the end of the spectrum defined by greater state support, it makes progressively less sense for the state to subsidize higher marginal levels of caretaking instead of other goods. At the upper end of the state-support spectrum, subsidizing more caretaking may actually be counter-productive for both the recipients of care, since it may retard their developing the level of autonomy needed to function well in society, and the caregivers, who may never get to pursue other opportunities in life. Although family members may still decide to perform this higher level of caretaking for dependents, they should do so without state subsidization.

At any point below the upper end of the spectrum, the state may legitimately support caretaking over other pursuits of citizens because of its critical importance to the health of the polity and its close connection to human dignity. This is not to say that other pursuits are not valuable; indeed, many should also be supported by the state, given the availability of resources. This is only to say that there are compelling reasons for the state to support caretaking responsibilities.

The Supportive State and Family Privacy

I have argued against the view that the ideal families in a liberal democracy are those that are autonomous, in the sense that they do not require any support from the state. There is, however, another tenet of liberal thought that is related to the view that families should be autonomous, and that merits further consideration: the belief in family privacy. The conception that there are some areas of life, particularly those connected with the home, personal relationships, and family, that should be free from state intervention and control is central to liberal democratic thought, especially in its American incarnations. Indeed, one of the hallmarks of liberalism is the conceptual walls it draws between various realms, which limit the legitimate scope of state action (Walzer 1984, 315). How should we think about the boundary between family and state in our revised version of liberalism? Put another way, given that the supportive state significantly curtails and revises the notion of family autonomy, should it restrict or even jettison the tenet of family privacy?

The notion that there can and should be an unbreachable delineation between the public world and the private home is, as I have argued, a myth. Yet there still exists an important concern at the heart of the notion of family privacy that deserves continued respect, which harks back to the central liberal notion of autonomy. The view that dignity for humans requires the ability to be self-directing, in the sense of making important decisions about the course of their lives, is central to the justification for privacy generally. While recent liberal theory has generally conceived this decisional autonomy to attach to individuals, there are strong reasons to accord such autonomy to families as well. Doing so comports with the concrete historical concerns that motivated liberalism. The institutional reforms sought by early liberals focused more on loosening a range of social enterprises—conducting business, engaging in worship and religious life, participating in scientific inquiry, educating citizens—from the control of the government and elites than on ensuring the untrammeled freedom of individuals.[14] Ascribing decisional autonomy to families and other associations recognizes the important role that they play in the fabric of the liberal democratic society. Citizens do not live their lives as atomistic individuals who construct institutions from scratch as an exercise of their individual autonomy, as simplistic social contract reasoning might suggest. Instead, they live their lives in and through institutions that organize and give meaning to their lives. Because of this, in Tom Spragens' words, "[a]n embodied liberty, one that is not merely abstract and hypothetical, is to a greater extent than generally realized a function of flourishing, well institutionalized, and broadly autonomous civic enterprises" (Spragens 1999, 140).

Transmuting the current, blanket conception of family privacy into a zone of protection for families' decisional autonomy shifts the state's role. No longer is the appropriate behavior for the state to withdraw completely from the realm of family life (already an impossible goal); instead it is to ensure that families have the means and wherewithal to make important decisions for themselves. Like the old doctrine of family privacy, some of what this requires on the part of the state is forbearance in directing the decision making of families. Under this revised view, absent compelling reasons, decisions about the ways in which individual families function or the lives of their members should generally be left to the family itself.

Yet support for familial autonomy requires more than the state's forbearing from dictating family decisions. The state must also seek to ensure that families have the wherewithal to exercise this autonomy. Not only does this mean helping to ensure that families have the capacity to make important decisions about their family, it also means helping to ensure that families have some reasonable means to effectuate their decisions. While early liberals saw the threat to autonomy as coming from the state, much of today's threats of encroachment on decision making come from the market. The danger is not that the market will coercively compel or prohibit certain types of families or decision making in families, the way the state might prohibit family members from using birth control or prohibit the decision by loved ones to take a family member in a vegetative state off life support. Instead, the threat from the market comes from the risk that families will be so much at its mercy that they cannot exercise meaningful choice with respect to how to accomplish important activities such as caretaking. Rousseau's caution should be taken to heart: that it is essential for democracies "as regards wealth, that no citizen should be rich enough to be able to buy another, and none so poor that he has to sell himself" (Rousseau 1994/1762, 87). His injunction should be taken to prohibit not just literal sale into slavery but also the condition in which one is forced to sell the bulk of one's waking hours and to sacrifice the majority of one's family time in order to put food on the table and a roof over the head of family members, and to provide medical care if they should get sick.

A revised doctrine of family privacy should, therefore, focus on limiting coercion by the market, as well as creating resources and space to ensure decision-making autonomy for families. Measures that establish an upper limit on mandatory working hours, allow employees paid time off for caretaking, raise the minimum wage so that workers need not work more than full-time to keep their families out of poverty, and enable workers to work flexible hours are some of the many measures the state can use to prevent this encroachment (Gornick and Meyers 2003). These measures allow families the institutional space to make important decisions and to accomplish important tasks without being completely beholden to the market.

Conclusion

Revising liberal political theory to take into account the fact of dependency in the lives of citizens transforms this theory in important ways. It changes the central questions that liberal theory asks from simply considering how resources should be fairly divided among citizens to how flourishing citizens can best be supported and nurtured. It also expands the goods that the state must take into account to include caretaking and human development. Further, it fundamentally transforms the role of the state. No longer can the state simply protect citizens' individual rights from violation by others; it must instead actively support the expanded list of liberal goods by ensuring that societal institutions facilitate caretaking and human development. The result is a more complex version of liberalism that must balance a wider range of goods than the current versions, but one that is also in a far better position to bolster human dignity and a flourishing polity.

Notes

1. I use the terms *liberal theory, liberal,* and *liberalism* throughout this chapter to refer to the Anglo-American line of political thought stretching from John Locke through John Stuart Mill and on to such recent thinkers as John Rawls, which

focuses on the importance of liberty, self-government, and the equal worth of citizens. This use of these terms is therefore broader than the use of the term *liberal* in common parlance to refer to those who hold political beliefs at the opposite end of the political spectrum from conservatives.

2. I develop this revision of liberal theory more fully in my book, *The Supportive State* (Eichner 2010).
3. As Thomas Spragens observed: "The goal was, and properly is, a political order in which all citizens are able to sail their own ships, as it were, and not to be either subservient crew members in the conduct of their own lives or adrift in boats with no rudders and luffing sails" (Spragens 1999, 122).
4. In addition to caring for children, a 2009 study by the National Alliance for Caregiving and the AARP estimated that there are 54.1 million American caregivers (23.5 percent of the adult population) who provide unpaid care to an adult aged 18 or older (AARP 2009, fig. 4). These caregivers are present in an estimated 28 million (24 percent of) US households (AARP 2009, fig. 1). The great majority of caregivers (86 percent) are helping relatives (AARP 2009, 18). By 2020, it is expected that 40 percent of the workforce will care for an elderly relative (Craver 2002).
5. As I discuss toward the end of this chapter, incorporating recognition of dependency also requires rethinking, although not discarding, state support for family privacy.
6. For communitarians, see Bellah et al. (1985); MacIntyre (1981); Sandel (1996; 1998); Taylor (1995); Walzer (1990). For feminists, see Rhode (1989); Smart (1989); Young (1990); Minow (1990); Hirschmann (1996, 157).
7. See also Macedo (2000, 169).
8. Some critics have contended that Engels' portrait of Manchester overstated the extent to which family ties eroded, because it understated the extent to which families actively resisted capitalism's corrosive effects (e.g., Humphries 1982, 199).
9. See Weissman (2007), citing relevant studies.
10. Martha Fineman does an excellent job of both laying out and dispelling the myths of individual and family autonomy that circulate in popular discourse (Fineman 2004).
11. The term "residual responsibility" was coined by Duncan Lindsey (Lindsey 1994, 202).
12. I describe these issues more thoroughly elsewhere (Eichner 2010, 39–43); see also Gornick and Meyers (2003).
13. Despite being the wealthiest country in the world, the United States has one of the highest rates of child poverty of any industrialized country. Over 16,000,000 US children—more than one in five—were poor in 2012. Of these children, 40 percent lived in extreme poverty. Children of color are disproportionately represented in this group (Children's Defense Fund 2014, 22).

    Further, although most families with children have parents who work full time, and most such children spend long hours in non-parental care settings, experts have deemed most daycare settings in the United States not to be developmentally enriching. More than half of daycare facilities in the United States provide care that is poor to mediocre. Only roughly one in seven provides care that has been deemed developmentally enriching (studies cited in Eichner 2010, 40–1). The combination of its high child-poverty rate and other factors caused one UNICEF report to rank the United States as second to last overall among the twenty-one wealthy countries ranked in terms of children's well-being (UNICEF 2007, 2).

14. In Thomas Spragens' words, "When liberal theorists and political leaders eulogized liberty, they had in mind not so much a concern with freeing individuals from social control generally but a concern with freeing these important social enterprises from the control of political authorities and social elites" (Spragens 1999, 138; see also Walzer 1990, 23).

References

AARP and National Alliance for Caregiving. 2009. *Caregiving in the US 2009.* <http://www.caregiving.org/data/Caregiving_in_the_US_2009_full_report.pdf>

Bellah, Robert, Richard Madsen, William M. Sullivan, Ann Scidler, and Steven M. Tipton. 1985. *Habits of the Heart: Individualism and Commitment in American Life.* Berkeley, CA: University of California Press.

Bendheim-Thoman Center for Research on Child Wellbeing. 2003. "Fragile Families Research Brief: Barriers to Marriage Among Fragile Families." <http://www.fragilefamilies.princeton.edu/briefs/ResearchBrief16.pdf>

Case, Mary Anne. 2001. "How High the Apple Pie: A Few Troubling Questions about Where, Why, and How the Burden of Care for Children Should Be Shifted." *Chicago-Kent Law Review* 76: 1753–86.

Children's Defense Fund. 2014. "The State of America's Children." <http://www.childrensdefense.org/zzz-child-research-data-publications/state-of-americas-children/index-1.html>

Craver, Martha Lynn. 2002. *Growing Demand for Elder Care Benefits.* Kiplinger Business Forecasts, 29 May.

DeWitt, Paula Mergenhagen. 1992. "Breaking Up Is Hard to Do." *American Demographics* 14: 52–7.

Dworkin, Ronald. 1985. *A Matter of Principle.* Cambridge, MA: Harvard University Press.

Eichner, Maxine. 2010. *The Supportive State: Families, Government, and America's Political Ideals.* New York: Oxford University Press.

Engels, Friedrich. 1975 [1844]. "The Condition of the Working Class in England." In *Karl Marx & Friedrich Engels: Collected Works,* Vol. IV, 304–598. New York: International Publishers.

Fineman, Martha. 2004. *The Autonomy Myth: A Theory of Dependency.* New York: New Press.

Galston, William. 1991. *Liberal Purposes: Goods, Virtues, and Diversity in the Liberal State.* New York: Cambridge University Press.

Gennetian, Lisa, et al. 2002. "Making Child Care Choices: How Welfare and Work Policies Influence Parents' Decisions." Manpower Demonstration Research Corporation (MDRC). <http://www.mdrc.org/publications/182/policybrief.html>

Goodin, Robert. 1985. *Protecting the Vulnerable: A Re-analysis of our Social Responsibilities.* Chicago, IL: University of Chicago Press.

Gornick, Janet, and Marcia K. Meyers. 2003. *Families that Work: Policies for Reconciling Parenthood and Employment.* New York: Russell Sage Foundation.

Gruber, Jonathan, and Brigitte Madrian. 2002. "Health Insurance, Labor Supply, and Job Mobility: A Critical Review of the Literature." National Bureau of Economic Research, NBER Working Paper no. W8817. <http://www.nber.org/papers/w8817.pdf>

Hirschmann, Nancy. 1996. "Rethinking Obligation for Feminism." In *Revisioning the Political: Feminist Reconstructions of Traditional Concepts in Western Political Theory,* edited by Nancy J. Hirschmann and Christine Di Stefano, 157–80. Boulder, CO: Westview Press.

Humphries, Jane. 1982. "The Working-Class Family: A Marxist Perspective." In *The Family in Political Thought,* edited by Jean Bethke Elshtain, 197–222. Amherst, MA: University of Massachusetts Press.

Kessler-Harris, Alice. 2001. *In Pursuit of Equity: Women, Men, and the Quest for Economic Citizenship in Twentieth-Century America.* New York: Oxford University Press.

Kittay, Eva Feder. 1999. *Love's Labor: Essays on Women, Equality, and Dependency.* New York: Routledge.

Lee, Sunhwa. 2007. "Keeping Moms on the Job: The Impacts of Health Insurance and Child Care on Job Retention and Mobility among Low-Income Mothers." Institute for Women's Policy Research. <http://www.iwpr.org/publications/pubs/keeping-moms-on-thejob-the-impacts-of-health-insurance-and-child-care-on-job-retention-and-mobility among-low-%20income-mothers/at download/file>

Lindsey, Duncan. 1994. *The Welfare of Children.* New York: Oxford University Press.

Lovell, Vicky, Elizabeth O' Neill, and Skylar Olsen. 2007. "Maternity Leave in the United States: Paid Parental Leave is Still Not Standard, Even among the Best US Employers." Institute for Women's Policy Research. <http://www.iwpr.org/publications/pubs/maternity-leave-in-the-united-states-paid-parental-leave-is-still-not-standard-even-among-the-best-u.s.-employers>

Macedo, Stephen. 2000. *Diversity and Distrust.* Cambridge, MA: Harvard University Press.

MacIntyre, Alasdair. 1981. *After Virtue: A Study in Moral Theory.* Notre Dame: University of Notre Dame Press.

Madrian, Brigitte. 2006. "The US Health Care System and Labor Markets." National Bureau of Economic Research, NBER Working Paper no. 11980. <http://www.nber.org/papers/w11980>

Mill, John Stuart. 1991 [1859]. *On Liberty and Other Essays,* 1st ed. Oxford: Oxford University Press.

Mincy, Ronald. 1990. "Raising the Minimum Wage: Effects on Family Poverty." *Monthly Labor Review* 113: 18–25.

Minow, Martha. 1990. *Making All the Difference, Inclusion, Exclusion, and American Law.* Ithaca, NY: Cornell University Press.

Minow, Martha. 1997. "All in the Family and in all Families: Membership, Loving, and Owing." In *Sex, Preference, and Family: Essays on Law and Nature,* edited by David Estlund and Martha Nussbaum, 249–76. New York: Oxford University Press.

Nussbaum, Martha. 2000a. *Women and Human Development: The Capabilities Approach.* New York: Cambridge University Press.

Nussbaum, Martha. 2000b. "The Future of Feminist Liberalism." *Proceedings and Addresses of the American Philosophical Association* 74: 47–79.

Olsen, Frances. 1985. "The Myth of State Intervention in the Family." *University of Michigan Journal of Law Reform* 18: 835–1121.

Rawls, John. 1971. *A Theory of Justice.* Cambridge, MA: Harvard University Press.

Rawls, John. 1993. *Political Liberalism.* New York: Columbia University Press.

Rhode, Deborah L. 1989. *Justice and Gender.* Cambridge, MA: Harvard University Press.

Rimer, Sarah. 1998. "Blacks Carry Load of Care for Their Elderly." *New York Times,* 15 March. <http://www.nytimes.com/1998/03/15/us/blacks-carry-load-of-care-for-their-elderly.html>

Rousseau, Jean Jacques. 1994 [1762]. "The Social Contract." In *Discourse on Political Economy and the Social Contract,* translated by Christopher Betts, 43–168. New York: Oxford University Press.

Sandel, Michael. 1996. *Dermocracy's Discontent.* Cambridge, MA: Belknap Press.

Sandel, Michael. 1998. *Liberalism and the Limits of Justice,* 2nd ed. New York: Cambridge University Press.

Schenk, Lynn Rep. 1993. Statement in Congressional Record. 139 Cong. Rec. H366-03. 3 February.

Smart, Carol. 1989. *Feminism and the Power of Law.* London: Routledge.

Spragens, Thomas. 1999. *Civic Liberalism.* Lanham, MD: Rowman and Littlefield.

Taylor, Charles. 1995. "Liberal Politics and the Public Sphere." In *New Communitarian Thinking,* edited by Amitai Etzioni, 183–217. Charlottesville, VA: University Press of Virginia.

UNICEF. 2007. *Child Poverty in Perspective: An Overview of Child Well-Being in Rich Countries.* Available at: <http://www.unicef-irc.org/publications/pdf/rc7_eng.pdf>

Walzer, Michael. 1984. "Liberalism and the Art of Separation." *Political Theory* 12: 315–30.

Walzer, Michael. 1990. *Spheres of Justice: A Defense of Pluralism and Equality.* New York: Basic Books.

Weissman, Deborah. 2007. "The Personal Is Political—and Economic." *Brigham Young University Law Review* 2(3): 387–450.

Young, Iris. 1990. *Justice and the Politics of Difference.* Princeton, NJ: Princeton University Press.

7

Privacy, surveillance, and care ethics

Marilyn Friedman

Is the privacy of Americans wrongfully violated by the American government's massive electronic data collection programs? Can care ethics handle this question? [1]

Recently it has come to light that the National Security Agency (NSA) of the US government is collecting and storing data about most or all electronic and telephone communications by Americans and many others. The electronic surveillance covers emails, cellphone calls, and internet searches. A value that is often invoked to defend the massive surveillance programs is national security (Miller 2013). Security in this context is meant especially to include safety from terrorist attacks. A typical argument has it that the data we gain from surveillance programs might include citizen communications to people with known or suspected ties to terrorist groups. The communications might also include information about actual plans for terrorist attacks. It is sometimes claimed that surveillance programs, which have been in existence covertly for several years now, have already succeeded in helping the government to avert several planned terrorist attacks.

It is argued *against* massive data collection programs that they invade the privacy of individuals (Shane 2013). Data are collected and stored regarding individuals about whom there is as yet no probable cause to suspect wrongdoing. The data are apparently stored in a way that makes them accessible to later analysis by both government employees and employees of private firms that contract with the government to do this sort of security work. One sort of abuse that might arise with these programs is that those with access to the data might reveal them for improper purposes such as destroying someone's political career.

The massive government surveillance programs thus present us with a conflict of values: security versus privacy. This discussion will pay only modest attention to that dilemma. What this discussion will focus on is the treatment that care ethics seems to give to each of those values in its own right. How does care ethics deal with the value of (national) security, including intelligence programs aimed at preventing terrorist attacks? How does care ethics handle the value of privacy? Are any special concerns raised for care ethics by the apparent individualism of (personal) privacy?

This discussion aims to show that care ethics can give full attention to the values of both security and privacy, that government surveillance programs do not constitute a challenge, or counterexample, to the adequacy of care ethics. Care ethics is as normatively adequate as any other ethical system for dealing with the problem of assessing surveillance programs. The way is then cleared for a discussion elsewhere of how care ethics would balance the two values. I do not show that care ethics is *superior* to other ethical systems in dealing with surveillance programs. My approach is thus a modest one.

First, a caveat. The conflict between security and privacy could arise for any society. However, local norms and cultural practices might shape the debate in distinctive ways. This discussion will focus only on security and privacy in a specifically American context.

Security

How does care ethics assess the moral value of national security and the surveillance programs that aim to promote it? In discussing this topic, I shall set aside two issues. First, I will not explore the legal or constitutional status of the surveillance programs. Second, I will assume that surveillance programs are *effective* in contributing to national security, that they make the United States at least somewhat safer than it would be otherwise. I am seeking grounds for a care ethical account of how to assess *morally* the value of (national) security.

Surveillance programs are one governmental response to the threat of terrorism. The issue of terrorism takes us immediately to the question of how to cope ethically with violence and war. Violence cannot be ignored globally. It is in ample evidence around the world these days. Many different groups of people are currently at risk of being the victims of aggression and violence.

Care ethics is one perspective for thinking about how to cope with aggression, violence, and war. As Virginia Held observes, care ethics resists violence and urges peaceful means of resolving disputes (2006, 139). Care ethics has always presented itself as an alternative to mainstream ethical frameworks, an alternative that promotes thinking about theoretically neglected or underappreciated aspects of moral life and moral orientations. Moral theory, like all areas of philosophy, has been historically developed mostly by men. War has long been characterized as a masculine endeavor. It seems that, still today in the United States at any rate, men in general are more likely than women in general (with exceptions in both groups, of course) to include military action among the range of options they are ready to take seriously as a proposed solution to aggressive first strikes against the United States by other groups. Care ethics represents an alternative to this perspective, an alternative advanced especially by members of those groups that have not historically manifested their moral agency through military action. In this way, care ethics persists in its earliest orientation, which is to embody peaceful moral options that might otherwise have been under-represented (cf. Ruddick 1989).

Although care ethics is opposed to the aggressive initiation of violence and the unjustified use of violence anywhere, questions remain over how best to respond to unjustified violence initiated by others. Many people believe that some forms and instances of unjustified violence can be stopped only by the use of military strikes carried out by victim nation-states or their allies. If this is true, then military action needs to number among the options that care ethics would consider when figuring out how to respond to unjustified violence.

However, regardless of whether a large-scale threat of force is to be met with a peaceful reaction or military retaliation, one needs to know what the dangers are. Peace-oriented though it might be, a care ethical perspective should be at the very least open to gaining information about the existence and nature of threats facing those whose care is in question. It should be noted that surveillance programs are not themselves forms of active military engagement. Indeed, one of the potential advantages of effective surveillance programs is to reveal threats of violence before they materialize, thereby allowing time for the use of non-violent preventive measures.

It is plausible to assume that US society faces at least some level of terrorist threat today. This assumption need not take the Hobbesian form of expecting a "war of all against all" as if in a state of nature. Also it does not require supposing that terrorism is the only or even the overriding global concern today or that the United States is an innocent terrorist target (more on this later). All one has to suppose is that there are *some* agents in the world today who are motivated to engage in large-scale violent attacks against the United States. Even if the odds for an American of being the victim of a terrorist attack are extremely small, still the means of attack are especially frightening. Explosives tear bodies apart. Terrorist attacks are also random and arbitrary, making it all but impossible for the ordinary person to know how to avoid them.

Intelligence efforts in the abstract, apart from their possibly violent military uses, are data-gathering exercises. They seek information about current and future threats. Efforts of this sort are in themselves not wrongheaded. One can be a pacifist and still accept the idea that simply trying to find out what threats of violence may arise in the future is a legitimate endeavor.

However, surveillance programs are carried out by agencies that are part of the government's military complex. The intelligence that surveillance programs provide could easily be used in some cases to rationalize undertaking military action that might or might not be justified. In evaluating surveillance programs, it is therefore important to consider their military uses. This suggests the need for a critical dialogue about government programs for intelligence gathering. Programs for data collection need not and should not preclude public criticism or debate about how the data will be used and whether the programs involve morally unacceptable means or consequences.

Fiona Robinson's book, *The Ethics of Care: A Feminist Approach to Human Security* (2011), is a useful place to start searching for care ethical perspectives on the security interests that massive surveillance programs are aimed to protect. To be sure, Robinson's book is "not primarily a work of security studies" (2011, 15). Her approach leads her away from strictly national security interests and toward "human security" interests. These are the welfare interests of ordinary people (46–7). Robinson wants to get beyond the "state-centrism and military focus" of conventional notions of (national) security (14). National security, as Robinson explains it, pertains to military security as understood in international relations. This sort of security involves the use of force and violence regarded as legitimate (7). Security in this sense is protection against threats of violence committed usually by other states (6–7).

Although Robinson aims her discussion away from national security, her book proves useful for focusing on national security after all, and on whether care ethics can give adequate weight to the value of national security. I discuss three of the many relevant sets of issues in her book. First, Robinson argues that, in the prevalent thinking about national security, women and children are conceptualized as "victims," "dependent," and "vulnerable." Robinson challenges this conceptualization. Women do assert agency and, at any rate, everyone is dependent at some stages of life at least (2011, 10–11, 56–7, 94–100). Second, Robinson argues that understanding security should begin with understanding practices of care at the levels of family, neighborhoods, ethnic groups, and so forth. Damaged care relations should be recognized as fundamental in disrupting people's security (10–11, 28, 44–6, 55–60). People won't have a sense of security in their everyday lives unless they are immersed in *"networks of care and responsibility"* (44, italics in original). Government security issues such as the threat of terrorism distract us from the real security problems of ordinary people, such as poverty and inadequate healthcare (11–13). Focusing on state security practices sustains a status quo that perpetuates such problems (14).

Third, Robinson maintains that the caring practices on which people depend globally are often carried out by women and are construed in "feminized" terms that "isolate men from these roles" and contribute to the "construction of hegemonic forms of masculinity that are associated with violence" (2011, 9, 22, 34–9, 57). This masculinizing might carry with it an unjustified enhancement of masculine power and authority in general. In the remaining parts of this section, I discuss the first and second concerns. The next section deals with the connection between security and males or masculinity.

Victims

Robinson claims that national security interests are portrayed in ways that overemphasize women and children as victims. This does not seem to me to be a widespread problem, if it is a problem at all. Instead it seems widely understood that the victims of a terrorist attack would include anyone who was at the wrong place at the wrong time—people of any gender, age, class, race, religion, or other identity. In the terrorist attack of 11 September 2001, many members of elite financial firms, thus including many successful businessmen, are known to have been among the victims. A terrorist threat and attack can be directed against those who are "constructed" as strong, invulnerable, independent, and masculine just as easily as it can be directed against those who are constructed as weak, vulnerable, dependent, and feminine.

Even if victims of terrorism were excessively portrayed as women and children, this by itself would provide no reason to reject security as a value that is offered to justify mass surveillance programs. At most the policy directive that would follow from erroneous data about terrorism's victims would be to correct the data.

Human Security

Robinson observes that caring relations are integral to security in people's lives. She takes "care seriously as the ethical and practical basis of human security" (2011, 6). Robinson argues that human security should be understood in ways that go beyond a focus on the state and the military (14). The focus of attention should be directed to society and people's everyday needs (15). Robinson is right that human security is disrupted by damaged everyday relations of care and these disruptions should be socially recognized as crucial.

So far, this is not an argument to devalue or disregard national security. Both forms of security can be jointly valued. Elevating the importance of human security does not require downplaying national security. Human security and national security both seem crucial and intertwined. Sometimes national security may even operate as the independent variable that can impinge on human security.

However, Robinson goes on to argue that the attention given to national security obscures the foundational human security problems, which are care-based (2011, 13). Also, she suggests, it reinforces existing power relations which may promote "cultures of militarism" and "violent solutions to social and political conflict" (48–9). The state may thus be contributing to care-based, human insecurities.

Robinson portrays national security issues as being centered only on states (2011, 47, 61). Terrorist attacks, however, are more complicated than that. Terrorist attacks might well have states as their ultimate, indirect targets. However, terrorist attacks usually operate directly against intermediate targets, which are ordinary people and neighborhoods *within* states (Primoratz 2013). Terrorism directly targets ordinary people as a way of indirectly influencing larger political groups or entities such as states. Thus, it is not simply states, as formal bureaucratic entities removed from the people, that are the targets of terrorism. Terrorism randomly attacks—and terrorizes—the ordinary people of a society. Anyone at any time could be a target. A terrorist attack can explode in any neighborhood, causing havoc in lives that previously had a high degree of human security. Both national security and human security are threatened by terrorism.

At the same time, Robinson's focus on the connection between caring relations and national security does point toward a different care-based connection that is extremely important to national security. Someone might argue that the attacks of 11 September 2001 constituted retaliation against the United States for damaged forms of international caring exhibited by the US toward peoples elsewhere, in the years prior to that date. A terrorist attack can be a reaction to past policies or practices of the state that is now targeted by terrorists. Perhaps past bad treatment by the United States of other peoples promoted resentment, resistance, and violent reaction by those peoples. Perhaps because Americans in the past, or still yet today, oppressed or violated the rights of people elsewhere, those people are now rising up to defend themselves. These suggestions call for us to identify the sorts of caring, including "human security," that should infuse international relationships, especially by powerful affluent nations such as the United States toward the poor nations and peoples of the world.

Here is one small example of an uncaring US policy. As I write this text, the news media are reporting that US government agencies, seeking to buy clothing at low prices, are buying them from overseas suppliers that impose harsh and dangerous working conditions on their employees (Urbina 2013). The conditions include "padlocked fire exits, buildings at risk of collapse, falsified wage records and repeated hand punctures from sewing needles when workers were pushed to hurry up." The countries in which these conditions allegedly prevail included "Bangladesh, the Dominican Republic,

Haiti, Mexico, Pakistan and Vietnam" (Urbina 2013, A1). Thus it would be no surprise to find that people in countries outside the United States blame the US government as well as US corporations and US consumers for acting in ways that support trade policies that brutalize workers in other parts of the world. The foreign victims and critics of those policies might well be tempted to retaliate by supporting movements of violent protest against the United States. In order to help forestall such violent reactions, it would be quite appropriate to use care ethics as a framework for thinking about how the United States and its citizens should improve their international trade policies so as to treat workers elsewhere with care and justice.

However, the road to just and caring international policies by the United States toward all other peoples is a slow road. National and corporate interests stand in its way. During the time that it would take for our international treatment of others even to approach remotely a level of equal recognition and respect, the United States would likely still be vulnerable to terrorist threats from other groups. Also, some of those threats might be coming from forces that are themselves unjust. There is no reason to assume that all non-US actors who engage in terrorism against the United States are morally abiding persons or agents who use violence only in legitimate self-defense against injustice and oppression. In addition, some terrorist threats against the United States might be domestic and might not constitute retaliation against US policies abroad. In that vein, we should not forget Timothy McVeigh and his bombing of the Alfred P. Murrah Federal Building in Oklahoma City in 1995, a bombing that killed 168 people, including nineteen children who were in the daycare center that was housed in the building.

Furthermore, even if a terrorist attack constitutes understandable retaliation against the United States, it nevertheless targets innocent persons who do not deserve that treatment. Terrorist attacks have a collective dimension and are indiscriminate in their impact. The members of a society, and/or its internal communities, suffer terrorist attacks together. Terrorism differs from targeted assassination, which is by definition targeted at particular persons (although it may certainly involve the "collateral" killing of innocents). A terrorist attack at a particular location harms anyone who is in the vicinity, regardless of whether or not they are a perpetrator of the alleged past wrongs that the terrorist might be trying to avenge.

Thus, even if past bad American treatment of other peoples had indeed spawned or bolstered a terrorist movement, it would not be true that every single American alive today shared equally in the responsibility for that past bad treatment. Young American children of today, to take the most obvious example, do not share in responsibility for any past bad treatment of people elsewhere—unless "shared responsibility" is treated as an ascribed metaphysical status that has nothing to do with a person's actual behavior (and I reject that definition of "responsibility"). So long as we conceptualize responsibility for wrongdoing as limited to someone's actual behavior and intentions (including culpable omissions), then young children, simply as children, are not responsible for the behavior of their elders and should not be punished for that behavior. Yet terrorist attacks against the United States, designed precisely to terrorize civilian populations, might well put young American children at risk of harm just as much as they would endanger culpable government or corporate officials who might have perpetrated wrongs against the states or peoples who would now seek to retaliate.

Preventive measures would protect, among others, young children who could well be the innocent victims of such attacks. Defending today's generation of children is a special responsibility that falls on their elders. Also, if terrorist acts constitute retaliatory violence, they do so without due process of law. Even a wrongdoer is not morally required to accept passively just any violence that is inflicted on her or on other members of her community without due process of law and without a legitimate verdict of her guilt. These considerations suggest that, even if the United States has acted uncaringly or unjustly in ways that spawned terrorist threats against itself, the country as a whole is nevertheless entitled to defend itself against those threats.

National security against terrorism appears to require a division of moral labor, with different people using different moral frameworks for different purposes. Virginia Held suggests the idea of different moral frameworks for the different branches of the US government (Held 1984). Analogously, different groups of persons should work on different *security*-related goals. Some thinkers and policy-makers should focus on how the United States can improve the caring quality of its international treatment of peoples elsewhere so as to engage with them all in a spirit of caring and justice. At the same time, other thinkers and policy-makers should focus on defending the United States against possible terrorist threats. Self-defense should go on even if those threats constitute retaliation for past bad treatment by the United States of other societies. Collecting information, in the abstract, that might lead to awareness of terrorist threats is a legitimate part of that self-defense framework. (Whether massive electronic surveillance in particular is a legitimate means of that self-defense is still an open question.)

Security, Men, and Masculinity

The third issue raised by Robinson that I shall consider is that caring practices are construed as women's work and separated from male roles, a conceptualization that contributes to the "construction of hegemonic forms of masculinity that are associated with violence" (2011, 9). Security is one such form of masculinity. The implication of Robinson's discussion seems to be that this form of masculinity should be abolished as far as possible.

There is no doubt that recognized caring practices, such as childcare and elder care, are feminized while security practices are masculinized. The latest slang exhortation to political leaders in the United States is to "man up." However, what if security work, apart from its masculine associations, were a good thing in itself to promote? Daniel Engster, for example, agrees that security is important and that care ethics supports this. He argues that a caring government must provide for the security needs of its people because this is something individuals cannot do effectively on their own (2007, 72, 80). If national security activities are valuable and needed, then at first glance, they should not be eliminated even if masculinized.

However, the harmful masculinized associations should not be forgotten and need to be weighed in the balance. Robinson outlines some of these harmful side-effects. For one thing, "hegemonic forms of masculinity license men's neglect of caring responsibilities" (2011, 23). For another thing, the "masculinist 'cultures' of violence that support militarism as an ideology" are related to the cultural devaluation of care (38). In addition, these practices are connected in turn to social norms that "perpetuate" men's violence against women (37–8). Robinson urges us to regard all forms of violence as being on a continuum "that includes both intimate violence and militarized violence sanctioned by states and international organizations" (23).

Robinson's comments prompt the following line of reasoning. National security is a dominant or hegemonic form of security. National security is culturally portrayed as masculine or with masculine associations. National security is sanctioned and highly valued. Men, typically regarded as masculine, gain social prestige and power from that association. The prestige and power that men as a group derive from their association with national security promotes side-effects that are problematic. One side-effect is that men neglect their caring responsibilities. A second side-effect is that the aura of legitimacy that surrounds military violence extends to other forms of male violence that are illegitimate. A third side-effect, not mentioned by Robinson but discussed by Iris Young (see below), is that the masculine associations of national security promote uncritical public acceptance of government policies that might be illegitimate. I discuss these three side-effects in turn.

Care Neglect

Joan Tronto joins Robinson in being concerned that national security work, which Tronto includes under the label of "protection," enables men to avoid doing care work (Tronto 2013). Tronto is in agreement with Robinson that the sort of masculinity that is dominant in US culture excludes care work (67–70). On Tronto's account, men engage in forms of activity that are regarded as more important than caring, and because of these alternative activities, they are socially excused from doing care work (30–3). The two most prominent alternative activities are protection and production (33). Protection is the alternative of interest here. Protection includes police work and military protection (74–5). These masculinized protection activities are socially accepted as licenses allowing their practitioners to avoid doing their fair share of care work.

Tronto challenges this arrangement for two reasons. First, she argues that, in a democracy, everyone who can do so should be assigned responsibility for care work (2013, 7, 11–12, 30). It is wrong for men to avoid doing care work. Second, Tronto argues that the dominant model of masculinity is actually mistaken in portraying male protectors as not engaged in care work (68–79, 91–4). Protection is a kind of care; indeed, a kind that is "essential for living well." It is a "critically important" form of care (93–4).

However, Tronto's two reasons operate at cross-purposes. If protection is indeed a form of care—and I agree with Tronto that it is—then men (and women) who do protection work are actually not avoiding care work at all. They are bearing a share of the care work that is "essential for living well." Indeed, some forms of protection work involve risks to life and limb (think of firefighting and combat) that often make those forms of protection a *fair* share of care work, if not more so. There are certainly problems with protection work, but failing to involve care is not in principle one of them.[2]

Granted, as Tronto argues, protection work is not *labeled* as care work. It is not socially regarded as care. However, this is a different issue. In that case, protectors would not be failing to fulfill their caring responsibilities. The problem would lie in the societal failure to recognize that protectors *were* fulfilling their caring responsibilities. To correct that problem, everyone would need to conceptualize protection work differently. However, the protectors would not need to change the type of work they do. If protection is care work, then those who do an extensive amount of it (as a full-time job, say) do fulfill their democratic caring responsibilities.

Tronto points out convincingly that protection is conceptualized as not feminine. People who do protection work do not do what is regarded as a feminine form of care (2013, 68–70). Tronto often seems to be arguing more specifically that everyone's responsibility in a democracy is to do a share of *feminized* care work. However, she is not clear on why everyone has the responsibility to engage in that specific form of care work.

Tronto does not argue that everyone has a responsibility to engage in *each kind* of care or each kind of socially necessary work. She does not argue that people who do feminized care work have the additional democratic responsibility of doing protection or production. In addition, protection may require or be done best when done as a full-time occupation. Protectors may not have the time or energy to shoulder substantial feminized care work responsibilities. (The reverse may be true of feminized care work as well.) If feminized care work and protection (masculinized care work) are both among the necessary activities for social well-being, as Tronto plausibly claims (2013, 93–4), then engaging in either one should discharge someone's democratic responsibility to engage in care work. Thus, any part of the work of national security and protection, however masculine it might be *thought* to be, is not vulnerable to the criticism that it excuses the people who engage in it from fulfilling democratic responsibilities of care. National security work is already a form of caring.

Violence

A second problematic side-effect of masculinized national security that Robinson suggests is that the aura of legitimacy surrounding male military violence extends to male domestic violence (2011, 9, 23). In Robinson's view, the root of the problem seems to be the cultural devaluation of care. She writes that the devaluing of care is what may sustain "cultures of violence" from "family to transnational level" (24). Put more carefully, Robinson is not saying that the legitimation of male domestic violence is a side-effect of legitimized military violence; rather, both are at least associated with, and perhaps are products of, the devaluation of care.

However, Robinson's observations suggest a causal claim about the connection between military violence and domestic violence. High-status, legitimized military violence, and military activity in general, may well bolster to some extent the societal toleration for domestic violence in some cases. Military work elevates the social status and expands the moral leeway of those who are associated with it. We are culturally accustomed these days to honoring military heroes for their exploits. People who are not actual soldiers may nevertheless fancy that they acquire some military cachet by buying camouflage clothing and playing videogames that simulate military conquests. One key point is that soldiers trained to seek control of interpersonal situations and to use violence if necessary to do so may well have trouble avoiding violence when returning to civilian life and dealing with persons they cannot control.

Anything that promotes illegitimate violence is a serious problem. However, this does not entail that legitimate violence, sometimes perhaps the only option for self-defense against aggression, must also be curbed. If we can differentiate legitimate from illegitimate violence, either conceptually or by example, then we should be able to articulate this distinction in social discourse and work to permit the former while diminishing the latter. This is not to say that abolishing illegitimate violence will be easy. It comes with its own obstacles and complexities. For returning veterans, for example, there are issues such as post-traumatic stress disorder, brain trauma, and recently increasing suicide rates among "elite" troops (Shanker and Oppel 2014). A plausible working strategy is to press, loudly and clearly, the distinction between legitimate and illegitimate violence and to oppose the latter wherever possible. This strategy would allow care ethics to give at least some recognition to security as a value.

Protection Logic

Iris Young offers a third interpretation of what is wrong with the cultural masculinization of protection or security. For Young, protection is culturally understood in terms of a "logic" of gendered associations (2003, 16). According to this logic, the protector role is masculine and the protected are in the role of women and children. (Whether the protectors are male and the protected are female is not really the point.) The masculinized protector has a great deal of practical leeway, such as being allowed to use violence against enemies. Meanwhile, the protected do not get to exert any protective agency, let alone violence. Instead the protected occupy a subordinate status in which they are expected to be grateful for protection and obedient toward the protectors (16–19).

Young is concerned that this gendered model of protection, when applied to national security, prompts citizens to take up the feminine role and become docile, accepting gratefully and uncritically whatever its government says it does to protect them, including the surveillance of citizens (2003, 20–1). Young explicitly does *not* argue that public officials should *not* try to protect people. She is not opposed to protection as such. In her view, the central questions have to do with how much power officials should have, whether the procedures are fair and follow due process, and whether citizens can easily review official policies and hold officials accountable (23). Young argues that the masculinist logic of protection endangers democracy by abolishing the equality that leaders and citizens should have in making policy decisions and in holding leaders accountable (27).

What Young rejects is not protection as such, but rather the gendered associations that confer legitimacy on authoritarian and non-democratic ways of implementing protection. Young's approach yields mixed results for our investigation. On the one hand, it suggests that seeking intelligence about possible security threats could be legitimate. On the other hand, however, it rules out non-democratic and abusive ways of collecting intelligence data. Abuses would include the absence of any of the following: probable cause, due process, democratic consent, and government accountability.

Young treats the gendered associations and the political abuses as a package. It seems to be her view that the masculinizing of the protector role automatically carries a public toleration of abuses. The protector as masculine is automatically given free rein to act as he sees fit. Some questions arise, however. Does the masculinizing of protection always have these effects? Does the American public really monolithically accept abuses as the price of protection? The masculinizing of protection has not dampened all opposition. Criticisms of security policies have emerged in public debates under the administrations of both President George W. Bush and President Barack Obama. While the members of a protection regime probably *want* uncritical loyalty from the public, there nevertheless remain critics among the protected public who will not be silenced. Critics are not necessarily "feminized," or docile, subjects of protection.

This suggests that the lens of masculinity may not be the key to discerning the extensive ill effects of protection that Young fears. Focusing on masculinity might be a distraction from the main problems. National security programs should be scrutinized directly for their fairness, due process, and democratic accountability. Some programs might be legitimate while others are not. Programs that are masculinized should not be summarily dismissed on that ground alone, until they are found to involve actual abuses.

To sum up, I have considered a number of reasons why security might be a problematic value for care ethics and have argued in each case that there is still reason to take security seriously. However, these conclusions are only part of the story. The next question is whether massive electronic surveillance is a legitimate means of promoting security.

Privacy

One value commonly invoked to challenge the mass surveillance programs is that of privacy. Ordinary people may well want most of their telephone and electronic communications to other specific persons to occur without intruders. There are at least two reasons why care ethics might not be able to give serious consideration to the value of privacy. First, care ethics usually takes on the feminist critique of the distinction between a public and a private sphere and the associated ideas of a realm of privacy and a right to privacy. Feminists have been especially concerned to make sure the right to privacy does not manifest itself in practices that shield from the reach of justice various historic harms and wrongs inflicted by men on women and children in the so-called private domain (MacKinnon 1989).

Second, feminist care ethicists in particular would probably share the widespread feminist criticism of individualism (Robinson 2011, 50, 90) and the concept of privacy seems individualistic on the face of it. Privacy may seem to be about individuals secluding themselves from others or denying access to themselves or to information about themselves. So the question about whether care ethics supports the moral importance of privacy is importantly a question about how care ethics handles the apparent *individualism* of privacy.

Public/Private

First consider the feminist rejection of the distinction between public and private spheres. Catharine MacKinnon, for example, objected to the concept of privacy and a split between public and private, or domestic, aspects of human life. Her argument is that the legal enforcement of this split has insulated the so-called private sphere from legal scrutiny, thereby allowing men in that sphere free rein to maintain social control and act in abusive and violent ways toward women and children (1989, 184–94). The so-called private sphere has centered heavily on the activities and practices of family, sexuality, and reproduction. Differentiating a so-called private sphere from the public sphere, according to this argument, has been especially bad for women and children.

Efforts are underway to try to correct the legal abuses of past practices of a right to privacy. Domestic violence and abuse can be criminalized and police and law enforcers can undergo training to respond to domestic violence in ways that aim to protect victims rather than perpetrators. Granted, these efforts to date have not ended domestic violence. However, there is probably no type of action that is completely prevented by being criminalized. For our purposes, what is important is that the concept of privacy is not what is doing the work of shielding domestic abusers from law enforcement.

Ideally, the distinction between public and private is a distinction based on certain important features of interpersonal treatment. Mill's harm principle, however much additional elaboration it needs, is still a relevant starting point toward one way of articulating a public/private distinction that would meet feminist concerns. Any activity in which one person threatens, harms, or wrongs another is "public" in the sense of being a legitimate activity for government scrutiny and control. Behavior that does *not* threaten, harm, or wrong others should be treated as presumptively private. That is, it should be treated prima facie as beyond the legitimate reach of government regulation unless there are good reasons to overrule this presumption. Domestic abuse is certainly a good reason for the state to regulate what abusers might want to keep private.

A private realm of some sort, limited by a harm principle, is valuable among other things for the freedom it affords people—certainly including women—to try out, if they wish, new ways of acting, living, protecting themselves, interrelating with others—and caring for others.[3] Anita Allen argues that women have interests in privacy. For example, they have interests in preventing government intrusion into many situations involving sexuality and reproduction (1988, 35–53 and *passim*). The intrusions into privacy that were long allowed by anti-sodomy statutes provide just one example. Also, a victim of domestic violence can benefit from specific protections of her privacy (Kristiansson 2013). For example, she may want privacy in the sense of non-disclosure regarding the new address to which she has moved to avoid an abuser. Or she may want privacy in the sense of confidentiality regarding what she tells a therapist about the abuse she has suffered.

Individualism

The second potential stumbling block for valuing privacy from a care ethical perspective is that privacy might be overly individualistic. Samuel Warren and Louis Brandeis (1890) offered an early, individualistic statement to the legal community about the right to privacy. They called it "the right to be let alone." This limited formulation might be taken to suggest that privacy is simply about disconnecting from other persons. It could seem to be a right to be isolated, to avoid human companionship, to live in solitude.

By contrast, care ethics, since its inception, has foregrounded the importance of interpersonal relationships and challenged individualistic conceptions of persons and their moral interests. Human beings are raised, develop, and gradually become adults in the context of interpersonal relationships and human societies. The attributes that characterize human beings arise from, and are often constituted by, human sociality. Recent ethical theory, including the ethics of care, has paid special attention to the various roles played by interpersonal relationships in morality and in the emergence of moral personality. In the view of many, this attention to relationality offsets a narrow individualism that had previously characterized moral theory and normative political theory.

At least some defenders of care ethics have emphasized interpersonal relationships ahead of personal individuality. For example, Virginia Held observes that care ethics treats persons as if they were "deeply affected by, and involved in, relations with others" and "at least partly constituted by their social ties" (2006, 46). Fiona Robinson regards a "relational ontology" as the "philosophical starting point" of care ethics (2011, 29). In Robinson's view, human identity and subjectivity develop through "mutual constitution" among human beings and "relations of interdependence and dependence are a fundamental feature of our existence" (4).

There are at least two relevant responses to this concern. First, an emphasis on individuality is not necessarily bad for women. Anita Allen differentiates between, on the one hand, accounts of the value of privacy that emphasize the creation and enhancement of personhood and, on the other hand, accounts that emphasize the creation and enhancement of relationships (1988, 37, 43–8). Allen agrees that to defend privacy in terms of its enhancement of personhood is indeed to rest one's argument partly on individualism. However, Allen regards the individualistic aspect of privacy as beneficial for women. She claims that privacy "can enable moral persons to be self-determining individuals" (44). Privacy can promote self-reflection and self-development, which help an individual to develop a sense of her own perspective different from that of the group, and a sense that she is entitled to moral respect for her own sake (44–5).

The second response, also argued by Allen, is that it would be a mistake to think that the only value of privacy lies in its individuality. The point of privacy is to prevent *unwanted* intrusion by others—intrusion affecting one's self and one's possessions, information about oneself, and unwanted intrusion into one's *relationships*. Thus, Charles Fried (1968, 475) claims that privacy is needed as a context for developing relationships of friendship and love. James Rachels (1975) argues that the ability to control access to ourselves and the dissemination of information about ourselves enables us to shape our interpersonal relationships in varied ways, allowing some persons to be very close while keeping others less close. These points are especially relevant to the NSA surveillance programs which particularly target interpersonal communications such as emails and telephone calls.

Anita Allen observes that privacy has a point only in light of the "social character of human existence." Separation makes sense only if there are others to whom one is connected in relationships. In the context of social relationships, she argues that privacy enables individuals to become "morally individuated," but also to develop the "character, personality and skills" that enhance the "*social* participation and contribution" that individuals make to group life (1988, 48, italics mine). Thus care ethics can value privacy for both its individuality and its relationality. Individuality does not preclude relationality and is therefore not a problem in principle for care ethics.

To be sure, care ethical systems differ in the degree to which they emphasize values for individuals. Daniel Engster, for example, claims that a caring government will guarantee rights to individuals against actions by the military or police that are unfair, unwarranted, arbitrary, or abusive (2007, 80). One reason he gives is that arbitrary government actions might interfere with the ability of individuals to care for themselves or others (80). Engster makes clear that his care ethics values "the care of individuals over group values and goals" (99). Individual dependency is what draws human beings together in groups, and it is as individuals that we claim care from others (99). Engster writes that "the group exists in care theory to support individuals and not the other way around" (99). Engster's care ethics thus supports individualistic concerns.

Virginia Held's care ethics, as noted earlier, contrasts with that of Engster on the question of individualism. Held writes that care ethics "conceptualizes persons as deeply affected by, and involved in, relations with others; to many care theorists persons are at least partly constituted by their social ties" (2006, 46). She claims that our "embeddedness in familial, social, and historical contexts is basic" (46). This is to see the person as an "embodied nexus of relations" (48).

On the question of individualism, the difference between Engster's care ethics and Held's care ethics seems to be one of degree. Held's approach gives more emphasis than does Engster's to relational aspects. At the same time, even Held makes concessions to individuality. She writes, for example, that "we are not prisoners of our upbringing and circumstances" (2006, 48). She allows that as a self develops, it becomes a "moral subject shaping her identity and life and actions" (48). We are "both enmeshed in and capable of shaping such relations" (48).

In accepting both the relationality and the individuality of persons, care ethics can avoid having to contest privacy on the grounds of its individualism. Privacy has great value for both the individual as such and the relational aspects of individuals. The way is clear for care ethics to accept the value of privacy as a prima facie reason to oppose surveillance programs.

What are the abstract possibilities for reconciling the value of security with the value of privacy in the overall moral evaluation of mass surveillance programs? Are security and privacy in a winner-take-all or zero-sum contest for moral priority? Or might both values retain moral significance to some degree, even if one is more important than the other? If the last suggestion is possible, a compromise that incorporated consideration of both values would make moral sense.

Adam Moore recommends a balance between security and privacy for "normal" times in which there is no security emergency and no imminent threat (2010, chapter 10). The idea is to permit surveillance programs to occur but only in regulated and limited forms. Surveillance would require a showing of probable cause, a warrant issued by a judge, and "sunlight" provisions in the form of a requirement that there be some form of public accountability after the fact. The process must not be thoroughly secretive and different authorized persons must agree to the legitimacy of surveillance over particular persons or groups. I see no reason why care ethics could not sign up to an approach similar to this one. But this is an argument to be postponed for another occasion.

Notes

1. I am grateful to Daniel Engster and Maurice Hamington for very helpful comments on an earlier draft.
2. I am treating care as a form of activity, not as an emotion or attitude.
3. Granted women may be constrained in the private realm in practice by social norms and practices that limit their freedom. That is why I qualify my point with the expression "limited by a harm principle."

References

Allen, Anita. 1988. *Uneasy Access: Privacy for Women in a Free Society*. Totowa, NJ: Rowman and Littlefield.

Engster, Daniel. 2007. *The Heart of Justice: Care Ethics and Political Theory*. Oxford: Oxford University Press.

Fried, Charles. 1968. "Privacy." *Yale Law Journal* 77: 475–93.

Held, Virginia. 1984. *Rights and Goods: Justifying Social Action*. New York: Macmillan.

Held, Virginia. 2006. *The Ethics of Care: Personal, Political, and Global*. Oxford: Oxford University Press.

Kristiansson, Viktoria. 2013. "Walking a Tightrope: Balancing Victim Privacy and Offender Accountability in Domestic Violence and Sexual Assault Prosecutions." Part I. *Strategies: The Prosecutors' Newsletter on Violence Against Women*, no. 9, May.

MacKinnon, Catharine A., 1989. "Abortion: On Public and Private." In *Toward a Feminist Theory of the State*, edited by Catharine A. MacKinnon, 85–9. Cambridge, MA: Harvard University Press.

Miller, Zeke J., 2013. "President Obama Defends NSA Surveillance Programs as 'Right Balance'." *Time*, 7 June 2013. <http://swampland.time.com/2013/06/07/predident-obama-defends-nsa-s>

Moore, Adam D. 2010. *Privacy Rights: Moral and Legal Foundations*. University Park, PA: Pennsylvania State University Press.

Primoratz, Igor. 2013. *Terrorism: A Philosophical Investigation*. Cambridge: Polity.

Rachels, James. 1975. "Why Privacy Is Important." *Philosophy and Public Affairs* 4: 323–33.

Robinson, Fiona. 2011. *The Ethics of Care: A Feminist Approach to Human Security*. Philadelphia, PA: Temple University Press.

Ruddick, Sara. 1989. *Maternal Thinking: Toward a Politics of Peace*. New York: Beacon Press.

Shane, Scott. 2013. "No Morsel Too Minuscule for All-Consuming N.S.A." *New York Times*, 2 November, 1, 10–11.

Shanker, Thom, and Richard A. Oppel, Jr. 2014. "War's Elite Tough Guys, Hesitant to Seek Healing." *New York Times*, 5 June, A1, 16.

Tronto, J. C. 2013. *Caring Democracy: Markets, Equality and Justice*. New York: New York University Press.

Urbina, Ian. 2013. "In Buying Cheap Clothes, US Flouts Own Counsel: Overseas Suppliers Offer Low Prices, but Working Conditions Can Be Harsh." *New York Times*, 22 December, A1, 6.

Young, Iris Mariion. 2003. "The Logic of Masculinist Protection: Reflections on the Current Security State." In *Women and Citizenship*, edited by Marilyn Friedman, 15–34. New York: Oxford University Press.

Warren, Samuel, and Louis D. Brandeis. 1890. "The Right to Privacy." *Harvard Law Review* 4: 193–220.

8

Care, normativity, and the law

Rita Manning

Care ethics can provide a valuable conceptual and normative resource for many issues in law, but given the conservative nature of law in general, much work needs to be done before care ethics can explicitly play such a role. In this chapter, I survey the landscape of law, discuss two attempts to incorporate care ethics into the normative framework of law, and suggest other avenues for incorporating care ethics in law and legal reasoning. I close with some examples of care ethics in judicial decision making. In this final section, I will first show the way care is used in Justice Kennedy's decisions in *Lawrence* v. *Texas* (Lawrence 2003) and *United States* v. *Windsor*, the so-called defense of marriage case (Windsor 2013). These decisions show the value that a care ethics can bring to judicial decision making. I will then show how the failure to use care ethics illuminates what went wrong in an important healthcare case.

Normativity and the Law

Most discussions of normativity and law focus on the role of moral appeals in judicial reasoning. US law students are taught that they may only appeal to legal authority, and that such authority is largely exhausted by the following: constitutions (federal and state), statutes (including administrative regulations), case law, treatises, and public policy (Schauer 2012). Nowhere in this list does morality explicitly appear. Part of the reason for this lack can be found in the notion of judicial restraint—the idea that judges should interpret the law and resist imposing their own subjective views, including their moral views. Such restraint is often defended by an appeal to the role of the judiciary in a democracy—legislatures express the will of the people when they make law and are subject to dismissal if the people find their legislating problematic. Judges, especially federal judges, are immune to politics and thus from democratic constraints. If we think it is important to defer to the will of the people, while protecting individual rights, we will want our judges to defer to the legislature unless doing so is incompatible with their role as arbiter of the law and protector of individual rights.

There is, of course, a long and spirited debate about the role of morality in judging. Ronald Dworkin, for example, argues that judges cannot dodge appeals to morality, especially in hard cases (Dworkin 1977; 1986). While I am inclined to agree with Dworkin, it is important to recognize the reality that legal culture, as it is transmitted to law students, does not allow for an explicit role for moral considerations in judicial reasoning. However, I am also inclined to agree with legal theorists like W. J. Waluchow that, while moral reasoning plays no explicit role in judicial reasoning, it is embedded in all the other legal authorities that do play such a role (Waluchow 1994).

Hence, rather than argue for adding moral appeals to the list of legal authority, I think it is a more promising strategy to look at the ways that moral perspectives, including care ethics, might play a valuable role within the accepted legal authorities, and within normative conceptions of judging.

Care and the Law: Some Preliminary Comments

Care ethics should not be confused with an ethics that applies only to caretaking practices. While many of the examples of ideal caring come from maternal practice, care ethics is a perspective that can be usefully applied in a wide variety of settings and practices, including law. Care ethics has not yet been adopted by legal theorists or judges, with some few exceptions, but I would argue that this is because of its recent articulation as a normative theory, not because of its irrelevance to law. I begin with a brief description of care ethics.

Care ethics, as all moral theories, begins with ordinary moral intuitions and social practices. While it can be traced back to the moral sentimentalism of David Hume and his colleagues in the British Sentimentalist school, Shaftesbury, Hutcheson, and Smith (Hume 1993/1777; Shaftesbury 2000/1711; Hutcheson 2003/1725; Smith 2010/1759), it did not receive systematic theoretical attention until the 1980s, when feminist moral philosophers and moral psychologists began to take seriously the moral experience of women (Gilligan 1982; Noddings 1986; Ruddick 1989; Baier 1987; Slote 2003). I begin here with my own elaboration of the theory (Manning 1992).

Not all care theorists think of care as a virtue (Held 2005), but I think the best way to understand care is as a virtue that guides our interactions with others, and has implications for our social policy, practices and institutions. In our actions, and as we create and maintain policies, practices, and institutions, care ethics focus on four central processes: moral attention, sympathetic understanding, relationship awareness, and harmony and accommodation.

Moral attention involves an awareness of the details that might make a difference in our understanding and response to the particular situation at hand. Moral attention is in the service of sympathetic understanding, which involves being open to sympathizing and even identifying with others, and becoming aware of what they want and need. In responding to others, caring persons look to satisfy their needs in ways that will preserve their sense of competence and dignity while at the same time addressing their needs or alleviating their suffering.

Care ethics assumes a relational account of persons. Our interests and our identities are constituted, in large part, by our relationships with others. Thus, care privileges communities as well as individuals. Attending sympathetically involves the obligation to nurture and extend the relationships that are supportive of human flourishing. Finally, care ethics involves accommodation and harmony. The desire to nurture networks of care requires trying to accommodate the needs of all, including oneself. It is not always possible, or wise or morally defensible, to do what everyone thinks they need, but it is important to give everyone concerned a sense of being involved and considered in the process. When we do this, we have a better chance of preserving the harmony that supports communities in which humans can flourish. Some communities may be stable and harmonious, but oppressive to those at the bottom. An ethic of care would be opposed to such societies because they involve superficial harmony at the cost of treating some as though they do not deserve the same care as others.

While care ethics is much more nuanced than some other moral theories, it is still action guiding in the same way that all virtue theory is action guiding. The development of caring involves cultivating key dispositions, especially empathy. Reasonable self-concern is also important, both because one is deserving of care and because effective caring is impaired when one doesn't take adequate care of oneself. In interactions with persons one knows reasonably well, a person with a well-developed empathic response can often be guided merely by attending to the details of the situation.

When one is not so familiar with the person or persons, or when one is developing guidelines for an institutional setting, one needs rules based on generalizations about the best way to be caring in interactions with others. These rules function to set a moral minimum and some reasonable expectations about how others will behave. The rules will specify some actions as beyond the pale, as incompatible with a genuinely benevolent motivation. At the same time, support and encouragement should be given to help people to exceed this minimum and offer genuine caring support to others. Thus, institutions should be sensitive to the need to develop and sustain models of ideal caring practices. Finally, the conditions for developing empathy should be encouraged, while conditions that undermine empathy should be avoided.

Caring for others often takes place in settings that make it extremely difficult if not impossible to be our best caring selves. An ethic of care provides both a moral and political ideal. It is a moral ideal as it describes a way to structure one's moral interactions with others. It is a political ideal as it provides a powerful critique of existing institutions.

Care ethics can provide these two ideals for law. I begin with the first. Since the law is often focused on relationships between persons who are not intimates and are appealing to law to provide the assurance that their interactions will be recognized and supported by law, we can look to the role of care ethics in setting moral minimums for all to follow. But many legal interactions will take place face-to-face and here sympathetic understanding has a role to play. Care as a political ideal provides guidance about how to structure legal institutions and the institutions that gain much of their force and efficacy through the law.

Robin West and Carrie Menkel-Meadow

Robin West and Carrie Menkel-Meadow are two of the lone voices in the legal academy who argue for the importance of care ethics in the law. Menkel-Meadow focuses primarily on a process of legal dispute resolution and the legal education that would facilitate such a process. West is more concerned with legal theory and how such theory could be structured to avoid harms to women. She argues that only an integration of care and justice can protect women from such harms (West 1999).

West holds a relational view of the self, but also argues that an excessive focus on others is neither caring nor prudent. She shares with many care ethicists the view that care is best exemplified in caring interactions between intimates and that maternal caring is the paradigmatic example. In contrasting the traditional role of the judge as impartial arbiter of the rule of law, she describes the caring judge as a maternal figure.

> As the tree provides shade not with its erect trunk but with its gracefully curved branches, the mother provides care, protection, warmth, comfort and love through the interwoven, interdependent strength of the circle of care, not through the independent linearity of the erect, principled, morally upright pillar of strength. (1999, 31)

Second, West sees both justice and care as virtues, and as equally necessary in doing legal justice.

> The work of doing legal justice—of remaining true to a judicial oath, of applying the law, of treating like cases alike, of insisting on institutional consistency, and so on—must be in the service of values which are life affirming... (1999, 49)

> Justice is not the *result* of the accurate application of law, the ascertainment of which requires the censoring of compassion. Rather, justice must *inform* our ascertainment, and hence our application of law . . . And the capacity for justice . . . must in turn be informed by our capacity for compassion. (1999, 48)

West uses examples of judging to illustrate how both care and justice are necessary. *DeShaney* (DeShaney 1988) involved a lawsuit by a mother against the County for its failure to protect her 14-year-old son, Joshua, from the severe battering inflicted by his father. The majority ruled that the state's failure to protect individuals from harm inflicted by private individuals does not violate the Due Process Clause. She writes of Justice Blackmun's dissent that

> Justice Blackmun was quite right, in *DeShaney*, to implicitly insist, in his dissent, that the just outcome in that case must be grounded in a compassionate response to Joshua's plight . . . The Court's failure in *DeShaney* . . . [is a failure to see that] justice, divorced from compassion is lethal. (West 1999, 49)

West also argues that the law should take the "gendered harms" to women as seriously as it takes harm to men, and she conceptualizes some of these harms as involving a commitment to justice with the exclusion of care, or a commitment to care to the exclusion of justice. She focuses particular attention on reproductive issues in law to illustrate both appropriate and inappropriate uses of care ethics (1999, 9, 96–8, 100–38).

Carrie Menkel-Meadow appeals to care ethics in defending a fundamental change in legal focus. The law, she writes, must "develop theories, strategies, and programs for encouraging . . . obligations (laws?) and behaviors to deescalate conflicts and search for better and more peaceful solutions to a myriad of human difficulties and 'injustices'" (2012, 83).

This solution will require that we interact in a caring way, "promoting the possibility of mutual understanding, empathy, sympathy, and 'fellow-feeling'" (2012, 85). Any change to the model of law "as defined by fights, struggles and 'winning' rights" (79) will require legal education that involves the conscious inculcation of the virtue of care. Menkel-Meadow makes the following suggestions for changes in legal education:

> Can we in a law school environment teach such *processes* as:
>
> 1. How to approach each other with *grace, generosity and true curiosity*, instead of the competitive adversarial mode so common now in legal discourse? Our language and orientations to each other must be trained to be "non-violent" in our daily lives, as well as in our legal ones?
> 2. How to *listen to learn* from each other about our differences, commonalties and where we can come together?
> 3. How to *solve the problems* of allocation of resources, material and human, in equitable ways?

4. How to *create new forms of human collaboration* to work together to literally make the world a better place? (2012, 107)

It is encouraging to read the very insightful and important work that West and Menkel-Meadow are doing in applying care ethics to legal theory, but there is much more work to be done. In the next section, I will suggest some avenues for continuing this work.

Finding Care in Legal Authority

Constitution

Constitutions play a fundamental role in the United States, and they change very slowly. Constitutional interpretation, on the other hand, is an ongoing activity. While there are a variety of views about such interpretation, we can arrange them on a continuum with strict interpretation (e.g., Justice Scalia's originalism; Scalia and Garner 2012) on one end and loose construction on the other. Care ethics is unlikely to prove persuasive to strict constructionists largely because they will claim that it does not appear in the writings of the founding fathers. Those who see the Constitution as a living document which provides a blueprint for resolving our current problems would be much more likely to find care ethics congenial. Justice Cardozo, for example, noted that when trust is the standard, one should be "held to something stricter than the morals of the market place" (*Meinhard* v. *Salmon*, 1928), and care ethics helps us to think through precisely what that stricter standard might be. Akhil Reed Amar, a constitutional scholar, argues that constitutional interpretation should take place against the backdrop of what he calls eleven unwritten constitutions, including a feminist constitution (Amar 2012). There is certainly room to explore care ethics here.

Public Policy

Appeals to public policy are often made in consequentialist terms, but this catch-all category is fertile ground for other moral perspectives, including care ethics.

Statutory Law

Statutes can be grouped in terms of doctrinal areas (e.g., property, contracts, criminal law, torts) and policy areas (e.g., health law, environmental law, family law) and there are moral notions embedded in each area. Criminal law, for example, rests on a deontological framework as it sorts liability in terms of mens rea consideration. Justifications of punishment rest on retributive and deterrence models. Restorative justice would benefit greatly from an analysis in terms of care ethics. Family law is understandably rich in moral appeals and can profitably be mined for its inclusion of care ethics. This model might then be extended to other areas of the law which have implications for families, such as immigration law.

Care and Case Law

Justice Kennedy's Use of Care Ethics in Lawrence and Windsor

Justice Kennedy wrote the majority opinion in the case of *Lawrence* v. *Texas* in 2003. The court held that the Texas statute that made it illegal for persons of the same sex to engage in sexual conduct was an unconstitutional denial of due process. Jason Pierceson describes Justice Kennedy's view in *Lawrence* as a variety of liberalism that he calls "rich liberalism." Under this view, "the individual as more socially situated and reliant on the state and society to develop fully as an individual. It differs from other versions of liberalism in emphasizing positive, rather than negative liberty" (2005, 34). I think that a better way to view Justice Kennedy's reasoning in these decisions is to see him as invoking an ethic of care. In both cases, Justice Kennedy invokes a relational ontology and notes the importance of protecting relationships and not just individual liberty interests. This is striking when noting that in both cases the constitutional framework was liberty interests. In *Windsor*, the Court ruled that the Defense of Marriage Act (DOMA) was an unconstitutional deprivation of the equal liberty of persons that is protected by the Fifth Amendment. In *Lawrence*, the court ruled that the petitioners' right to liberty under the Due Process Clause (Fourteenth Amendment) gives them the full right to engage in private conduct without government intervention and that the Texas statute furthers no legitimate state interest which can justify its intrusion into the individual's personal and private life.

We can see care ethics in Justice Kennedy's majority opinion in *Lawrence*:

> The statutes do seek to control a personal relationship that, whether or not entitled to formal recognition in the law, is within the liberty of persons to choose without being punished as criminals... adults may choose to enter upon this relationship in the confines of their homes and their own private lives and still retain their dignity as free persons. When sexuality finds overt expression in intimate conduct with another person, the conduct can be but one element in a personal bond that is more enduring. The liberty protected by the Constitution allows homosexual persons the right to make this choice... (Lawrence 2003)

Here Justice Kennedy prioritizes the personal relationship over the liberty interest of individuals, but liberty and personal relationship are not unrelated.

On Justice Kennedy's view, the very reason that this liberty interest is protected by the Constitution, and other interests might not be, is because of the importance of the personal relationship and personal bond.

Justice Kennedy's majority opinion in *United States* v. *Windsor* (Windsor 2013) makes a similar appeal to the importance of relationship, family, and community:

> DOMA's principal effect is to identify a subset of state sanctioned marriages and make them unequal. The principal purpose is to impose inequality, not for other reasons like governmental efficiency. Responsibilities, as well as rights, enhance the dignity and integrity of the person. And DOMA contrives to deprive some couples married under the laws of their State, but not other couples, of both rights and responsibilities. By creating two contradictory marriage regimes within the same State, DOMA forces same-sex couples to live as married for the purpose of state law but unmarried for the purpose of federal law, thus diminishing the stability and predictability of basic personal relations the State has found it proper to acknowledge and protect. By this dynamic DOMA undermines both the public and private significance of state sanctioned same-sex marriages; for it tells those couples, marriages are unworthy of federal recognition. This places same-sex couples in an unstable position of being in a second-tier marriage. The differentiation demeans the couple, whose moral and sexual choices the Constitution protects, see *Lawrence*, 539 U. S. 558, and whose relationship the State has sought to dignify. And it humiliates tens of thousands of children now being raised by same-sex couples. The law in question makes it even more difficult for the children to understand the integrity and closeness of their own family and its concord with other families in their community and in their daily lives.

One criticism of my claim that Justice Kennedy was making an appeal to care ethics in these two decisions is that he failed to make this appeal in other cases.[1] Perhaps the most infamous case that comes to mind is *Gonzalez v. Carhart* (Gonzalez 2007) where the court held that a state ban on a certain type of abortion procedure was not an unconstitutional violation of Fifth Amendment privacy rights. There Justice Kennedy makes two glaring errors, both of which were central in the court's argument. The first was an inclusion in the decision of a graphic, emotionally loaded description of fetal distress as a necessary part of the abortion procedure (the so-called partial-birth abortion, or dilation and extraction) that was the central issue in this case. The second was Justice Kennedy's claim that some women "come to regret their choice to abort the infant life they once created and sustained," and that severe depression and loss of esteem can follow. Rather than see these two claims as a failure to apply an ethic of care, I think we can view them as a failure to apply this ethic correctly.

The first failure is that Justice Kennedy focuses so much attention on the fetus that he fails to see that pregnant woman and their doctors are also crucially affected by the choice of this procedure. Their doctors want the freedom to use the procedure that is most protective of the lives of their maternal patients, and the women themselves have an interest in surviving this procedure with their lives and health intact. Hence Justice Kennedy is guilty of a failure of empathy—he focuses on the fetus (the "near and dear") to the exclusion of these other parties. The second failure is that he asserts a questionable empirical claim whose plausibility depends on an outmoded view about the role of women as primary caregivers whose very identity is constructed through their caregiving activities. While he made mistakes in both cases, these cases can be construed as mistakes in applying care rather than a failure to use a care perspective. This is not the case for my next case, where the Court's failure was a failure to apply anything like a care ethic. Indeed, this case is an example of a failure to apply any moral perspective fairly and consistently.

Moore *v.* Regents of the University of California

Moore v. *Regents* (Moore 1990) is useful for illustrating the way care ethics can be brought to bear in the multiple doctrinal and policy areas involved in this case: property, contracts, tort, and health law. *Moore* was a ruling at an early stage of litigation, with few facts in evidence, and therefore the court assumed the facts as described by Moore in its ruling. In this section, which is a critique of *Moore*, I shall make the same assumption, though a fuller analysis of the moral issues in this case would require a substantial review of all the relevant facts.

Moore was a decision by the California Supreme Court in 1990, and the US Supreme Court denied certiorari in 1991 so Moore essentially remains the law of the land. In *Moore*, the court held that, while Moore did have a claim against Dr Golde and the UC Regents for a violation of informed consent, he had no property interests in the bodily tissue removed by Dr Golde under cover of the defective consent.

John Moore was diagnosed with hairy cell leukemia in 1975 and sought treatment from Dr Golde at the UCLA Medical Center. Dr Golde did various tests, some of which involved drawing blood, and strongly recommended that Moore undergo a splenectomy (spleen removal), to which Moore consented. Unbeknownst to Moore, Dr Golde had recognized, before recommending the surgery, that Moore's tissue, including his spleen, was potentially valuable both for his own academic research and for commercial use. Dr Golde never told Moore about this. Between 1976 and 1983, Moore made several trips to UCLA from his home in Seattle to have various fluids and other samples, including skin, bone marrow, and sperm, collected, under the misrepresentation by Dr Golde "that such visits were necessary and required for his health and well-being, and based upon the trust inherent in and by virtue of the physician–patient relationship..." (Moore 1990, 126). In fact, these tissue withdrawals were primarily for Dr Golde's research and financial interests. In the meantime, the UC Regents patented the cell line that Dr Golde developed using Moore's tissues, naming Dr Golde, and Shirley Quan, a UCLA researcher, as inventors. They then made arrangements with Genetics Institute, Inc. and Sandoz Pharmaceuticals Corp. for commercial development of the cell line and products to be derived from the cell line. Both Golde and the Regents benefitted handsomely from these financial arrangements. Golde became a paid consultant whose remuneration included common stock. Genetics Institute agreed to pay Golde and the Regents at least $330,000 over three years for exclusive access. Sandoz joined the agreement in 1982 and the payment to Golde and the Regents was increased by $110,000.

How the Court used Moral Perspectives to Decide Moore

While the court appealed to case law to guide its decision about the failure of informed consent, it noted that there was no law that guided its decision about whether to extend the tort of conversion to this case. The court appealed to both patient autonomy and the effects on "innocent" researchers of allowing patients a right to their body parts (Moore 1990, 143). While it was couched in the language of public policy, this argument involved an implicit appeal to and application of the two moral theories that are most often appealed to in Anglo-American law: deontology and consequentialism. In *Moore*, the concern for patient autonomy is expressed in terms of the foundational value of protecting patients' decisions about their own body parts. This is a quintessentially Kantian appeal (Kant 1993/1785). The other policy concern expressed by the court is that "innocent" researchers will face unlimited and unexpected tort liability. This can be explicated in both Kantian and consequentialist terms. The Kantian argument is that one should only face liability when one is in some way guilty or at least able to foresee such liability. Failure to limit liability in this way treats the innocent researchers as mere means to advance an end that is not their own. There is also a straightforward consequentialist appeal here. The *Moore* majority is concerned that holding researchers liable in this way will undercut academic research and the "infant biotechnology industry" (Moore 1990, 143). The concurrences are also couched in moral language, and include substantive concerns that can be explicated in terms of moral theory.

How the Court Might Have Applied Moral Theory in Moore

My discussion in this section will proceed in three parts. In section 1, I will discuss the case using a Kantian framework. Section 2 involves a consequentialist analysis. In the closing section, I will apply care ethics.

1. A KANTIAN ANALYSIS

In his dissent, Justice Broussard points out that in this case the court need not settle the issue of whether one's rights over one's body parts end when they are removed from one's body because in *Moore* the deception and the treatment of Moore as a mere means begins while the body parts are still in his body, since the defendants began the plan to use his tissue for research and financial gain before the splenectomy (Moore 1990, 150). They compounded this failure to treat him as an end in himself by telling him that his health required the collection of further body tissue that could only be done at their facility in Los Angeles. This required that he make frequent trips from his home in Seattle. The majority thus failed to offer a consistent Kantian analysis of this case because they failed to consider Moore's interest in his body parts while they were still in his body. In so doing, they acquiesced in the policy that allows researchers to treat humans as a crop to be harvested at will. Further, the court was insufficiently attentive to the fact that the treating physician's and researchers' deception extended to involving Moore in supporting the cost of their harvesting of his tissue by making many trips from Seattle to Los Angeles. In so doing, the treating physician and researchers were dismissive of Moore's status as an end in himself.

This was not the only failure here. They also failed adequately to consider the "innocence" of researchers. If it is wrong to treat someone as a mere means, and exemplary to treat someone with respect, then actions, policies, practice, and institutions are to be praised or blamed by appeal to how they treat persons. We can now ask: how innocent are the researchers? If this reference is to the doctor, researchers, and institutions named in *Moore*, the majority agrees that they are at least liable for the failure of fiduciary duty and the failure to disclose which began while the body parts were still in Moore's body. The court further describes the failure to disclose as a violation of patient autonomy, a value deeply rooted in Kant's view of humans as ends in themselves. If the reference to "innocent" researchers includes future researchers, we can ask what policies and practices would ensure that they would indeed be innocent. Here, I would argue that treating patients whose body parts are used in research as ends in themselves and never merely as means requires both disclosure and at least the option of being consulted about their future use in commercial endeavors. In refusing to recognize Moore's claim to his tissue, the court foreclosed this latter possibility. If patients have no property interest in their cells after their removal, then no patient will be able to assert control over their use.

2. A CONSEQUENTIALIST ANALYSIS

One of the constraints of applying a consequentialist analysis in *Moore* was that the decision was written at a very early stage of the litigation—the court was merely determining whether the plaintiff had stated a cause of action. Thus we do not have the evidence and argument that would have emerged if this were an appeal of a motion at the end of the trial. Still, in its discussion of whether the tort of conversion should be extended to this case, the court did adopt an analysis that can be characterized as consequentialist.

In *Moore*, the court balanced the interest in patient autonomy against the following interest: "we not threaten with disabling civil liability innocent parties who are engaged in socially useful activities, such as researchers who have no reason to believe that their use of a particular cell sample is, or may be, against a donor's wishes" (1990, 143). The court ultimately refused to extend the tort of conversion in this case because "the theory of liability that Moore urges us to endorse threatens to destroy the economic incentive to conduct important medical research" (146).

The first question we can ask here is whether the court adequately considered the consequences likely to follow from a decision to extend the tort of conversion. In defense of its prediction of the dire results of such an extension, the court cites the Office of Technology Assessment that "[u]ncertainty about how courts will resolve disputes between specimen sources and specimen users could be detrimental to both academic researchers and the 'infant biotechnology industry'" (Moore 1990, 143).

I would argue that the outcomes consistent with the extension of the tort of conversion are numerous, but in considering the consequences of extending the tort of conversion to this case, the court assumes as the only real possibility a world in which researchers have no access to human tissue, and the infant biotechnology industry is strangled in its crib. Moreover, in refusing to extend the tort of conversion, the court closed the door on promising policy alternatives.

While the court might have been insufficiently attentive to the possibilities involved in extending the tort of conversion in this case, the court is not completely indifferent to patients like Moore. They simply argue that they have adequately addressed concerns for the autonomy of patients by allowing the tort of failure to disclose to go forward.

This is an inadequate remedy. A refusal to extend the tort of conversion would affect the cause of action that the court affirmed in this case: fiduciary duty and duty to inform. If researchers and physicians are faced with a conflict between what is best for their patients and their own financial and research interests, the patient is at risk. This risk is not sufficiently addressed by allowing failure to disclose as a cause for action. As Justice Mosk points out, this remedy will not solve the problem because there are serious obstacles to winning such an action (Moore 1990, 179). A patient has to show that, were it not for the failure to disclose, he or she would not have had the procedure. In this case, one wonders whether Moore would have refused the splenectomy, given that he was being treated for hairy cell leukemia, a pretty frightening illness for any patient. Second, the patient needs to show not only that he or she would have refused the procedure in question, but that any reasonable patient in a similar situation would also refuse. Finally, the patient has to show an injury. As one critic points out, if conversion is not a cause of action, it is not clear what injury Moore suffered beyond the money spent on airfare (Corrigan 1992). If the damages under the theories of fiduciary duty and duty to disclose are small and the likelihood that they will be assessed is remote, there is no reason to suppose that clinicians and researchers will be deterred when the temptations of academic renown and financial reward conflict with good patient care.

3. A CARE ANALYSIS OF *MOORE*

Care is a virtue that guides our interactions with others, and has implications for our social policy, practices, and institutions. Caring communities are characterized by the centrality of trust. Persons in caring communities are committed to being morally attentive and sympathetically understanding, and they are also responsive to the need to build and maintain networks of care. They trust that they will benefit from a reciprocal caring attitude from others in their community. Their social practices and institutions support such caring interactions.

We can contrast caring communities with the world of the market. The world of the market is characterized by the centrality of justice, which is usually fleshed out in Kantian and consequentialist terms. Market transactions are characterized by the need to constrain persons in their interactions. Contracts must be enforced, property rights protected, and potential victims shielded from various harms.

These models are not meant as descriptions of the world. Rather, they are ways of thinking through how we want our practices to be structured. As an aspirational model, there is much to recommend the caring community. However, I would agree with West that the most comprehensive moral assessment in the legal arena involves both care and justice.

The *Moore* court did not have care ethics available as a well-developed and articulated moral perspective, since care ethics had not yet emerged as a body of systematic legal scholarship. It did, however, have available the moral capacity that underlies care: the ability to empathize. Heidi Li Feldman provides a reason why the court might have benefitted from engaging empathy in her discussion of the centrality of virtue theory as a foundation for negligence: "Due care or consideration for other people's safety is a species of benevolence, part of caring about other people generally" (Feldman 2000, 1440).

Failure of Empathy

One of the things that I find striking about *Moore* is the failure to pay moral attention and apply sympathetic understanding to Moore's plight, contrasted with the court's concern about "innocent researchers." We see this in the failure of the court to consider alternatives that might be more sensitive to the plight of Moore and patients similarly deceived by those charged with their care. One might explain this in terms of a failure of empathy. Martin Hoffman describes two ways in which empathy can fail that are relevant here (Hoffman 2000). First, he notes that one can be empathically over-aroused when one is confronted with someone who is suffering, and this "can move observers out of the empathic mode, cause them to be preoccupied with their own personal distress, and turn their attention away from the victims" (10). Moore was a victim in two ways: he was afflicted with a frightening illness and he was betrayed by the doctor who was supposed to be caring for him. Judges are human, and perhaps this response to his suffering is part of the story. Philosophers might describe this move as "psychologizing" or "ad hominem" but I think it is important to note that arguments can go wrong in two ways: in terms of content and motivation. If we never pay attention to motivation (conscious or otherwise) in assessing arguments, we miss details that may turn out to be crucial.

Hoffman describes familiarity as another way empathy can fail. It is natural to feel more empathy for those with whom one can identify. A person with a potentially deadly disease is someone no one wants to identify with. Doctors and researchers, on the other hand, are the educational and social equals of judges, so some identification with them and their issues is to be expected.

Care and Transactions in Human Tissue

It is helpful here to look more generally at cases of transactions of human tissue. First, we can distinguish between types of tissues: renewable tissue (e.g., blood), organs for transplantation, biological materials that can create human life, and tissues that would otherwise be discarded after medical procedures. Second, we can distinguish between two different medical settings: clinical and non-clinical. I begin with organs for transplant.

Francis Kane, Grace Clement, and Mary Kane argue that live kidney donations, for example, are seldom motivated by a sense of justice—they are not given to strangers merely because doing so is thought to be a demand of justice (Kane et al. 2008). Rather, "the offer of a live kidney nearly always comes from within a relationship already established" (176). This suggests that framing live organ donation in terms of caring communities better captures our intuitions about such gifts.

Reproductive technology is another instructive example. In a discussion of third party international egg donation, Carmel Shalev rejects a market model in favor of a care model, in part because reproductive technology is connected to maternal practice, which is a practice that, at its best, is a model for care ethics:

> The relationship between the women who collaborate as mothers in third-party reproduction practices is one of mutual interdependence and vulnerability. Ideally, they would be connected in a web of seeing and responding to each other's needs. (Shalev 2012, 154)

So far, our examples support framing tissue donation in terms of care ethics. Giving a live organ or an ovum that might result in the birth of a human child are examples that naturally fit this model. But what about less intrusive donations that have a less momentous function? Consider biobanks (collections of biological materials (e.g., blood and/or tissues) and personal data gathered from large numbers of people), for example. Judit Sándor cautions that even in this case framing the issue in the language of banking is problematic:

> The widely used term "biobank" not only blurred the boundaries between the human rights based norms in the field of biomedical research and the commercial legal norms, but have [*sic*] also contributed to the transformation of biomedical disciplines into new commerce-oriented fields. (Sándor et al. 2012, 4)

One might argue that all these examples (live kidney donation, ovum donation, and biobanking) illustrate the important insight that care ethics can provide because such an ethic better captures our moral intuitions about how a morally sensitive person would behave in these cases.

Care ethics also suggests a resolution to the tension between the interests of patients like John Moore and researchers. Consider, for example, Donna Gitter's discussion of PXE International, which is a patient group that successfully negotiated with researchers and commercial ventures to develop and market genetic tests for pseudoxanthoma, a serious genetic disease (Gitter 2004). As a result of PXE's efforts, such a test has been developed and is available to prospective parents for a modest fee (GeneDx 2013). In this case, prospective parents created a network of care with researchers and all have benefitted through PXE's efforts to actively recruit participants for research and to raise money and awareness about this orphan disease.

Care and the Failure of Dr Golde

We can now apply care ethics to John Moore's treatment by his physician. The court focused on the clinical setting in the first part of the opinion where the primary issue was the failure of consent. The issue of conversion was treated by the court primarily in terms of justice—whether Moore had a property interest in his cells. However, this analysis fails to fully capture our intuitions about what was wrong with Dr Golde's treatment of Moore. Care ethics provides valuable insight here. Moore was especially vulnerable because he was acutely ill. He depended on his doctor to care for him during this medical crisis. His doctor instead treated him like a tissue farm. This is a fundamental failure on the doctor's part to be attentive and sympathetically understanding of Moore's status as a patient in need of care. Dr Golde also failed to recognize the relationship of physician and patient that calls up a duty to make the patient's health the central focus of the relationship. Given the high bar for damages for a failure to disclose, the court's decision here places patients in a clinical setting in a difficult position. When they most need to be able to trust their physician, they are most at risk of a conflict between what is best for them and what will further the treating physician's research and financial goals.

One might suggest that the considerations of justice expressed in terms of Kant and consequentialism can do all the work here. While I agree that they are both powerful ways to guide our decision about this case, they are insufficient by themselves because they fail to capture our intuition that Dr Golde's failure in John Moore's case was not just a failure to treat him with respect or to consider the consequences of his behavior for Moore and all future patients, but a fundamental failure of care. Here we can appeal to Bernard Williams' insightful discussion of the drowning wife (Williams 1981). If one comes upon two people drowning in a lake and one of them is one's wife, one ought to save one's wife, simply because she is one's wife. The demands of care require such a response to the needs of intimates. If one reflects on the justice of choosing one's wife (that doing so could be justified in terms of a lottery principle, or that such a motivation could maximize utility), one is having "one thought too much" (18). Similarly, patients will find it difficult to put their trust in the physician who needs to be prodded in terms of duty to put patients' needs first.

Caroline Forell and Anna Sortun offer a similar analysis of what went wrong with Moore's treatment at the hands of Dr Golde and suggest that we need a new remedy in the law, a statutory tort of betrayal of trust:

> Such affirmative misconduct is an extraordinary transgression, involving exploitation and deceit. It is an outrageous abuse of the doctor–patient relationship that in no way resembles the negligence claim of lack of informed consent. Betrayal, disloyalty and taking advantage are at the heart of the Moore allegations and merited a specific remedy for the dignitary injury apart from, and instead of, lack of informed consent. (Forell and Sortun 2009, 591)

This is not the only legal remedy that has been suggested for Moore, but it is instructive insofar as it illustrates how care ethics can shape our views about the possibility and plausibility of legal remedies.

Conclusion

In this chapter, I have argued that care ethics can be a valuable resource for theorizing about the law and for teaching the next generations of law students. While the law is often explicated and developed through the lens of deontology and consequentialism, there are valuable insights that these perspectives fail to capture. Care ethics is a necessary corrective. It assumes a better grounded understanding of personal identity as relational, it includes empathy as a primary moral disposition, and it can make sense of concerns about the importance of community. Though law is in many ways a profoundly conservative institution, there are many doctrinal and policy areas that could benefit from a thoroughgoing care ethics analysis.

Note

1. This objection was offered by Maxine Eichner in an earlier discussion of this chapter.

References

Amar, Akhil Reed. 2012. *America's Unwritten Constitution: The Precedents and Principles We Live By*. New York: Basic Books.

Baier, Annette. 1987. "Hume: The Women's Moral Theorist?" In *Women and Moral Theory*, edited by Eva Feder Kittay and Diana T. Meyers, 37–55. Lanham, MD: Rowman and Littlefield.

Baier, Annette. 1995. *Moral Prejudices: Essays on Ethics*. Cambridge, MA: Harvard University Press.

Corrigan, Anne T. 1992. "Note: A Paper Tiger: Lawsuits against Doctors for Non-disclosure of Economic Interests in Patients' Cells, Tissues and Organs." *Case Western Reserve Law Review* 42: 565.

DeShaney. 1988. *DeShaney* v. *Winnebago County Department of Social Services* (489 US 189).

Dworkin, Ronald. 1977. *Taking Rights Seriously*. Cambridge, MA: Harvard University Press.

Dworkin, Ronald. 1986. *Law's Empire*. Cambridge, MA: Harvard University Press.

Feldman, Heidi Li. 2000. "Prudence, Benevolence, and Negligence: Virtue Ethics and Tort Law." *Chicago-Kent Law Review* 74: 1431–66.

Forell, Caroline, and Anna Sortun. 2009. "The Tort of Betrayal of Trust." *University of Michigan Journal of Law Reform* 42: 557–609.

GeneDx. 2013. <http://www.genedx.com/test-catalog/disorders/pseudoxanthoma-elasticum-pxe/> (accessed 11/11/2013).

Gilligan, Carol. 1982. *In a Different Voice*. Cambridge, MA: Harvard University Press.

Gitter, Donna M. 2004. "Ownership of Human Tissue: A Proposal for Federal Recognition of Human Research Participants' Property Rights in Their Biological Material." *Washington and Lee Law Review* 61: 257–345.

Gonzalez. 2007. *Gonzalez* v. *Carhart* (500 US 124).

Held, Virginia. 2005. *The Ethics of Care: Personal, Political and Global*. New York: Oxford University Press.

Hoffman, Martin. 2000. *Empathy and Moral Development*. Cambridge: Cambridge University Press.

Hume, David. 1993 [1777]. *An Enquiry Concerning the Principles of Morals*. Indianapolis, IN: Hackett.

Hutcheson, Francis. 2003 [1725]. *An Inquiry into the Original of Our Ideas of Beauty and Virtue*. Indianapolis, IN: Liberty Fund.

Kane, Francis, Grace Clement, and Mary Kane. 2008. "Live Kidney Donations and the Ethic of Care." *Journal of Medical Humanities* 29: 173–88.

Kant, Immanuel. 1993 [1785]. *Groundwork for the Metaphysics of Morals*. Indianapolis, IN: Hackett.

Lawrence. 2003. *Lawrence* v. *Texas* (539 US 558).

Manning, Rita. 1992. *Speaking from the Heart: A Feminist Perspective on Ethics*. Lanham, MD: Rowman and Littlefield.

Meinhard. 1928. *Meinhard* v. *Salmon* (249 N.Y. 458; 164 N.E. 545).

Menkel-Meadow, Carrie. 2012. "Toward a Jurisprudence of Law, Peace, Justice, and a Tilt Toward Non-violent and Empathic Means of Human Problem Solving." *Harvard Unbound* 8: 79–108.

Moore. 1990. *Moore* v. *Regents of the University of California* (51 Cal.3d 120).

Noddings, Nel. 1986. *Caring: A Feminine Approach to Ethics and Moral Education*. Berkeley, CA: University of California Press.

Pierceson, Jason. 2005. *Courts, Liberalism, and Rights: Gay Law and Politics in the United States and Canada*. Philadelphia, PA: Temple University Press.

Ruddick, Sara. 1989. *Maternal Thinking: Toward a Politics of Peace*. Boston, MA: Beacon Press.

Sándor, Judit, Petra Bárd, Claudio Tamburrini, et al. 2012. "The Case of Biobank with the Law: Between a Legal and Scientific Fiction." *Journal of Medical Ethics* 38(6): 347–50.

Scalia, Antonin, and Bryan A. Garner. 2012. *Reading Law: The Interpretation of Legal Texts*. Eagan, MN: West Publishing.

Schauer, Frederick. 2012. *Thinking Like a Lawyer: A New Introduction to Legal Reasoning*. Cambridge, MA: Harvard University Press.

Lord Shaftesbury. 2000 [1711]. *Characteristics of Men, Manners, Opinions*. Cambridge: Cambridge University Press.

Shalev, Carmel. 2012. "An Ethic of Care and Responsibility: Reflections on Third-Party Reproduction." *Medicine Studies* 3: 147–56.

Slote, Michael. 2003. *Morals from Motives*. New York: Oxford University Press.
Smith, Adam. 2010 [1759]. *The Theory of Moral Sentiments*. Chichester, UK: Capstone.
Waluchow, W. J. 1994. *Inclusive Legal Positivism*. New York: Oxford University Press.
West, Robin. 1999. *Caring for Justice*. New York: New York University Press.
Williams, Bernard. 1981. *Moral Luck*. Cambridge: Cambridge University Press.
Windsor. 2013. *United States* v. *Windsor* (133 S.Ct 2675).

9

Of medicine and monsters

Rationing and an ethics of care

Ruth Groenhout

An ethics of care is focused on care for vulnerable others, and on meeting the needs of those who need care. In the context of healthcare, this rather obviously leads to a patient-centered focus, and provides a perspective from which a number of healthcare-related issues can be analyzed. But when it comes to making decisions about the limits imposed by economic structures, and about either rationing resources or developing reasonable limits to care, it might seem that an ethics of care has little to say. Both rationing and drawing limits to care have been difficult issues for care theorists because they seem more like failures of care than concepts that can properly be included in an ethics grounded in care. But my argument in this chapter will be that an ethics of care does have the resources to address the question of rationing, and that developing those resources adds an important dimension to care as an ethical theory.

One of the tasks of any ethical theory is to delimit the realm of the morally required from the morally permissible. Placing limits on the amount of healthcare provided to those who need it requires us to have some sense of when, as a community, we are required to offer care, and when it is permissible to either fail to provide it, or to refuse to provide it. While different theories will locate these limits in different places, with (for example), utilitarians placing limits when the benefits of care are outweighed by total costs of providing care, or social contract theorists limiting care when it infringes on the autonomy of either the care recipient or the caregiver, the basic finitude of human resources and energy require that any reasonable theory have some way of making these distinctions.

This chapter argues that an ethics of care can and should provide guidance for thinking about limits. And in particular it focuses on questions of the quantity of care rather than the delivery of care or the quality of the care given, both of which have received more attention from care theorists.[1] In the case of healthcare, in particular, the almost unlimited capacity to develop newer and costlier technologies has produced a serious crisis for both funding and providing care in a reasonably equitable manner to all who need it. The sheer expense of medical technologies produces spiraling cost increases as professionals try to provide the best care possible for all their patients, and those increases in costs make it harder and harder to provide even basic care for many who need it. Obviously there are factors beyond technological changes that drive increases in healthcare costs, but newer technologies in particular generate a serious problem for the provision of healthcare.

Clearly there must be limits to the provision of medical care. Resources are not unlimited, and as a society we need to be able to spend the resources we have on a wide variety of needs—education, infrastructure, environmental protection—in addition to healthcare. Limits to what can be provided clearly need to be drawn, but the problem is determining where those limits lie. And that determination is particularly difficult from a perspective of care because of the nature of medical needs.

I have already indicated why limits are needed. The argument of this chapter begins by identifying why medical care poses a particularly difficult issue for care theory. I then adopt a distinction developed by Tove Petersen (2008) between care in interpersonal relationships and professional care relationships to argue that the expression of care in institutionalized settings needs to be conceptualized in ways that set limits to the care that can and should be provided. I add to Petersen's account of these differences the need for a procedural structure for developing guidelines for the provision of care. The points I will make in this section are then used to analyze the recent case of Sarah Murnaghan, a 10-year-old girl in need of a lung transplant. Her case is used both to illustrate the need to adopt a perspective informed by care when making decisions about access to scarce resources, and also to argue that care theory needs to adopt a procedural framework for this type of case in order to set ethically responsible limits in healthcare.

Limiting Care: Medicine as Monster

Healthcare is an arena that poses a serious problem for care theory precisely because of the fact that care theory begins with the moral imperative to care. As I reflected on the topic of this chapter, in fact, it occurred to me that healthcare generates a situation much like the utility monster[2] generates for utilitarian ethical theory (Nozick 1974). The utility monster, the problem of a single set of concerns that swamps every other moral consideration, represents a serious theoretical problem for any theory that defines the right in terms of the maximization of utility. Utilitarianism, if it is to be considered a worthwhile account of the ethical life, must have some way of dealing with utility monster problems. Just as the utility monster identifies a key weakness in utilitarianism, so too, I argue, does contemporary healthcare identify a key weakness in care theory. To the extent that the theory can address the problem without ad hoc or arbitrary emendations, to that extent it proves itself a worthwhile account of ethics (and, of course, to the extent that it cannot, to that extent it is shown to be problematic).

So why does contemporary healthcare represent the "utility monster" of care ethics? Start with the nature of healthcare. Medical care[3] is a need, not a luxury (except in certain non-paradigm cases such as cosmetic surgery) and it is needed for the most basic aspects of life. It protects from illness (in the case of vaccines), it cures sickness and damage, and it saves people who are close to death. These are vital and, frequently, urgent needs. Denying medical care, then, involves denying individuals access to treatment or care that could alleviate severe pain and prevent physical harm or even death, or treatment that could cure or ameliorate disease. I take it that the claim that most medical care is a necessity not a luxury is relatively uncontroversial. There is good research demonstrating that, for populations as a whole, there are a number of interventions that generate far greater health benefits for lower overall costs than many expensive medical treatments. If one were a utilitarian, this would be a decisive reason to refuse to provide some expensive interventions to provide resources for cheaper, more beneficial options—clearly this maximizes benefits and minimizes costs. From a perspective of care, however, the fact that there are less expensive interventions that increase the well-being of the population as a whole cannot end the discussion, since attentiveness to the particularities of individuals' lives requires that we continue to care about, and respond to, the needs of individuals. And those needs often call for expensive medical intervention.

Further, those who need medical care represent one paradigm set of cases of people toward whom care should be directed. Care theorists often highlight the way that vulnerability, physical need, and suffering generate empathy and so provide a grounding for an ethics of care (Noddings 1984; 1989; Manning 1992; Kittay 1999; Slote 2007). Because some or all of these are present in cases of those who need medical care, denying medical care to those who are vulnerable, suffering, and in serious physical need seems precisely what an ethics of care should prohibit, not mandate.

The fact that medical care is a critically necessary resource for some of the most vulnerable and needy among us sets the context for calling medical care the "UM" of care ethics, but what takes medicine into a separate realm from almost any other issue is the state of contemporary medical technology. There are medical responses available for a wide array of medical conditions, many of them very effective, and almost all of them very expensive. Organ transplants, new scanning technologies, machines that can keep a weak heart functioning while a patient waits for a transplant, bonding materials that can hold shattered bones together, pharmaceuticals that alleviate the worst symptoms of advanced cancers—all of these are available in the United States, and all for a very hefty price, both in terms of absolute dollars and in terms of commanding the resources of healthcare professionals, intensive care beds, and the like (Callahan 2009).

Len Fleck, for example, notes that just the newly developed technologies for heart care support, specifically implantable cardiac defibrillators and left ventricular assist devices, are projected to cost the healthcare system around $54 billion annually (Fleck 2009, 6). These are only two treatment technologies, and ones that focus solely on heart care. Furthermore, the various treatment modalities that Fleck identifies are now several years older, and newer and even more expensive options continue to appear. Meanwhile, in countries that have, so far, been able to control healthcare costs to some degree, the pressure to expand access to care and the use of new technologies is enormous. Canadian provinces in close proximity to the United States are especially affected by this dynamic, leading to higher costs and pressure to provide treatments that have not been approved by provincial oversight boards.

Even when treatments have not been shown to be effective, of course, they are often demanded by patients. Again, this is not surprising, since those demanding them frequently face seriously debilitating disease or death, and can hardly be blamed for grasping at straws. But this contributes, again, to spiraling healthcare costs. Insofar as medicine appears to offer the only glimmer of hope that a terminal patient may have, there will be constant and persistent demands even for treatment that has not been shown effective. The main problem generating unsustainable costs, however, is not ineffective treatment, but effective treatment.

Healthcare works, and it works well. As a result there is enormous pressure to provide it, and to develop even more of it. This produces a system, unfortunately, that is ultimately unsustainable because we cannot, collectively, afford to keep providing all the available care to as many as are currently receiving it, and yet there seems no way to set limits to the care that we feel is medically and morally required. Attempts to set limits to care are often portrayed by the media as draconian. How can we deny a dying patient, only seventeen years old, her last chance of survival by denying her a liver transplant (*NBC News* 2008)? How can patients dying of cancer be told that a medication that might save their lives cannot be provided because there are no funds for it (Cohen 2014)? Denying care (in the sense of treatment) in cases such as these seems the paradigmatic case of failing to care (in the sense used by care theory)[4]—and care is what an ethics of care says we must provide. But providing care at this level threatens to overwhelm many of the other central aspects of human life. Middle-class wages have essentially been flat for two decades because the soaring costs of insurance eat up the funds that might provide salary increases. Medicare costs are one of the major drivers of the national deficit. Countries with national healthcare systems have, up to this point, been able to keep their costs from rising as fast as the unregulated system in the United States, but as costly technology continues to become available, pressure keeps increasing on these systems to provide US levels of care.

Medical care, thus, functions as the UM of care ethics because medical needs threaten to swallow up every other moral consideration. Like the utility monster, medical needs are almost unlimited, and are, for the most part, vital for continued life or function of the individual. Attempting to limit access to medical care in order to preserve space for other concerns (education, libraries, etc.) is problematic because these other concerns are not life and death matters. While it seems obvious that healthcare cannot be the only good that is morally important, attempts to limit care in order to keep taxation levels reasonable, or attempts to define basic care while treating more expensive care as something people need to pay for out of pocket or through private insurance, are regularly described as immoral refusals of care because the people who are denied care are so obviously vulnerable, desperate, and in need of those resources. In the context of an account of ethics that makes care the heart of ethics, and ties care to vulnerability, medical needs seem to have turned into a monster ready to gobble up all the available caring resources, leaving none for anyone or anything else.

Limits and an Ethics of Care

Limits need to be set in medicine (Daniels and Sabin 2002). That, I think, is uncontroversial. The question we need to focus on here, then, is how to structure limits in ways that respond to the requirements of care. One way to begin thinking about how to set limits within a context of care is to think about the ways that caring people do make these sorts of decisions. Rather than starting with deontological principles of autonomy and basic respect for the dignity of all individuals, for example, a care theorist might instead draw on the sorts of considerations that healthy families go through when deliberating about how to provide care to all members of the family, especially when some have exceptional levels of need. Imagine, for example, that I am a parent with several children. One of my children has a serious learning disability and requires more of my attention and support than the others. It is, certainly, appropriate that I spend more time with that child than another, given the need to work with these learning challenges, but I would fail to be a caring parent if I devoted all my time and energy to just this one child. Although my other kids may not need the same level of support, I still need to spend time with them, make sure they are thriving in school, and simply be with them as a good parent would.

In other words, when there are multiple others toward whom I have duties of care, the fact that one has serious and demanding needs does not mean that as a caring person I automatically deny the others. Instead, as a caring parent, I need to balance the greater needs of the one against the legitimate needs of the others. Fairness requires that all my children be treated as much loved members of the family, and while they will not all be treated the same, and one will get more of my attention and resources, that does not mean that the one's greater need entitles him or her to all my resources.

More generally, while it is certainly true that care needs to take account of the level of neediness and vulnerability of those who need care, this does not entail that any single sort of neediness can legitimately claim all the resources. Instead, like any other moral system, a caring system will need to make decisions about what level of resource allocation is compatible with both a caring response to the more vulnerable party and a fair response to others who also have some claim on those resources.

From the perspective of care, there is no single formula that can identify exactly where the line must be drawn. A particularistic system cannot specify exact limits in advance, since it needs to maintain flexibility and openness to particular situations (Brandsen 2006). But we can note some features of any system that can be justified on the grounds of protecting and maintaining relationships of care.

First, care theorists should advocate limits that can be justified to the various individuals involved. That is, it must at least be the case that all the parties affected by limits, whether more or less needy, could see the system of distribution as relatively reasonable, rather than as irretrievably stacked against them (Hankivsky 2004). One way of thinking of this constraint is that it requires that all concerned have equal standing, in some sense. As Joan Tronto puts it, "all are equally eligible to be heard, about their status and concerns, in making assignments of responsibility" (2013, 108). I would add that all are also equally eligible to be heard in making claims about their need for the available resources.

The requirement that limits be justifiable, however, cannot be interpreted as the need for all affected to actually find those limits justified. Ideally one might hope for that outcome, but in the real world, with serious issues at stake, and (in the case of medical resources) sometimes lives at stake as well, it will not always be the case that all concerned are able or willing to see any limits on their access to healthcare as justified. Limits instead must be such that they are justifiable (pushing care theory, in Daniel Engster's term, toward rational caring (2007)) and structured in such a way that they are open to revision and responsive to legitimate challenges (Tronto 2013).

Determining reasonable limits and adequate structures of openness and accountability are both iterative and interrelated processes. What counts as reasonable generally varies from perspective to perspective, and limits that affect me personally are often felt as far more onerous than limits that affect another. Later in this chapter I will return to some of the considerations that determine reasonability in limiting access to healthcare, but first the issue of open and responsive procedures is worth examining a bit more carefully.

In general (though not always), in systems where there is a great deal of local control and ownership, and where the administrators are generally acknowledged to be fair and looking out for the good of all, it is easier (though never automatic) to achieve something like a sense of equity. But as systems get bigger, administrators more distant, rules more abstract and absolute, people's willingness to accept differential levels of access to resources becomes weaker. When those denying me access to care are faceless, unknown bureaucrats, and when those who (supposedly) have a greater need for resources than I do are anonymous strangers, I am far less likely to trust the system, and far more likely to do everything I can to game it in my own favor.

This is a feature of social systems that makes sense within the framework of an ethics of care. Relationships really do matter. They are not merely abstract forces that one mentions in a philosophical treatise, but real forces that change how social systems work (Tronto 1994). The relationships in which people stand, both the nature of the relationship in terms of the various roles people play, and the nature of the relationship in terms of social capital that has been built up or squandered, change the structure of what sorts of systems are acceptable to participants. The more abstract, the less trust, the more the only acceptable system of distribution must be one of impartiality and equality. This suggests that the more systems of distribution of healthcare become large-scale, principles-based systems of distribution, to that same extent the rules will have to be the same for all concerned, the level of care to which individuals have access will need to be largely equal, and the expectation should be (if we are reasonable) that all will demand access to the same level of care when possible. This has the positive result of ensuring rules that apply equally to all, the negative result of producing a one-size-fits-all system that lacks the capacity to respond to particularistic circumstances.

This conclusion—that large-scale systems of distribution need to be relatively impartial and egalitarian—may seem to be a rejection of the particularity and attentiveness to the individual that care theory builds into its account of ethics. As a number of theorists have argued in recent works, however, developing social policies and principles that are generally impartial and egalitarian is not contrary to an ethic of care, but can instead be a requirement of providing for the care of citizens in any decent (and caring) society (Hankivsky 2004; Held 2006; Engster 2007; Tronto 2013). An ethic of care advocates creating structures of "collective caring," in Engster's phrase, in order to ensure that care is provided fairly, adequately, and accessibly for all, and for many issues this requires large-scale social structures for the delivery of care, as we find in the case of medical care.

There are a number of reasons why providing care at the level of social structures requires principles applied in fair and egalitarian ways. One reason is the simple need to address imbalances of power. When systems have built-in flexibility to respond to particularistic needs, people who are generally privileged in society will tend to demand and receive more than their fair share of any resources, and their demands will be felt (by them and often by others) as appropriate.[5] Any system of social provision of care that prioritizes empathetic responsiveness to particularistic needs without setting limits and structures for ensuring fairness will be vulnerable to perpetuating this type of inequity because it responds to felt needs, and the built-in inequities of the system will correspond to inequalities in people's sense of need and/or entitlement. For large-scale systems of distribution, then, fair and egalitarian principles are not contrary to care, but actually support and protect it.

Medical care is the sort of care that needs large-scale social systems for distribution. It is highly technical and requires specialized training and facilities for adequate delivery, and the need for any particular sort of treatment or intervention is unpredictable and varies enormously from person to person. Fair and caring provision of medical treatment thus seems to be precisely the sort of case that requires some form of distributive principles. Because medical care is so important, and because the systems that provide it are large and complicated, it is also the sort of system that generates the suspicion of bureaucracy, the sense of unfairness that large-scale bureaucracies naturally generate. And, as argued earlier, the sheer cost of medical care requires that limits be drawn, limits that will be experienced by those who face them as unfair and burdensome. So what can an ethics of care offer in terms of responding to these foreseeable structural issues?

There are at least two requirements, I would argue, that should structure principles that are derived from care. The first may not seem particularly compatible with an ethic of care at first sight, since I will argue that a fair system of distribution should be generated by experts in the field. As part of my argument for this I would like to utilize a distinction made by Tove Petersen (and others, but Petersen makes it clearly, and applies it specifically to the healthcare context).

Petersen notes that an ethics of care needs to be capable of distinguishing between what she terms interpersonal relationships of care—personal relationships between family members, friends, personal connections, and the like—and professional relationships of care. In the latter camp she includes the various caring professions—nursing, medicine, and education, for example (2008). Her focus is on nursing as a caring profession. Nursing is a profession profoundly at risk for demanding overly altruistic responses from practitioners (a variation on the UM problem I discussed above). Petersen's analysis of how care should function in this context makes a number of important points, only one of which I am going to develop here.

Petersen notes that a central part of nursing care involves care that responds to the needs of a particular other. But the sort of particularistic care that a nurse should offer is not like the infinite responsiveness to one particular other that one finds in, for example, the thought of Levinas. Instead, the particularistic care that nurses offer is a particularism rooted in professional and theoretical knowledge. Nursing education develops skills and expertise that allow nurses to respond to a patient in ways that are appropriate to that particular patient, and to do so in ways that non-professionals are unable to do. That is at least one of the excellences that constitute nursing expertise. "Particularism," then, in the context of nursing care, does not require that one particular patient be allowed to make unlimited demands on a nurse's care. Instead, care is particularized for patients because of the nurse's specialized knowledge and expertise, both with the medical issues involved and with how various types of patients respond to various types of treatment protocols.[6] Taken in this way, professional attentiveness to particularity will be the practical expression of expert knowledge applied to particular cases and issues.

Petersen's point can be broadened, I would argue, to include issues that go beyond the professional care offered to patients or clients. In the case of medical treatment decisions, and particularly decisions involving scarce resources and enormous expense, we can follow Petersen's lead in arguing that attentiveness to particularity in a professional context should not be interpreted as trying to provide unlimited care. Instead, the attentiveness to particularity that is appropriate to professional caring contexts is a particularity of expertise and experience, based on theoretical knowledge of the conditions and contexts within which care needs to be given.

If that is the way that professional particularity is understood, then, in the context of allocation decisions we will need structures of decision making generated by expertise. What this means is that in cases where a resource is both scarce and expensive, the policies we adopt for distributing the resource need to be developed by experts on the subject. Obviously there are other considerations as well in cases of this sort. To avoid entrenching implicit bias, for example, it is also important that those who develop policies are representative of a wide range of class and privilege (and this may not always coincide with subject-area expertise) and certainly other considerations may play a role here, too. My point is not to generate a complete set of considerations for those who set policies in this type of situation, but merely to note that among their qualifications care theory would include professional expertise and experience. Care in a professional context is not best interpreted in terms of empathic responsiveness to a particular other, but is, instead, a reason for developing principles that give all potential recipients of care a fair and measured set of explicit and well-grounded principles of distribution. Particularly in a context such as healthcare where the level of technical complexity is so high, expert knowledge is needed to generate reasonable principles for the straightforward reason that non-experts often cannot adequately assess many of the factors that must be considered.

Once principles are proposed, however, they must be contestable. Principles that aim to create structures of care cannot be implemented in an absolute top-down fashion. The responses of those who receive care are vital (though not definitive) for evaluating whether or not care is adequate (Noddings 1984), and any large-scale system will need structures that allow feedback, criticism, and proposals for change when those receiving care consider it to be badly structured (Tronto 2013). But given the nature of medical care, when principles or rules are challenged, the challenge needs to be directed at the rules, not at the fact that specific individuals don't receive the care that they want and perhaps need. Again, though this might seem paradoxical in the context of care, it is not. A system of distribution that establishes limits to when care can be provided will sometimes not provide care to those who need it. And that refusal will generate demands for access to what has been denied. If the system of distributing care is unfair, those who complain should be allowed to make that case and argue for changes. But if their complaint is simply that (under an arguably fair system of distribution) they did not gain access to the needed care, this in itself is not always unjust.

In the same way that caring families set up rules so that every member gets their time to be treated as special and their time to do chores as well, and just as the rules are necessary to make sure that those who complain loudly don't get away with demanding unfair treatment, in the same way, challenges to systems of distribution need to address the rules involved, not focus specifically on particular cases to the exclusion of others.

Both of these basic principles help to limit the UM features of medical care, because both start from within systems that assume limited resources. The problem with always focusing on individual cases is that it generates the assumption that surely the right resources are available somewhere (and in individual cases it often is possible to scrape together resources), leading to the assumption that any denial of care is unacceptable... and generating the UM situation. Developing caring structures requires the rejection of magical thinking in favor of a clear recognition of what is actually available. Given those resources, then, developing rules that try to be fair to all, and allowing those rules to be challenged when necessary, are integral parts of a caring system.

An Illustrative Concluding Case: Sarah Murnaghan's Lung Transplant

One of the most intractable arenas of limited resources and deep need in contemporary medicine is organ transplantation. In a chapter of this length it is not possible to resolve all the issues that the scarcity of organs raises, but a few points can be made in illustration of the issues raised above. In order to focus this discussion, I would like to consider a specific case—the recent case of Sarah Murnaghan—and use that case to focus on some specific issues raised in the earlier discussion.

Murnaghan's case appears to be a classic tale of a little girl rescued from an evil bureaucracy (Welch and Asher 2013). Ten-year-old Sarah needs a lung transplant due to cystic fibrosis, but there is a good chance that she will not receive a pair of lungs because she is not on the adult registry. As a 10-year old, she is limited to the children's registry. Keeping her on that list (and off the adult list) is the United Network for Organ Sharing, otherwise known as UNOS, with its rules that give priority to recipients for adult lungs who are 12 years and older. Her parents sue Kathleen Sebelius, the Health and Human Services Secretary, and the judge rules that Murnaghan must be placed on the registry, calling the rule discriminatory towards children, arbitrary and capricious, and an abuse of discretion (Norman and Millman 2013). Sebelius is described as a "one-woman death panel" by right-wing opinion pieces (Orient 2013). Murnaghan's placement number on the organ recipient list is changed by direct order of the judge in the case, and she receives not one, but two lung transplants. (The first is unsuccessful.) Reports of the case almost universally treat it as a triumph that Murnaghan received the transplant.

From the perspective of care ethics, should we accept the framing of this issue? Is it the case that when a 10-year-old who needs a lung transplant is able to jump forward on the recipient list due to a judge's ruling, care for the individual has triumphed over rigid, legalistic principles? Based on the earlier discussion, I am going to argue that this way of framing the issue gets it deeply wrong. While there are reasons for regularly reviewing the criteria for how recipients are placed on organ lists, and while there may be reasons for changing the criteria for younger children in particular, the judge's ruling in this case is problematic for a number of important reasons, and needs to be challenged. Both of these issues illustrate the points made in the earlier section—that an ethics of care needs a procedural account of principles and processes in the context of medicine, and that without such an account it falls prey to the "utility monster" problem almost automatically. I will begin with this last point.

The Murnaghan case clearly illustrates how a caring focus on an individual in need, without consideration of fair principles of distribution, generates a UM problem in the context of medicine. The judge who decided this case was faced with a 10-year-old girl who would die without a lung transplant. Her exclusion from the list of adult recipients appeared to be something close to a death sentence, given the scarcity of child donors of vital organs. Those who had excluded her from access seemingly had done so for what sound like bureaucratic reasons: Sebelius argued that it was not her place to second-guess the committee charged with setting standards for access to the registry, an argument that seemed perverse to the judge. Faced with a deeply needy and vulnerable individual, the judge did what (it seems) a caring judge should do—he insisted that Sarah should have access to the adult organ registry immediately.

So long as our focus is on one individual's emotional response to another in need, this case seems an open-and-shut case of acting in a caring way. The problem comes when we broaden our focus to all the individuals involved in a case of this sort. Sarah is not the only person desperately needing a lung transplant. There are currently just under 1,600 people in the United States waiting for a lung transplant, many of whom will not get one in time (Government Transplant Data). When the Murnaghan case went to trial, there were four other adolescents needing lung transplants in the same health center that cared for Sarah. Insisting that she be placed on the adult registry, as the judge decided to do, was a good thing for Sarah, obviously, but not so good for those patients she jumped ahead of. The two sets of lungs that she received were a life-saver for her, but they would have been a life-saver for at least one other person, and possibly two. These other people are nameless and faceless to us, both because medical confidentiality prohibits any healthcare system from disclosing identifying information about patients, and because it is not always possible to identify the recipient who would have suited a particular donated organ, given the complexity of matching blood types and the like. But they are not nameless and faceless to their families, and certainly their hopes and fears for their own futures are meaningful in much the same way as Sarah's. The problem is that, for the judge in the case, only one person appears as an individual. Other people affected by his ruling are faceless and anonymous, persons in the abstract, perhaps, but not actual individuals needing a caring response.

When a personalized sense of care becomes the central focus for our responses, in the way that it seems to have become the central focus for this judge's ruling, the result is an inability to recognize that even difficult limits may sometimes be justified by a concern for the fair provision of care for all the people involved in the system. Further, when decisions about providing care are made on the basis of an emotional response to the need of another, an already scarce resource may be used in ways that provide only limited assistance to those who receive it. The median survival rate for recipients of double lung transplants is 6.6 years (NIH) and only about 55 percent of patients survive five years after a transplant (Allday 2012). The sicker a patient is, the more unlikely she or he is to experience a long-term benefit from a transplant, since co-morbidities diminish positive outcomes. But the sicker a patient is, the closer to death, the more she or he tugs at our heart strings, and the more our empathetic response is to try to provide any chance at survival that she or he might have. The result is a system that tries to provide enormously expensive treatments, using resources that are in extremely short supply, to those who may benefit very little, if at all, because their condition is already so serious.

Organ recipient regulations are set up, in part, to circumvent this dynamic, and eligibility for lung transplants in particular requires that there be no other major organ damage in the recipient. But if we follow the lead of the judge in this case, and focus on a particular patient with complicating factors, but one who could, conceivably, gain a few more years of life with a lung transplant, we will find ourselves transplanting organs into those patients whose need we see most clearly, generating only marginal benefits while healthcare costs skyrocket.

Further, basing decisions about who is to receive organ donations on perceptions of an individual's need can produce paradoxically problematic results in other ways as well. Regulations for listing patients on registries for organs distinguish among different classes of people in order to protect one or another group. In the case of lungs, children are separated from adults precisely because there are so many more adults in serious condition than children. If the two registries were combined, the statistical chance of any child receiving a new set of lungs would diminish because more adults would qualify for the available child-sized lungs. It is precisely to protect children's access to lungs that separate registries have been set up, and the judge's ruling removing age constraints for listing on a registry will, if followed in the long term, be harmful to children like Sarah who need a transplant (Halpern 2013).

Both of these considerations indicate that making decisions about placement on organ recipient registries is not something that should be done by people unfamiliar with the complexities of evaluating suitability for transplant recipients, or by people who do not have a good understanding of the various factors at issue in transplantation. A piecemeal approach to organ transplantation will result in increased costs but lower benefits, serious inequities that may harm the very types of persons we are trying to help, and (though I have not developed the point here for reasons of time) all the inequities associated with allocation decisions made on the basis of emotional appeal, including tendencies to show illegitimate preferences for already privileged classes of patients.

The first of these three problems, the factor of increased costs and decreasing benefits, is directly relevant to the UM problem. Fair rules for organ recipients balance the chance of success and the seriousness of various individuals' situations as best they can. But they necessarily also limit people's access to needed care. Fair rules do not ensure that everyone gets an organ, unfortunately, and they cannot do so. But interventions such as the judge's in the Murnaghan case do not ensure that everyone gets access either—they simply ensure that some people are allowed to jump the queue, rather than accepting that even with fair principles, some individuals will not receive the care they desperately need. And while principles can at least make sure than no one is denied arbitrarily, interventions and individual decisions about allocations both result in unfairness and increase the costs and inefficiencies in the system, resulting ultimately in far worse outcomes than the original system.

A second point can be made, however, about the Murnaghan case. One of the issues that generated a separate set of lists for children and adult recipients was a simple concern for making sure that transplanted organs were appropriately sized for optimal results. Children's smaller bodies do better with smaller organs; adult bodies do better with adult-sized organs. But as commentators have pointed out, if the main concern for allocation is physical size, then age is a fairly poor proxy for actual measurements of size (Ladin and Hanto 2013). If the guidelines cite age as a factor, but are actually designed to regulate body size, then there is good reason to change the regulations. Body size, after all, can be as easily measured as age, so there is no need to use age as a proxy, and a significant cost to doing so. If, on the other hand, the guidelines already take such issues into account, as other commentators claim, then proposals for change may be misguided (Egan and Sweet 2013).

I do not know how these considerations will play out in the case of guidelines for organ recipient registries in the future, but considerations of this sort are clearly worth raising. And this generates another way in which we might approach the Murnaghan case. When allocation principles are perceived to be inappropriate or unfair, they can and should be challenged. Nothing I have said so far should be taken to indicate that I think that the Murnaghan parents were wrong in trying to change guidelines they perceived to be unfair. That sort of challenge is entirely appropriate, in fact, so long as the concern is directed at the guidelines themselves and the criteria they put in place. Guidelines can be unfair to particular demographics, due to a wide range of reasons. And from the perspective of care, it is vital that those who live with the effects of principled systems be able to challenge the system when it appears to burden them unfairly. This type of challenge is precisely what differentiates a responsive system from the sorts of absolutist, legalistic principles that many care theorists rejected in the first place.

But the point to note here is that the challenge needs to be directed at problematic aspects of the principles. Professional care, under conditions of limited resources, must always allow for appeals when the principles themselves appear to be unfair. But appeals based on the problematic nature of the principles themselves need to be distinguished from appeals based on an individual's need for the particular resource, since all the individuals waiting for lungs have the same desperate need. Appeals go wrong precisely when the care offered ceases to be professional care and becomes particularistic care in the sense that is (sometimes) appropriate for interpersonal relationships.

Resource allocation is a particularly difficult moral issue, especially in the context of healthcare. For proponents of an ethics of care, that difficulty is multiplied by the fact that care theory does make the emotional response of care central to ethical analysis. But taming the utility monster is possible, I think, if we respect the particularities of specific relationships in which people stand, recognizing that professional relationships exhibit care in specifiably different ways from, say, family relationships. An ethics of care still requires attentiveness to particularity, but how that attentiveness is practiced makes an enormous difference for how care is provided to those who need it.

Notes

1. My thanks to Maurice Hamington for calling my attention to this distinction. Among the care theorists who have addressed questions of limits to and requirements of quality of care and care delivery are Joan Tronto, Eva Feder Kittay, and, unsurprisingly, Maurice Hamington himself.
2. The utility monster (UM) is a theoretical being capable of absolute maximal happiness (or utility, or preference satisfaction, depending on the variety of utilitarianism at issue). Because the monster is capable of experiencing the absolute maximal amount of happiness, its happiness trumps that of any other beings, and (by utilitarian definition) the right policies become those that channel all resources and all action toward the satisfaction of the UM. Diverting anything elsewhere, by definition, diminishes overall happiness, and so is contrary to what morality demands.
3. I will be using healthcare, medicine, and medical care as largely interchangeable terms in this chapter. There are reasons for separating them in many contexts, but for the purposes of this chapter the differences are not salient.
4. And the fact that I use the same word in both cases again underlines the close connection between medical care and ethical care.

5. I take it that some variant of this concern is one of the reasons Martha Nussbaum has been generally critical of an ethics of care. Her work with women's groups in some Indian provinces has made her aware of the way that systems of privilege can leave some groups of people expecting far less than is their due, others expecting more. When both the privileged and the disempowered accept the rightness of their station in life, the privileged will demand, and feel justified in demanding, more than their share.
6. This discussion summarizes several issues raised in Petersen's discussion in *Comprehending Care* (2008), predominantly in chapter 8. Petersen also discusses the dangers of this type of particularism in entrenching structures of class and race privilege, an obviously important issue, but one that I set aside here to focus on her discussion of particularism and expertise.

References

Allday, Erin. 2012. "Lung transplant patients face tough odds." *SFGate*, 31 October. <http://www.sfgate.com/health/article/Lung-transplant-patients-face-tough-odds-3998899.php>

Brandsen, Cheryl. 2006. "A Public Ethic of Care: Implications for Long-Term Care." In *Socializing Care*, edited by Maurice Hamington and Dorothy C. Miller, 205–26. Lanham, MD: Rowman and Littlefield.

Callahan, Daniel. 2009. *Taming the Beloved Beast: How Medical Technology Costs Are Destroying our Health Care System*. Princeton, NJ: Princeton University Press.

Cohen, Elizabeth. 2014. "Company Denies Drug to Dying Child." *NBC News*. <http://www.nbcnews.com/id/28393752/ns/health-health_care/t/teens-family-sues-cigna-over-denied-transplant/#.U0a5vShOg99>

Daniels, Norman, and James E. Sabin. 2002. *Setting Limits Fairly: Can We Learn to Share Medical Resources?* Oxford: Oxford University Press.

Egan, Thomas, and Stuart Sweet. 2013. "Rationing Lung Transplants." *New England Journal of Medicine*, 21 November. <http://www.nejm.org/doi/full/10.1056/NEJMc1311946>

Engster, Daniel. 2007. *The Heart of Justice: Care Ethics and Political Theory*. Oxford: Oxford University Press.

Fleck, Len. 2009. *Just Caring*. New York: Oxford University Press.

Government Transplant Data. <http://optn.transplant.hrsa.gov/data/>

Halpern, Scott D. 2013. "Turning Wrong into Right: The 2013 Lung Allocation Controversy." *Annals of Internal Medicine* 159(5): 358–9.

Hankivsky, Olena. 2004. *Social Policy and the Ethic of Care*. Vancouver: UBC Press.

Held, Virginia. 2006. *The Ethics of Care: Personal, Political, and Global*. New York: Oxford University Press.

Kittay, Eva Feder. 1999. *Love's Labor: Essays on Women, Equality, and Dependency*. New York: Routledge.

Ladin, Keren, and D. W. Hanto. 2013. "Rationing Lung Transplants—Procedural Fairness in Allocation and Appeals." *New England Journal of Medicine*, 15 August. <http://www.nejm.org/doi/full/10.1056/NEJMp1307792>

Manning, Rita. 1992. *Speaking from the Heart: A Feminist Perspective on Ethics*. Lanham, MD: Rowman and Littlefield.

NBC News. 2008. "Teen's Family Sues Cigna over Denied Transplant," 26 December. <http://www.nbcnews.com/id/28393752/ns/health-health_care/t/teens-family-sues-cigna-over-denied-transplant/#.U0a5vShOg99>

NIH. <http://www.nhlbi.nih.gov/health/health-topics/topics/lungtxp/risks.html>

Noddings, Nel. 1984. *Caring: A Feminine Approach to Ethics and Moral Education*. Berkeley, CA: University of California Press.

Noddings, Nel. 1989. *Women and Evil*. Berkeley, CA: University of California Press.

Norman, Brett, and Jason Millman. 2013. "Sarah Murnaghan Lung Transplant Case: Sebelius Ordered to Make Exception on Transplant." *Politico*, 5 June. <http://www.politico.com/story/2013/06/sarah-murnaghan-lung-transplant-ruling-kathleen-sebelius-92299.html>

Nozick, Robert. 1974. *Anarchy, State, and Utopia*. New York: Basic Books.

Orient, Jane. 2013. "A Death Panel of One: A Dying Girl Exposes a Cold and Callous Government Bureaucracy." *Washington Times*, 10 June. <http://www.washingtontimes.com/news/2013/jun/10/a-death-panel-of-one/>

Petersen, Tove. 2008. *Comprehending Care: Problems and Possibilities in the Ethics of Care*. Lanham, MD: Lexington Books.

Slote, Michael. 2007. *The Ethics of Care and Empathy*. London: Routledge.

Tronto, Joan. 1994. *Moral Boundaries: A Political Argument for an Ethic of Care*. New York: Routledge.

Tronto, Joan. 2013. *Caring Democracy: Markets, Equality, and Justice*. New York: New York University Press.

Welch, Chris, and Zain Asher. 2013. "With Just Weeks Left, Sarah Fights the System for Life-Saving Pair of Lungs." *CNN Health*, 27 May. <http://www.cnn.com/2013/05/27/health/pennsylvania-girl-lungs/>

Part III

Care Ethics, Non-Western, and Subaltern Cultures

10

Towards a feminist ethics of *ubuntu*

Bridging rights and *ubuntu*

Amanda Gouws and Mikki van Zyl

Currently we are facing the moral failure of neoliberalism to deliver justice to the world's people, and increasingly, essential services are being privatized, with care labor needing to be accessed through the market. Using the notion of care, both as ethical concept and as gendered labor, we investigate moral discourses prevalent in South Africa today.

When looking at the production of moral philosophies, feminist knowledge was marginalized (Held 1990) in much the same way as African moral theories have been marginalized (Arnfred and Ampofo 2009). In practice, for example, the dominance of the human rights framework as a universal moral paradigm that is based on an individualist ontology has eclipsed relational ontologies such as a feminist ethics of care and *ubuntu*.

We propose a feminist moral theory from the South by bridging rights and *ubuntu* to synthesize a southern feminist relational ethic of justice. This places us in a "double jeopardy"—bridging the fractures between dominant moral discourses emanating from the North with moral discourses embedded in heteropatriarchies from Africa. Hence our engagement with a feminist ethics of care faces the difficulties of "translation"—a need to explain oneself (Comaroff and Comaroff 2012, 114)—first from South to North, and second from feminist discourses to patriarchal ones.

Centering ourselves in Africa means we also speak critically to the dominant Northern discourses of rights and justice, gender and care, and propose how the synthesis of principles from a feminist ethics of care, together with *ubuntu*, can contribute to substantive gender equality as framed in the South African Constitution.

We agree with the guiding concepts of equality and dignity deriving from the liberal democratic framework established in the SA Constitution, but we argue that a synthesis of *ubuntu* and an ethics of care can provide a better framework for achieving justice. While we focus on gender justice, we believe our synthesis is transferable to other inequalities, since it addresses both material injustices and injustices of recognition. Justice is a well-used term, and therefore can be ambiguous. It is best explained by a phrase coined by Judith Butler (2004, 8–9) around the concept of what is a "livable life." She argues that this requires not only the material means of survival, but also recognition from others as equals. We argue that livable lives depend on receiving adequate care over a lifetime, and in caring for others. We concur with Daniel Engster (2005), who defines care both as actions which secure the well-being of others and as the basis for a moral and political theory. He suggests that caring is not only about meeting needs and developing capabilities, but also means doing it in an attentive, respectful, and responsive way. He concludes that caring is a fundamental human value based on our dependencies on one another.

We also understand human society as relational and interdependent, and therefore argue that justice perspectives need to take into account this relationality. It does not mean that the individual is set apart from the community, nor does it mean that the individual is subjected to community will, but that all individuals are situated in a community—the location where individuals develop their unique qualities and contributions to the community for the public good. They also receive support and are sanctioned to behave in ways that are not harmful to the community. Care therefore becomes the symbol for communal relationships representing reciprocal responsibilities as well as a source of dignity and equality. Hence we argue that an ethic of relational justice as embodied in *ubuntu* and a feminist ethics of care is more appropriate for the achievement of equality and dignity. In a society riven with deep inequalities, concepts of justice need to integrate relational understandings of our mutual dependencies on, and reciprocal responsibilities to, each other. For the majority of individuals to thrive, the whole society needs to flourish. We believe a Southern feminist ethic of care synthesized from *ubuntu* and a Northern feminist ethics of care is one avenue to shift dominant liberal democratic perspectives of individual rights to achieve equality and dignity. We focus on gender equality as a key trope for achieving a more egalitarian, respectful and caring society.

Care in an African Context

In pre-colonial, colonial, and post-colonial times in Africa, care has always been considered a "women's issue." What form the care took—whether it was in extended family formations, nuclear families or single-headed households, and involved care for children, the sick, people with disabilities or the aged—women were responsible for arranging it or doing it. This connection between women and care has become so naturalized that care is seldom viewed as political. Care, however, is a political issue that is constructed through the way the state regulates and administers its subjects and through the discourses it constructs around care issues. But care is also practical and who provides and how care is provided is deeply embedded in what the political context allows. Care therefore needs to be viewed as contextual, but rooted in political understandings of rights, needs, and, in the South African context, the discourse of *ubuntu* (people can only be human through other people).

How political discourses unfold is directly related to how identities are constructed under certain state forms and how these states construct regulations of rule to administer their citizens. We first look at pre- and post-apartheid state formation to show what possibilities there are for care to be viewed as a relational concept, as embodied by a feminist ethics of care and *ubuntu*. In the post-apartheid society in current sociopolitical conditions of high levels of violence, specifically gender-based violence,[1] HIV infection, and the neglect of children,[2] the care burden on women increases in magnitude. We interrogate how the contemporary South African state can ensure justice for those in need of care as well as those doing the caregiving.

Post-apartheid State Formation

The process of colonization in Africa and specifically British colonial administrations created a bifurcated citizenship consisting of citizens (those with access to rights) and subjects (those Africans who lived under customary law) (see Mamdani 1996). Citizens had rights, but subjects were regulated through the process of codification of African customary law that included pacts with traditional leaders (chiefs and headmen) to the exclusion of women. Codified customary law represented an alliance between colonial authorities and African male elders around access to land and resources that were controlled by men. The negative consequences of codified customary law included the reinforcement of patriarchal norms and the entrenching of male bias, leading to a more rigid division between the public and private spheres, and rendering women outside the benefits of the law (see Gouws 2013). These conditions of bifurcation were inherited and reinforced by the apartheid state.

Manicom (1992, 449) has argued that state formation is central to the construction of the domestic as private. The structuring of domestic or household forms and relationships in South Africa was a consequence of state regulations and various state measures under apartheid. It not only defined what was private but also defined and structured the very terms on which domestic struggles took place. The construction of women as subjects of the state was produced under different state policies and practices infused with gender meanings.

When the colonial state reorganized productive relations (through, for instance, migrant labor of men) it meant a change in reproductive relationships and power relations between African men and women. In pre-colonial times, production was organized along gender and generational lines and mediated by customary practices such as *lobola* (bride price) and the regulation of marriage, fertility, and familial forms (Manicom 1992, 450). Through the state's policies and practices, citizens were constructed as objects of rule infused with normative gender meanings that facilitated and reproduced the construction of subordinate social and political identities. The recording of the "native" as head of the household inscribed gender, and encoded men's authority over women. In the process of construction, "native" as a category of rule was viewed as a masculine one. "Native" women, on the other hand, were linked to reproduction, as a sexualized construct and a social problem, not as carers (Manicom 1992, 456).

Because care is so closely connected with women's reproductive capacities, how women are regulated and administered by the state also determines the form that women's caregiving work will take. For women living under customary law, caregiving for children took place in the extended family and was also closely connected to care for physical needs such as cooking and cleaning, which were women's responsibilities. Fetching firewood and water was also women's work and still is for rural women in the post-apartheid state.

The apartheid state was deeply nationalist and patriarchal, and developed its relations of rule according to a racial hierarchy that benefitted whites. As with liberal societies, it located care in the private sphere and enforced the division between the public and private sphere through its policies. Nationalist rule as well as its opposition, in the form of liberation movements, confined women to the sphere of reproduction—as "mothers of the nation" (see Hassim 2005).

Many African women who moved to urban areas became engaged in dual caregiving locations. Women who became domestic workers cared for the children and families of the white labor force (colonial administrators and white households under apartheid), and still had to care for their own households (see Cock 1980). In the (white) employers' households, care was considered a service to be paid for with very exploitative wages for very long hours that took the form of personalized care.[3] In the context of both types of households, care was still confined to the private sphere with very little recourse to the law for caregivers, who were dependent on the goodwill of their employers for any benefits. Caregiving in their own households was made invisible as part of a woman's marital obligations.

The transformation of the apartheid society to a democratic society opened spaces for claims as rights-bearing citizens and opened new spaces for political contestation around issues of rights. One of the greatest challenges for the post-apartheid state was the social inclusion of millions of citizens who had been socially and economically excluded, marginalized, and oppressed.

The Post-apartheid State in a Global Context

The post-apartheid state can be categorized as a state of late colonialism (see Barchiesi 2011) that locates social inclusion in the nexus between citizenship and work, at a time of accelerated globalization processes which have decreased waged employment in neoliberal capitalist environments. Barchiesi (2011, 6) argues that the democratic transformation occurred at the same time as the ensuing of a deep crisis in waged employment, which amplified social marginality in a global trend toward the declining centrality of the labor contract, causing millions of people to end up in "precarious" labor situations. Precariousness can be understood as not having an income, or having a minimal income from waged work. The consequences of this phenomenon are articulated by Barchiesi (2011, 21) as follows: "Precariousness, being outside waged work, or living in-between waged and unwaged activities ceased therefore to be seen as conduits for meanings and strategies. They became conditions of uprootedness and speechlessness." In South Africa these conditions have created the largest gap between rich and poor globally with a Gini coefficient of around 0.7 (OECD 2013, 18).

Conditions of precariousness impact caring in different ways. On the one hand, they may initiate caring that arises from shared oppression, but on the other hand, they undermine not only people's abilities to care for one another, but also their ability to look after themselves. Caring relationships become destabilized, thereby exacerbating inequalities and impairing people's dignity. For the majority of African women in the post-apartheid state—who are uneducated or have low levels of education, and are mostly excluded from waged work or in low-wage categories of labor such as domestic work—globalization and the structural adjustment of economies required by international monetary institutions have deepened social exclusion and poverty, and increased the care burden. The unemployment of the male waged worker has also deepened women's care burden in the face of a lack of resources for caregiving.

In these economic conditions, under democratic rule, concepts of citizenship framed people as rights-bearing and rights-claiming individuals. For women, gender justice became embedded in the liberal notions of equal opportunity and law reform intended to include women into the body politic.

Social transformation shifted from a focus on structural social change, poverty, and inequality, to a focus on an abstract "ungendered" individual citizen under liberal rule—a citizen who is also assumed to be male.

Barchiesi (2011, 14) argues that the late colonial state attempted to gain African workers' acquiescence by legalizing trade unions, regulating employment conditions, and introducing new social provisions with the aim of bestowing on African working-class families the respectability linked to a male breadwinner. In countries like South Africa, social and labor reforms were confined to a small minority of regular wage earners that excluded women, rural workers, and casual employees. Local political elites thought that the relations of rule could be established through the creation of a modern, male, waged working class who would be responsible and governable (Barchiesi 2011, 15). Even where special measures have been introduced to deal with racial disadvantage, such as affirmative action and black economic empowerment, African men have benefitted more than women (see Burger and Jafta 2010, 20).

By linking work to citizenship on the assumptions that the citizen and the worker are male, the imaginary of liberal democratic citizenship reinforces the public/private divide to the exclusion of care work. The invisibility of women's positions under conditions of precarious labor relations makes the huge burden of women's care work similarly invisible. Precarious labor conditions, rising prices of basic necessities, and the crisis of a subsistence economy force women in post-colonial societies into the informal economy or sex work, where income is unstable, and also disperses the burden of care to different generations of women. For example, grandmothers often care for grandchildren or those with HIV-related illnesses, never being free from a care burden until they die. The profound ambivalence of love and duty may bring joy at the same time as potential harm, where a strict division of labor comes at the expense of self-care. Neoliberal governmentality encourages self-help, community development, and decentralized capacity building for those on the periphery of the labor market, rather than offering state intervention (Barchiesi 2011, 17).

With high unemployment[4] and precarious labor conditions, the state has become the main source of capital accumulation for the ascendant black middle class (see Southall 2013, 34) who can afford outsourced, privatized services. Aspiring to personal service in their households, members of the middle class in the post-apartheid state often suffer from what Tronto (2006, 12) calls "privileged irresponsibility" when it comes to care delivered as a "private service" by others. Here women's care work is presumed and people feel entitled to such care. This also makes people blind to the traditional division of labor in the household (whether care work is done by a wife or another woman who takes over a wife's caring duties).

Privileged irresponsibility is rarely visible. For the middle class and the ruling elite who are in positions of superiority, there is no need to consider their role or responsibility in maintaining a system where care workers are exploited. Tronto (2006, 12) calls this the "peculiar ignorance" of the beneficiaries of the system. Privileged irresponsibility is possible because of the liberal state's focus on individualism and autonomy as markers of individual independence, because work is viewed as a constituent aspect of citizenship but care is not.

A Feminist Ethics of Care—Autonomy and Relationality

To the extent that citizens are able to claim rights (as in the case of the working male individual citizen), they are viewed as authentic citizens. But given the way that women's subjectivities have been constructed under the post-colonial liberal democratic state, rights claiming may be limited in contexts of marginalization and violence that render women "vulnerable" and "dependent."[5] A discourse of needs based on vulnerability has overtaken a discourse of rights in the post-apartheid state. Needs are antithetical to politics and a discourse of needs is not about needs satisfaction but about *needs interpretation* (Fraser 2013, 54).

A rival discourse of needs interpretation would be based on a feminist ethics of care. As Buker (2006, 55) argues, the ethic of care challenges two basic assumptions of liberal theory. First, it challenges the public/private split, and second, it challenges individualism as the source of moral authority that liberalism has located in the individual's consciousness. A feminist ethic of care relocates a portion of this moral authority in the collective political community, situating it in relationality or relationships between people and between the state and citizens.

Care is juxtaposed with the liberal notion of autonomy on the assumption that care is social (Clement 1998, 21). Since all humans are socially constituted and at some points are vulnerable and dependent, care and autonomy are not mutually exclusive (Urban Walker 2006, 148). Both caregiver and care recipient need a certain amount of autonomy, otherwise the ethic of care will be deficient. A certain amount of self-determination is needed so that caregiving is controlled, but not necessarily controlling the care recipient (Clement 1998, 22).

Liberal autonomy defines the individual in minimalist terms, focusing on self-determination, self-reliance, and independent, abstract self-maximizing, atomistic individuals (MacDonald 2010, 203). As a political capacity in liberal democratic states, individual autonomy is viewed as something that should be ensured or encouraged by the state. Liberal autonomy abstracts people from their contingent and external relations with other people (203). It often involves objectification of other human beings—othering—and the exercise of power and control over them in the fear of dependence (Jordan 1997, 54).

Autonomy must be understood as relational, social in nature, contingent or processual, and exercised in practice. Even with the liberal notion of autonomy, others will form part of the exercise of autonomy. For example, intersecting identities of race, class, gender, ability, etc., play an important role in the extent to which autonomy can be exercised. Relational autonomy does not necessarily imply dependency but can work to transform (and de-stigmatize) dependence (MacDonald 2010, 204). As MacDonald (2006) as well as White and Tronto (2004) argue, relational autonomy focuses on relationships, context, contingency, and constraint but does not look to narrow down autonomy. Relational autonomy is contextual. This contextuality should be expressed in public.

Since feminist care ethics center the self in a web of social relationships, it follows that the moral self is conceived through relations of empathy, concern, and care. In contrast, "the man of reason" is in a moral dilemma pitted between "what is good for myself" and "what is good for everyone else"—yet in actuality the other is not a generic "everyone," but a specific flesh and blood other (Held 1990, 47). Thus according to feminist ethics, we are ineluctably bound into relationships with others—not only relatives, friends or colleagues, but also social groups through gender, class, and race affinities. Hence the self in feminist ethics is a "relational self" (Held 1990, 339), and how we respond emotionally to others who are embodied and specific is inescapably moral (Jaggar in Held 1990). In contrast to moral maturity being conceived through individual independence and autonomy, feminist ethics regard moral maturity as the ability to sustain relations of mutual empathy and intersubjectivity. Furthermore, it is this concept of self in relation to others that underpins a feminist ethical praxis to end the oppression, subordination, and abuse of others, particularly of women and girls (Friedman 2000, 205).[6] Held (2006, 3) argues that an ethics of care is situated within care practices, and expressed through values of care. This leads to the characterization of a caring relationship which was described by Tronto (1993) as attentiveness, responsiveness, responsibility, competence, and integrity. Through these practices and values it is possible to set standards for practices of care, both social and political, and when approaching political aspects of care, justice is centermost.

Therefore, in summary, the critical elements for a feminist ethic of care revolve principally around relationality, which is expressed through personal affective relationships situated in a concrete context. Further, an ethic of care demands embodied care practices which are responsive to others' needs, ranging from the private to the public realms. In South Africa, *ubuntu* may create the bridge between community and public.

Ubuntu as an Ethic of Care

The concept of self in a communitarian philosophy stands in stark contrast to the Hobbesian conception of self as a person who springs fully formed from nature as a rational, independent, self-determining individual who enters into social contracts with others (Held 1990). This reified being is without ancestry and has apparently reared himself (*sic*) (Di Stefano in Held 1990, 326). In *ubuntu*, ancestry, kinship, and community are woven into the self through myriad social and affective bonds.

These bonds are expressed through care for each other, where allowing another to suffer is seen as part of the process of dehumanizing both the other as well as oneself. Thus failure to care is inimical to *ubuntu*, positioning care as a central feature of *ubuntu*. Through the aspects of caring for one another and belonging in a community, *ubuntu* sees people bound together in relations of mutual respect and dignity, where one's humanity is diminished by acts of greed or deeds of oppression.

What is *Ubuntu*?

There are a number of commonalities as well as differences between feminist conceptions of self and their relationality to others and the Southern African communitarian worldview of *ubuntu*, which has parallels throughout sub-Saharan Africa (Metz and Gaie 2010). Most people in South Africa, even whites, know about *ubuntu*. But as an indigenous African philosophy and worldview, it is more likely to be believed and practiced by black people. However, like any belief system commonly held by people—who are fallible and inconsistent—the question remains as to the extent to which beliefs are translated into actions. Below, we argue that a distinction should be made between "*ubuntu*-talk" and "*ubuntu*-do."[7] For example, a Northern "belief" in personal liberty may be interpreted individualistically; I may believe in personal liberty but behave in a way which denies someone else their personal liberty, resulting in the hypocrisy of "one set of rules for me and another set for you"—a recipe for social injustice.

The first feminist to link a feminist ethics of care and *ubuntu* was Sandra Harding (1987), who noted the similarities between an ethics of care and African values of relationality. *Ubuntu* has been described by a variety of authors from different backgrounds since 1846. Until the second half of the twentieth century it was mostly regarded as a human quality, after which some authors started representing it as an African humanist philosophy (Gade 2011; 2012; Metz 2011). This brings to mind the distinction that ethics of care theorists make between care as moral theory and care as labor or praxis.

Authors from a range of positionalities have written on *ubuntu*. Christian Gade (2012), a Danish philosopher, noting that most academic discussions of *ubuntu* have been produced by non-indigenous Africans, focuses on how people of African descent understand *ubuntu*. To the question "What is *Ubuntu*?" Gade (2012) elicits two different answers from South Africans of African descent: *ubuntu* as the moral quality of a person, or *ubuntu* as a philosophy or worldview which sees all humans as interconnected. (When we asked non-academic Africans of our acquaintance what they understood by *ubuntu*, they all referred to it as a particular way of being: generous and caring and rooted in community.) Thus *ubuntu* is based on the perception that to be a person (human) we are bound into community through relationships of care and obligation. In the first view, *ubuntu* is emphasized as the moral conduct of a person, and the second is a philosophical discourse based ontologically on the ineluctable interdependence between people. The responses showed further variations about persons, with some people believing that all people may be considered persons commanding equal dignity and respect (similar to the human rights framework), and others believing there were conditionalities to being considered a person. The latter group believed that one is not merely a person by being born, but must achieve personhood through contributions and obligations to the community (Gade 2012).

Self and Other

An emphasis on achieving *ubuntu* also led to some interpretations which framed white people as others; white people were not considered persons because they did not behave with respect or recognize the dignity of Africans (Gade 2012). Therefore, in contrast to the human rights framework where all humans are considered equal, mechanisms for othering exist in some interpretations of *ubuntu*, based on a person's conduct towards others.

This emphasis on the aretaic dimension—related to Northern virtue ethics, but because of its relational ontology not equated to it—consolidates an understanding that *ubuntu* does not exist outside its embodiment in human practices. Nonetheless, the idea that a person needs to achieve *ubuntu* can be seen as promoting a "normative" conception of a person, and will inevitably be historically and culturally specific. A normative conception of who qualifies as human potentially constructs an other, where the distinction plays into existing power hierarchies in society, such as privileging some persons on the basis of, for example, unequal social status, gender inequalities, and age differences. A further challenge around normative conceptions of a person based on categories such as race, gender, or other intersectional issues is related to the danger of essentializing identities. Yet, Metz (2011) argues that using *ubuntu* communal social principles, the connectedness between individuals' humanity overcomes the distancing and objectification of the other. Philosophical arguments around *ubuntu* assert that, in a communitarian ethic, the other must be engaged, in order to maintain everyone's humanity. However, in practice, *ubuntu* has relied on normalized discourses of patriarchal and gerontocratic hierarchies, othering people with low status, young people, women, and gender non-conforming people (Gouws and Van Zyl 2014; Marais 2012). Therefore, like other ethical frameworks, *ubuntu* falls short in the implementation of its rhetoric of equality and dignity.

Ubuntu and Justice

Many writers focus on *ubuntu* as a philosophy, rather than practice (Mbiti 1990/1969; Metz 2007; 2011; 2012; Ramose 1999; 2002), positioning *ubuntu* as an ethical framework of relational justice. Comparisons between liberal democratic and *ubuntu* discourses of justice show the former as adversarial, whilst African systems focus on restorative justice.[8] The principles of the Truth and Reconciliation Commission (TRC) exemplified this approach and spurred much investigation in South Africa into the links between *ubuntu* and justice (Bohler-Muller 2005; 2006; Cornell & Van Marle 2005; Gade 2013; Keevy 2009; Mokgoro 2003). This enterprise immediately engaged the human rights framework on which the South African Constitution is based. Some interpretations foreground arguments for *ubuntu* to be interpreted as an egalitarian philosophy in line with the Constitution. But at the same time, Bohler-Muller (2005) and Keevy (2009) are critical of how African customary law has been encoded to entrench gender inequalities, pointing to the differences in how women's human dignity is valued between *ubuntu*-talk, and *ubuntu*-do.

On another point, Metz (2011, 534) defends *ubuntu* against criticisms from jurists, human rights advocates, and political theorists who reject *ubuntu* as being too vague to apply in a legal context. He proposes that "*ubuntu* is the 'underlying motif of the Bill of Rights'." Using the concepts of "identity" and "solidarity" to characterize how individuals are bound into community through empathy for others, he argues that human dignity is a foundational value for both the human rights framework and *ubuntu*. However, he says that the Kantian view of a person's worth—and therefore their dignity—is based on autonomy, while in *ubuntu* it relates to their capacity for community (541). Using a concept of dignity derived from *ubuntu*, he argues that violations of a person's dignity can be interpreted as human rights violations (547). He concludes by arguing that *ubuntu* can provide a foundation for a public morality in South Africa, and can be used to resolve current dilemmas of justice (559).

From an *ubuntu* perspective, when people damage humanity by the way they behave towards others, for example by committing crimes, these are viewed as being committed against the whole community rather than only an individual. This damages the humanity of both the perpetrator as well as the victim, which rends the social fabric. This conception of an individual's bad actions damaging the whole community emphasizes the interconnectedness between persons, and is also the basis for the imperative of reconciliation as exemplified by the Truth and Reconciliation Commission in South Africa. The TRC provided a prototype for how *ubuntu* can be integrated into the public and political spheres and institutionalized in the justice system as a relational ethic of care.

Ubuntu as Activism/Praxis

Archbishop Emeritus Desmond Tutu's formulation of *ubuntu* emphasizes both the ontological dimension as well as the aretaic—the importance of behaving in a caring way:

> *Ubuntu* . . . speaks to the very essence of being human. When we want to give high praise to someone we say, "*Yo, unobuntu*"; "Hey, so-and-so has ubuntu." Then you are generous . . . hospitable . . . friendly . . . caring and compassionate. You share what you have. It is to say, "My humanity is caught up, is inextricably bound up, in yours." We belong in a bundle of life. We say, "a person is a person through other people" . . . A person with *ubuntu* is open and available to others, affirming of others, does not feel threatened that others are able and good; for he or she has a proper self-assurance that comes with knowing that he or she belongs in a greater whole and is diminished when others are humiliated or diminished, when others are tortured or oppressed, or treated as if they were less than who they are. (Tutu 1999, 31)

Steve Biko, the Black Consciousness[9] activist, included *ubuntu* as part of his liberation ideology to restore Africa's humanity (Biko 1978; Oliphant 2008; Ratele and Botha 2014). Biko's concept of African culture included the concept that all humans have inherent value, but like Tutu, he asserts that oppression diminishes all humans. Therefore Biko argued that it is incumbent upon Africans to liberate themselves from "dehumanizing" colonial cultures, thereby "humanizing South Africa," and also to overcome "dehumanizing cultures" in other parts of the world (Oliphant 2008, 227). The concept of *ubuntu* which was finally incorporated into the Black Consciousness Movement was an amalgam with the liberal democratic principles of universal human rights (Alexander 2008). Thus the principles of *ubuntu* as caring for humanity are given as the *raison d'être* for activism against injustice, and must inform practices of struggle. Though *ubuntu* is practiced with reference to particular contexts, it is simultaneously presented as a universal ethic. Unlike an ethic of care, which distinguishes between the particularity of "caring for" as against the general "caring about," *ubuntu* sees caring as continuous from individual to stranger.

Though there was never a specific focus on women's liberation in the Black Consciousness Movement (O. Mangena 2008), it is seen as generically being able to lay the foundation for including *ubuntu* as part of gender activism (Ratele and Botha 2014). We acknowledge that *ubuntu* as practice is fluid and subject to change; however, when researching care for people with HIV-related illnesses in resource-poor communities, we found that the burden of care—*ubuntu*—was borne on the shoulders of women. Not only did women care for members of their own extended families, but also they did an enormous amount of volunteer (unpaid) home-based care for others in their communities (Gouws and Van Zyl 2014). Typical of care in neoliberal settings, this invisible cadre of care workers allows the state to eschew its responsibilities of care for people suffering from AIDS. Other African feminists have also pointed out that *ubuntu*-talk has seldom included gender issues (Keevy 2008; Manda 2007; F. Mangena 2013), but assert the strategic importance of incorporating an African discourse of value such as *ubuntu* into African feminist activism.

Therefore, we include activism against oppression as a political dimension of "caring" for our community, and emphasize the embodied dimensions of *ubuntu* through care practices (see also Mabovula 2011), but simultaneously insist on a feminist praxis in the struggle for gender equality.

Gender in a Southern Relational Ethics of Justice

Whatever the talk about *ubuntu* and gender equality, we need to assess gender practices as they are situated in and expressed through people's cultures. How does one make sense of the excessively high rates of gender-based violence in South Africa? Where is *ubuntu?*

Gender identities in post-apartheid South Africa have been shaped by factors such as the globalizing influences on culture, while the discourses on sex and sexuality have been foregrounded against a backdrop of gender-based violence and HIV and AIDS. Despite arguments that hegemonic masculinities across Africa are "diverse... dispersed, heterogeneous and fluid" (Ratele 2008, 532), the authors in *From Boys to Men* (edited by Shefer et al. 2007) show how "traditional" aspirations such as virility, being a breadwinner and head of household, and being heterosexual with a need for sex persist (Ratele et al. 2007, 126). Most African men still aspire to having authority over women and children, and when combined with gender-based violence and taking HIV risks (Sathiparsad 2007), hegemonic masculinities emerge as antithetical to an ethic of care—denying women relational autonomy, and thereby denying them dignity and justice. With the (invisible) gendered care burden on women's shoulders, it is apparent that *ubuntu* is deeply riven by gender inequalities.

An exacerbating factor is that rights are atomized: as victims of gender-based violence, women are construed as vulnerable/needy, and not seen as rights claimants. Perpetrators' rights are seen as trumping victims' rights, leading to communities perceiving that the state does not deliver justice, and participating in vigilante actions, often killing alleged rapists (Meth 2010). If care—as exemplified in *ubuntu*-talk—were a public value and politicized, the focus would shift to the empowerment of the survivors of violence rather than only punishing the perpetrators. It would move from autonomy and dependence to interdependence and relationality.

Both rights and *ubuntu* have failed women. However, as a Southern discourse, *ubuntu* still has currency in South Africa (Outwater et al. 2005; Ratele and Botha 2014; Praeg and Magadla 2014), and, as Lewis Gordon (2014) indicates, could be adapted as both a reinvention of tradition and a critique of Western modernity. We agree with Siphokazi Magadla and Ezra Chitando (2014) who suggest that opposing a "traditional" *ubuntu* with the "modernity" of rights in the Constitution will not open a space for addressing violent masculinities. Rather, we argue that *ubuntu* must be infused with a feminist ethic of care principles and feminist praxis to work toward dignity and equality, and especially gender equality.

As Hekman (1992, 1109) points out, while the idea of the pre-modern community rejects liberal individualism, it still writes a specific "script" for women—that of reproduction and caring. This is also her critique of communitarianism. While it improves the status of the subject to constitute it as embedded and embodied, the community of this subject is still a hierarchical one where women have less power than men. So, women are embodied in the pre-modern community but only as subordinate to men (Hekman 1992, 1116). The same is true of the pre-colonial community from which *ubuntu* derives, and this is why *ubuntu* needs to take on board a feminist ethic of care.

Drawing on liberal democratic values, the South African Constitution promises equality and dignity through human rights, yet as Mogobe Ramose (2014) argues, rights cannot be separated from their meaningful realization. However, we argue that the individualist and rationalist ontology of the human rights framework cannot address needs and responsibilities that arise in relationships with others. In a context of neoliberal globalization, it has not succeeded in delivering justice to marginalized, "needy" or "vulnerable" citizens. We argue that the relational principles of care embedded in both a feminist of ethic of care and *ubuntu* provide criteria for justice which do not render inequalities in society invisible, and provide an ethical framework of justice which exhorts action by individuals and institutions to care for individuals as well as others in society. If discourses of care or *ubuntu* supplant those of rights, a greater possibility exists for more people to have "livable lives."

Synthesis: a Feminist Ethics of *Ubuntu*

In order to recognize the origins of our relational ethic of justice, we call it a "feminist ethics of *ubuntu*." This acknowledges our lifelong praxis of feminism and our location in the South, and South Africa in particular. *Ubuntu* has legitimacy in Africa as an indigenous ethical framework of care, in contrast to Northern liberal frameworks such as human rights. *Ubuntu* is also at the core of a system of restorative justice, in contrast to the individualism of liberal adversarial justice systems. Feminism is renowned for its commitment to end gender and other intersectional inequalities, while a feminist ethics of care focuses particularly on the feminization of care, and how care as a philosophical construct has been devalued in the North. A feminist ethics of care also untangles care as praxis in the form of caregiving as labor, and addresses the private–public dichotomy, proposing ways to institutionalize care at the public level. Therefore we draw on the communality, relationality, and non-stigmatized notion of dependency from *ubuntu* and the relationality, gender equality, and praxis from a Northern feminist ethic of care to synthesize our Southern feminist ethics of *ubuntu*.

We interrogated care as a concept, arguing that both feminist ethics of care and *ubuntu* regard care as an ethical concept which expresses the quality of relationships between people. Moreover, we suggested that care is an ineluctable dimension of human relationships. Consequently, an analysis of care must address how power is deployed between people in their everyday lives, as well as how care is integrated into the polity—relationships between groups of citizens, and between citizens and the state. Second, from a feminist standpoint we argued that caregiving as labor is deeply feminized, racialized, and geopoliticized, thereby stigmatizing both those who are in need of care and those who provide care. Both a feminist ethics of care and *ubuntu* regard relationality and interdependency as ineluctable—therefore as discourses they destigmatize dependency. However, while *ubuntu*-talk is egalitarian, *ubutu*-do is shaped by normative ideologies of heteropatriarchy. A feminist ethic of care focuses on overcoming gender inequalities manifested in the feminization of care, suggesting that all humans recognize their own care needs and take responsibility for the care of others.

This ethical stance is promoted by both a feminist ethic of care and *ubuntu*. We argue for a situated ethics of care, which is qualified by "caring for" as well as "caring about"—that is, care needs to happen both at a particular and at a general level. This type of ethic is best encapsulated in the notion of *ubuntu* as a human quality of caring, which involves the feminist notion of an embodied labor of care—in other words, we eschew *ubuntu*-talk in favour of *ubuntu*-do. We also argue that care is integrated in activism that aims to address contexts of unequal power, and material conditions that are not conducive to care. These struggles would be aimed at, for example, gender inequalities and the feminization of dependency. Our location in the South reminds us daily of the interdependencies between people as they struggle to attain livable lives in the face of neediness and vulnerability caused by structural, physical, and psychosocial violence.

We assert that we are all situated in communities, some by default and others by "choice," whereby we conform more or less to the norms set by that community. This binds us into relationships of dependency with others, as well having responsibilities and obligations towards them. We subscribe to a view that, with an ethical norm of care, communities shape contexts where individual diversity may thrive. Hence, individual autonomy arises in a negotiated relationship between self and other. We argue for relational ethics which prioritize equality and dignity, but balance the needs of the individual against the needs of the community at a material level as well as at the level of recognition: that is, livable lives.

By justice we evoke the core values of equality and dignity in the liberal democratic South African Constitution, while recognizing that these ethical precepts are not achievable outside a recognition of the relationality between people. We support a justice system which is able to achieve a balance between individual needs and the communal good. As neoliberalism deepens inequalities between people, we propose a relational ethic of justice, which can support livable lives. The failure of our liberal justice system to deliver livable lives suggests that an equilibrium between individual rights and communal good may be more ably attained in a restorative justice system such as the one represented in *ubuntu*.

Both feminist ethics of care and *ubuntu* regard activism as necessary for the achievement of justice, and therefore we propose a relational ethic of justice that will require a transformation of the normative discourses of privilege and hierarchy, which perpetuate inequalities and erode people's dignity. We also insist that a feminist *ubuntu* must be built on an embodied praxis of care.

Conclusion

With this chapter we have attempted to illustrate that care does not happen in a vacuum: care work is a complex political issue which is based on performance and the discourses surrounding it. These are determined by the state's regulation of rule, as well as the social and political context, overlaid with different discourses of value.

States may facilitate or hinder how discourses about care become hegemonic, or how care becomes institutionalized as a public value. We have demonstrated these issues by looking at the liberal rights-based state of post-apartheid South Africa, showing that a liberal rights discourse is countered by a needs/vulnerability discourse that does not promote care or dignity, but rather victimhood. The political context of high levels of gender-based violence, HIV infection, and child neglect leads to an increased care burden on women.

We have shown that *ubuntu* and the feminist ethics of care share many similarities, such as relationality and the obligation to care. The concept of the self as an intersubjective being is what makes us human, where care is not confined to primary others, but extends to forming ourselves through others ranging from family to community, group, and nation.

There is much *ubuntu*-talk in masculinized arenas such as politics, philosophy, and some churches, but on the ground women are bearing the burden of caring for their families, friends, and communities through declining economic circumstances. Therefore the indigenous discourse of *ubuntu* is failing women's well-being and dignity, and requires activism to advance gender equality. We recognize that for political reasons to do with post-colonial and post-apartheid identity formation, *ubuntu*—and its other African variants elsewhere—is a tangible and "desirable" discourse of value in Africa, and provides a "different voice" from human rights for addressing care.

A relational ethic of justice requires a focus on restoring women's dignity and not positioning them as victims in need of "rescuing." It is important for women to be part of defining what is "wrong": that is, what is injurious to the community. In this regard, Nancy Fraser's (2007) concept of "parity of participation" becomes important. Communities should give women the space to articulate their concerns to the same extent that men can. When care needs are confined to the private and not made public through discourse, women's concerns will remain invisible. The extent of gender-based violence is a public phenomenon of which communities are very aware, and therefore a lasting solution can only be a communal one.

An *ubuntu* perspective on justice for women will require focusing on the power relationships between perpetrators and victims, in order to restore the humanity of both. But if *ubuntu* as care ethic is to overcome social inequalities, especially gender inequalities, it must be infused with feminist praxis. Feminist ethics of care theorists have shown how care may be made a public value, through addressing needs/vulnerability. Infusing standards of care developed in a feminist ethics of care into *ubuntu* can create Southern public discourses and practices of care that will trump rights talk.

Notes

1. The South African Police statistic for sexual offences in 2012 was 64,514, a statistic that is highly disputed by civil society based on the claim of high rates of underreporting of rape. The One in Nine Campaign argues that only one in nine rapes are reported (see One in Nine Campaign: <www.oneinnine.org.za>).
2. By 2015 at least 5.7 million children in South Africa could be orphaned, and 30 percent of children between the ages of 15 and 17 will have lost their mothers according to a Medical Research Council report (cited in Health Systems Trust 2014). Some of these children live in children-headed households or on the streets.
3. Strong bonds of love often developed between white children and their African carers.
4. "At the end of 2012 there were approximately 3.1 million non-searching unemployed and 4.5 million searching (official) employed (QLFS data). The strict (official) rate of unemployment was 24.9% and the expanded rate 35.9%" (Posel et al. 2013).
5. In 2009 the South African government created the Ministry for Women, Youth and People Living with Disabilities. These groups are now all called "vulnerable groups" and many policy documents refer to these groups as "vulnerable."
6. Domestic violence in South Africa is rife. Shelters in the Western Cape turn away on average twenty-three women a week who are in need of shelter space (see Commission for Gender Equality 2013). Many women who return to abusive environments are killed. In 2012 the average amount of money budgeted per woman per day for shelter accommodation in the Western Cape was R28. The average amount of money spent on keeping a perpetrator in prison per day amounts to more than R300.
7. Praeg and Magadla (2014) argue that many critical engagements with *ubuntu* fail to distinguish between historical *ubuntu* praxis and contemporary reinventions of post-colonial *ubuntu* philosophy.
8. See, for example, Urban Walker (2006) on care and restorative justice.
9. The Black Consciousness Movement arose during the 1970s in South Africa as a cultural and political liberation movement based on critiquing white racism and psychological oppression, and affirming the integrity of African culture. Steve Biko developed this cultural philosophy of black pride and resistance, which is still the cornerstone of much black activism today.

References

Alexander, N. 2008. "An Illuminating Moment: Background to the Azanian Manifesto." In *Biko Lives! Contesting the Legacies of Steve Biko*, edited by A. Mngxitama, A. Alexander, and N. C. Gibson, 157–70. New York/Basingstoke: Palgrave Macmillan.

Arnfred, S., and A. A. Ampofo. 2009. "Introduction: African Feminist Politics of Knowledge." In *African Feminist Politics of Knowledge: Tensions, Possibilities, Knowledge*, edited by A. A. Ampofo and S. Arnfred, 5–27. Uppsala, Sweden: Nordiska Afrikainstitutet.

Barchiesi, F. 2011. *Precarious Liberation: Workers, the State, and Contested Social Citizenship in Postapartheid South Africa*. New York: State University of New York Press.

Biko, S. 1978. "Black Consciousness and the Quest for a True Humanity." *Ufahamu: A Journal of African Studies* 8(3): 10–20.

Bohler-Muller, N. 2005. "The Story of an African Value." *SA Public Law* 20(2): 266–80.

Bohler-Muller, N. 2006. "Developing a New Jurisprudence of Gender Equality in South Africa." LLD thesis, University of Pretoria. Accessed 3 February 2014 at: <http://repository.up.ac.za/bitstream/handle/2263/25545/Complete.pdf?sequence=4/>

Buker, E. A. 2006. "Care and Order: State Reformation and the Feminization of Liberalism." In *Socializing Care: Feminist Ethics and Public Issues*, edited by M. Hamington and D. C. Miller, 49–68. New York: Rowan and Littlefield.

Burger, R., and R. Jafta. 2010. "Affirmative Action in South Africa: An Empirical Assessment of the Impact on Labour Market Outcomes." CRISE Working Paper no. 76. Accessed on 31 January 2014 at: <http://r4d.dfid.gov.uk/PDF/Outputs/Inequality/workingpaper76.pdf>

Butler, J. 2004. *Undoing Gender*. New York/London: Routledge.

Clement, G. 1998. *Care, Autonomy, and Justice: Feminism and the Ethic of Care*. Boulder, CO: Westview Press.

Cock, J. 1980. *Maids and Madams: A Study in the Politics of Exploitation*. Johannesburg: Ravan Press.

Comaroff, J., and J. L. Comaroff. 2012. "Theory from the South: Or, how Euro-America is Evolving Toward Africa." *Anthropological Forum* 22(2): 113–31.

Commission for Gender Equality (CGE). 2013. "Proposal for Reform: Combating Violence against Women and Children in the Western Cape by Increasing Access to Shelters and Improving the Quality of Services." Unpublished report, 29 November.

Cornell, D., and K. van Marle. 2005. "Exploring *Ubuntu*: Tentative Reflections." *African Human Rights Law Journal* 5: 195–220.

Engster, D. 2005. "Rethinking Care Theory: The Practice of Caring and the Obligation to Care." *Hypatia* 20(3): 50–74.

Fraser, N. 2007. "Feminist Politics in the Age of Recognition: A Two Dimensional Approach to Justice." *Studies in Social Justice* 1(1): 23–35.

Fraser, N. 2013. *Fortunes of Feminism: From State-Managed Capitalism to Neoliberal Crisis*. New York/London: Verso.

Friedman, M. 2000. "Feminism in Ethics: Conceptions of Autonomy." In *The Cambridge Companion to Feminism in Philosophy*, edited by M. Fricker and J. Hornsby, 205–24. Cambridge: Cambridge University Press.

Gade, C. B. N. 2011. "The Historical Development of the Written Discourses on Ubuntu." *South African Journal of Philosophy* 30(3): 303–29.

Gade, C. B. N. 2012. "What is Ubuntu? Different Interpretations among South Africans of African Descent." *South African Journal of Philosophy* 31(3): 484–503.

Gade, C. B. N. 2013. "Restorative Justice and the South African Truth and Reconciliation Process." *South African Journal of Philosophy* 32(1): 10–35.

Gordon, L. R. 2014. "Justice Otherwise: Thoughts on Ubuntu." In *Ubuntu: Curating the Archive*, edited by L. Praeg and S. Magadla, 10–26. Pietermaritzburg: University of KwaZulu-Natal Press.

Gouws, A. 2013. "Multiculturalism in South Africa: Dislodging the Binary between Universal Human Rights and Culture/Tradition." *Politikon* 40(1): 35–55.

Gouws, A., and M. van Zyl. 2014. "Feminist Ethics of Care through a Southern Lens." In *Care in Context: Transnational Gender Perspectives*, edited by V. Reddy, S. Meyer, T. Shefer, and T. Meyiwa, 99–123. Cape Town: HSRC Press.

Harding, S. 1987. "The Curious Coincidence of Feminine and African Moralities." In *Women and Moral Theory*, edited by E. F. Kittay and D. T. Meyers, 296–315. New Jersey: Rowman and Littlefield.

Hassim, S. 2005. "Nationalism Displaced: Citizenship Discourses in the Transition." In *(Un)Thinking Citizenship: Feminist Debates in Contemporary South Africa*, edited by A. Gouws, 55–70. Aldershot, UK/Cape Town: Ashgate/UCT Press.

Health Systems Trust. 2014. "South Africa: Number of Children Orphaned by AIDS to Increase." Accessed on 31 January 2014 at: <http://www.hst.org.za/news/south-africa-number-children-orphaned-aids-increase>

Hekman, S. 1992. "The Embodiment of the Subject: Feminism and the Communitarian Critique of Liberalism." *Journal of Politics* 54(4): 1098–119.

Held, V. 1990. "Feminist Transformations of Moral Theory." *Philosophy and Phenomenological Research* 50: 321–44.

Held, V. 2006. *The Ethics of Care: Personal, Political, and Global*. New York: Oxford University Press.

Jordan, J. 1997. "Clarity in Connection: Empathetic Knowing, Desire, and Sexuality." In *Women's Growth in Diversity: More Writings from the Stone Center*, edited by J. Jordan, 50–73. New York: Guilford Press.

Keevy, I. 2008. African Philosophical Values and Constitutionalism: A Feminist Perspective on Ubuntu as a Constitutional Value. Unpublished doctoral thesis, Faculty of Law, University of the Free State, Bloemfontein.

Keevy, I. 2009. "Ubuntu versus the Core Values of the South African Constitution." *Journal for Juridical Science* 34(2): 19–58.

Mabovula, N. N. 2011. "The Erosion of African Communal Values: A Reappraisal of the African Ubuntu Philosophy." *Inkanyiso Journal of Humanities and Social Sciences* 3(1): 38–47.

MacDonald, F. 2006. "Relational Group Autonomy: Ensuring Agency and Accountability in the Group Rights Paradigm." Paper presented at the annual meeting of the Canadian Political Science Association, June.

MacDonald, F. 2010. "Relational Group Autonomy: Ethics of Care and the Multiculturalism Paradigm." *Hypatia* 25(1): 196–213.

Magadla, S., and E. Chitando. 2014. "The Self Become God: Ubuntu and the 'Scandal of Manhood'." In *Ubuntu: Curating the Archive*, edited by L. Praeg and S. Magadla, 176–92. Pietermaritzburg: University of KwaZulu-Natal Press.

Mamdani, M. 1996. *Citizen and Subject: Contemporary Africa and the Legacy of Late Colonialism*. Princeton, NJ: Princeton University Press.

Manda, D. L. 2007. "The Importance of the African Ethics of Ubuntu and Traditional African Healing Systems for Black South African Women's Health in the Context of HIV and AIDS." Unpublished doctoral thesis, Department of Philosophy, University of KwaZulu-Natal, Durban.

Mangena, F. 2013. "The Search for an African Feminist Ethic: A Zimbabwean Perspective." *Journal of International Women's Studies* 11(2): 18–30.

Mangena, O. 2008. "The Black Consciousness Philosophy and the Woman's Question in South Africa: 1970–1980." In *Biko Lives! Contesting Legacies of Steve Biko*, edited by A. Mngxitama, A. Alexander, and N. C. Gibson, 253–66. New York/Basingstoke: Palgrave Macmillan.

Manicom, L. 1992. "Gender and State in the History of South Africa Ruling Relations: Rethinking State and Gender in South African History." *Journal of African History* 33(3): 441–65.

Marais, B. 2012. "Queering Ubuntu: The Self and the Other in South African Queer Autobiography." Unpublished master's thesis, Department of English, University of KwaZulu-Natal, Pietermaritzburg.

Mbiti, J. S. 1990 [1969]. *African Religions and Philosophy*. Oxford: Heinemann.

Meth, P. 2010. "Unsettling Insurgency: Reflections on Women's Insurgent Practices in South Africa." *Planning Theory and Practice* 11(2): 241–63.

Metz, T. 2007. "Toward an African Moral Theory." *Journal of Political Philosophy* 15(3): 321–41.

Metz, T. 2011. "Ubuntu as a Moral Theory and Human Rights in South Africa." *African Human Rights Law Journal* 11(2): 532–59.

Metz, T. 2012. "Developing African Political Philosophy: Moral-Theoretic Strategies." *Philosophia Africana* 14(1): 61–83.

Metz, T., and Gaie, J. B. R. 2010. "The African Ethic of Ubuntu/Botho: Implications for Research on Morality." *Journal of Moral Education* 39(3): 273–90.

Mokgoro, J. Y. 2003. "Constitutional Claims for Gender Equality in South Africa: A Judicial Response." *Albany Law Review* 67(2): 565–73.

OECD 2013. "OECD Economic Surveys: South Africa." Accessed 31 January 2014 at: <http://www.oecd.org/eco/surveys/South%20Africa%202013%20Overview%20FINAL.pdf>

Oliphant, A. 2008. "A Human Face: Biko's Conceptions of African Culture and Humanism." In *Biko Lives! Contesting Legacies of Steve Biko*, edited by A. Mngxitama, A. Alexander, and N. C. Gibson, 213–32. New York/Basingstoke: Palgrave Macmillan.

Outwater, A., N. Abrahams, and J. C. Campbell. 2005. "Women in South Africa Intentional Violence and HIV/AIDS: Intersections and Prevention." *Journal of Black Studies* 35(4): 135–54.

Posel, D., D. Casale, and C. Vermaak. 2013. "What is South Africa's 'Real' Unemployment Rate?" Econ3x3, *Politicsweb*. Accessed 31 January 2014 at: <http://www.politicsweb.co.za/politicsweb/view/politicsweb/en/page71639/page71639?oid=363205&sn=Detail&pid=71639>

Praeg, L., and S. Magadla. 2014. "Introduction." In *Ubuntu: Curating the Archive*, edited by L. Praeg and S. Magadla, 1–9. Pietermaritzburg: University of KwaZulu-Natal Press.

Ramose, M. B. 1999. *African Philosophy through Ubuntu*. Harare: Mond.

Ramose, M. B. 2002. "The Ethics of Ubuntu." In *Philosophy from Africa: A Text with Readings*, edited by P. H. Coetzee and A. P. Roux, 2nd ed., 324–30. Cape Town: Oxford University Press.

Ramose, M. B. 2014. "Ubuntu: Affirming a Right and Seeking Remedies in South Africa." In *Ubuntu: Curating the Archive*, edited by L. Praeg and S. Magadla, 121–36. Pietermaritzburg: University of KwaZulu-Natal Press.

Ratele, K. 2008. "Analysing Males in Africa: Certain Useful Elements in Considering Ruling Masculinities." *African and Asian Studies* 7(4): 515–36.

Ratele, K., and M. Botha. 2014. "Profeminist Black Men: Engaging Women Liberationists, Undermining Patriarchy." *BUWA! A Journal on African Women's Experiences*: 14–19. Accessed 3 February 2014 at: <http://www.osisa.org/sites/default/files/profeminist_black_men-_engaging_women_liberationists_undermining_patriarchy.pdf>

Ratele, K., E. Fouten, T. Shefer, A. Strebel, N. J. Shabalala, and R. Buikema. 2007. "'Moffies, Jocks and Cool Guys': Boys' Accounts of Masculinity and Their Resistance in Context." In *From Boys to Men: Social Construction of Masculinity in Contemporary Society*, edited by T. Shefer, K. Ratele, A. Strebel, N. Shabalala, and R. Buikema, 112–27. Cape Town: University of Cape Town Press.

Sathiparsad, R. 2007. "Masculinities in the Era of HIV/AIDS: The Perspectives of Rural Male Zulu Youth." In *From Boys to Men: Social Construction of Masculinity in Contemporary Society*, edited by T. Shefer, K. Ratele, A. Strebel, N. Shabalala, and R. Buikema, 181–94. Cape Town: University of Cape Town Press.

Shefer, T., K. Ratele, A. Strebel, N. Shabalala, and R. Buikema (eds.). 2007. *From Boys to Men: Social Constructions of Masculinity in Contemporary Society*. Cape Town: University of Cape Town Press.

Southall, R. 2013. "The Power Elite in Democratic South Africa: Race and Class in a Fractured Society." In *New South African Review 3*, edited by J. Daniel, P. Naidoo, D. Pillay, and R. Southall, 17–38. Johannesburg: Wits University Press.

Tronto, J. 1993. *Moral Boundaries: A Political Argument for an Ethic of Care*. London: Routledge, Chapman and Hall.

Tronto, J. 2006. "Vicious Circles of Privatized Caring." In *Socializing Care: Feminist Ethics and Public Issues*, edited by M. Hamington and D. C. Miller, 3–26. Lanham, MD: Rowman and Littlefield.

Tutu, D. M. 1999. *No Future without Forgiveness*. New York: Random House.

Urban Walker, M. 2006. "The Curious Case of Care and Restorative Justice in the US Context." In *Socializing Care: Feminist Ethics and Public Issues*, edited by M. Hamington and D. C. Miller, 145–62. Lanham, MD: Rowman and Littlefield.

White, J. A., and J. C. Tronto. 2004. "Political Practices of Care: Needs and Rights." *Ratio Juris* 17(4): 425–53.

11

Caring reciprocity as a relational and political ideal in Confucianism and care ethics

Maureen Sander-Staudt

In recent decades, a lively debate has developed around the question of whether a Confucian ethic shares enough similarities with care ethics to warrant their compatibility and potential collaboration. Authors have answered this question differently, with some arguing that Confucianism and care ethics are compatible (Li 1994) and others arguing that they are not (Star 2002; Yuan 2002; Herr 2003). The possible compatibility of Confucianism and care ethics is intriguing because it suggests that care ethics is not simply a Western or female ethic and that there may be a plethora of "different voices" in Confucianism and other moral traditions. More importantly, areas of compatibility would allow care ethics and Confucian ethics to build a synergistic social philosophy that more fairly supports the work of care, and serves as an alternative to liberal social contract theories which tend to privatize care responsibilities.

In this chapter I defend the idea that care ethics and Confucianism improve one another when they collaboratively conceptualize reciprocity as a moral and political ideal that is *not* rooted in the liberal presumptions of equality, rationality, independence, or the expectation of direct mutual advantage. I begin by reviewing the debate surrounding the possible affinities between Confucianism and care ethics, and introduce two strategies for making Confucianism more responsive to care ethics' sensitivity to sex and gender disparities. I then detail how reciprocity can serve in Confucianism and care ethics as a relational ideal that subdivides as a virtue, moral motivation, model for epistemic exchange, and political ideal. I conclude by showing that caring reciprocity admits to cultural variation, as demonstrated in its practical application to the question of what grown children owe their aging parents.[1]

The Compatibility of Confucianism and Care Ethics—Two Strategies for Union

Chenyang Li was one of the first scholars to highlight resemblances between care ethics and Confucianism so that they can "learn from and support one another" (Li 1994; 1999; 2000, 24; 2002). Li compares the concept of "care" found in the work of care ethicists like Nel Noddings and Carol Gilligan, with aspects of the Confucian concept of *jen*, which translates variously as benevolence, love, altruism, kindness, humanity, human-heartedness, magnanimity, compassion, or the best of men (Gilligan 1982; Noddings 1984; Li 1994). Li notes that the ontology of Confucianism, which rests on the "five-fold relations," is much like the ontology of care ethics in being fundamentally relational.[2] Li further observes that these ethics similarly emphasize a sense of reciprocity that demands that one care for others, and a system whereby the moral obligation to care is gradated so that we have a stronger obligation to care for those closer to us than those at a distance (Li 1994, 74, 76).

The Confucian concept of reciprocity, known as *shu*, is sometimes called the "Silver Rule" because it is a negative formulation of the Golden Rule, meaning that it proscribes against imposing on others what one does not want to be imposed upon oneself.[3] Although from a care ethical perspective this concept may seem limited in that it incorporates only a negative duty to refrain from harming others, Li notes that Confucius also taught that a person of *jen* who wishes to sustain or develop himself, does so by sustaining and developing others. Thus, the principle of *shu* in Confucianism creates an injunction to care for others.

Whereas Li is enthusiastic about the idea of developing a collaborative project between Confucianism and feminist care ethics, other philosophers object to this proposal, revealing that this collaboration can take more or less controversial forms depending upon what strand of a moral theory is emphasized. Critics of Li fall into two groups. The first group rejects the compatibility of Confucianism and care ethics because they differ significantly in their orientation to virtue and care (Star 2002). My focus in this chapter, however, is critics in the second group, who are concerned with questions about the proper role of women and children in the family. They speculate that because Confucianism is so thoroughly entrenched as a conservative and patriarchal ethic, a synthesis of Confucianism and care ethics will only perpetuate patriarchal oppression (Yuan 2002; 2005; Herr 2003; 2012).[4] This creates a challenge for any attempt to harmonize care ethics and Confucianism, because most versions of care ethics today are formulated as inherently feminist, meaning that they fundamentally challenge patriarchal assumptions and gender-based double standards that characterize traditional Confucianism. Theorists like Joan Tronto (1994), Eva Feder Kittay (1999), and Virginia Held

(2006) have developed feminist versions of care ethics that explore the moral significance of care without assuming that it is fitting for women to predominantly do the work of care. These and other theorists (Hamington 2004; Engster 2007) have developed political philosophies of care that are largely gender neutral, and which extend ideals of care to economic and political theory. If Confucianism is to be compatible with modern-day care ethics, then it must be responsive to objections that it is inherently and unavoidably a patriarchal moral theory.

Two strategies suggest themselves for a feminist care ethic seeking to mitigate the gender disparities characteristic of traditional Confucianism. First, traditional Confucian concepts may be revised to be more equitable in terms of sex and gender roles. Second, traditional Confucian concepts that potentially endorse gender and other forms of equity may be given greater prominence. Following the first strategy, Li posits that *ren/jen* is a virtue that can be interpreted in a gender-neutral way. This strategy seeks to achieve a more equitable ethic by altering masculine language. Additionally, we might convert the traditional five-fold relations to more gender-neutral and equalized renditions (e.g., spouse–spouse rather than husband–wife). Unfortunately, in most English translations of Confucian works, this strategy is currently compromised by the near-standard use of the ambiguous noun "man," rather than "human" or "woman," as well as the modification of this noun with the pronouns "he" and "him." This flaw may be attributable more to translators of Confucianism than to Confucianism itself, and is relatively easily fixed. But a larger problem may be that the motivation for this semantic transition is impeded by the way that classic Confucianism focuses on the perspectives and activities associated with men in training for administrative social roles. As a whole, Confucianism deals little with women and the actual daily work of care, which is of central significance in care ethics. A collaboration between care ethics and Confucianism must thus expand and reorient the Confucian emphasis on patriarchal administration of family and society, to focus more on the direct, hands-on practice of caring for the bodily and emotional needs of self and others.

But making this shift is not without challenges. For example, in comparing Confucianism, care ethics, and Christian ethics, Xiao Wei identifies a dilemma pertaining to role hierarchies that arises for a Confucian ethic that would be compatible with a feminist care ethic (Wei 2008). On the one hand, Confucianism is a hierarchical ethic that teaches that not all people deserve the same respect, love, or caring as do higher-ranking people (36). Confucianism instructs that people are born unequally, and that the superior man deserves the highest respect or love and caring, whereas women should always play the role of people who care (36, 41). On the other hand, a feminist care ethic endorses more egalitarian care relations between men and women, and seeks to dissolve sex- and gender-based hierarchies. Such an ethic asks "who is offering care and who is receiving care?" in the hopes of detecting and subverting relations that are asymmetrically reciprocated. Wei finds that Confucianism on its own is lacking a principle of justice for dealing with this problem, and for both theories, "the problem is to find a way to deal with conflicts of interest under the conditions of a market economy" (42). Wei's analysis suggests that it is not enough to merely shift our focus to the activities of care without asking why it is women and other subordinated groups who are primarily responsible for this work, and without making an argument for why such work ought to be more fairly distributed and reciprocated.

Wei's analysis importantly brings into focus how current market relations are activities that continue to be greatly based on sex and gender roles, such that women, "inferior men," and other disempowered people tend to perform the bulk of menial care labor without equal returns. The focus on the conditions of the market economy raises several important points for collaboration between Confucianism and care ethics. First, while there has been an increase in women in the paid workforce around the world, there has been little change regarding the expectation that care is largely the private responsibility of families, and most centrally, of women. Second, even if sex equality is achieved such that men and women equally have the choice to perform care work or not, a gender-based hierarchy could still persist whereby caregivers (male or female) are yet subservient to those who enjoy what Joan Tronto terms "privileged irresponsibility," thus retaining hierarchy and unbalanced reciprocity (Tronto 1994). Finally, the intersectional nature of caring hierarchies under market conditions means that such disparities are likely not only to be based on sex and gender, but also to be marked by unique configurations of class, profession, nationality, citizenship status, generational status, and much more. For these reasons, it is not enough that we merely revise Confucian concepts like *ren* to be more inclusive of women. Rather, it is also desirable to employ the second strategy for amending Confucianism and feminist care ethics—that of bringing greater emphasis to concepts such as "reciprocity" in both ethics, so that people who are engaged in the giving and receiving of care do so more equitably and with more adequate levels of give and take.

In stressing how sex-based social inequities are often overlooked in Confucianism, Wei herself overlooks the possibility that *shu* could be the needed principle of feminist justice that she finds lacking in Confucianism. For Li, the duty to reciprocate care recommended by *shu* extends to caring about the ways in which women have been subordinated to men, as well as other forms of disparity (2002, 8). Despite their misgivings about his larger project, some of Li's critics agree that the concept of reciprocity can more adequately harmonize Confucianism with feminist care ethics. For example, Ranjoo Herr argues that a Confucian model of the family can be compatible with feminist commitments once it is understood that reciprocity is a central thread of Confucianism (Herr 2012). Herr notes that the concept of *shu* is of equal importance to, and serves to constitute, the concept of *jen/ren* in Confucianism. She uses the reciprocal proscription of *shu* to argue against a universal sex-based division of labor because human beings are invariably diverse in their dispositions (343). For this reason, *shu* recommends that men be free to devote themselves to domestic work and women to public work, because prohibiting such activities runs contrary to negative reciprocity, by treating others in ways that cannot be self-condoned (343). While this is a promising start toward amending sex-based care hierarchies, to pursue the full promise of this second strategy as employed by Herr, it is necessary both to sketch the potential content of reciprocity more fully, and to examine the extent to which it can be used to arbitrate these and other caring hierarchies.

Reciprocity as Caring Virtue, Motivation, and Epistemic Exchange

Reciprocity is a concept that features heavily in many moral and political traditions because it governs ideals of appropriate exchange. Although Noddings and subsequent care ethicists have developed this concept explicitly, there has not yet been a sustained analysis of reciprocity in care ethics, perhaps because of how it has been associated negatively with social contract theory (Noddings 1984). In Kantian and Rawlsian contract theories, reciprocity serves as a prerequisite for citizenship, a motivation for otherwise disinterested social cooperation, and an expectation of mutual advantage. Because Confucianism and care ethics both refute that mutual disinterest, self-interest, and autonomy are the preconditions of moral relations, the substance of reciprocity in a Confucian care ethic differs substantially from the concept of reciprocity found in social contract theory.

To speak to the importance of reciprocity for a Confucian care ethic, both ethics agree that as a willingness to appreciate and return care that is given, reciprocity is generally a desirable condition for establishing caring relations that are just. Caring relations cannot and should not always be reciprocal, but a relationship that is not reciprocal when it could be, is only questionably just. Unlike care, reciprocity is not typically thought of as a purely emotional state, but like care, it is possible to understand reciprocity as many other things—a biologically rooted standard of justice, practice, motivation, principle, ideal, virtue, duty, etc.[5] I propose that reciprocity is best characterized as a relational ideal that incorporates all of the above, but which stops short of being a rigidly prescribed duty. Care ethics is a flexible moral theory that seeks to maintain relationships, so it makes room for reciprocity without elevating it to the status of an inviolable principle, an absolute duty, or a clearly delineated imperative. There will be exceptions and a need for contextual application of reciprocity. However, this does not mean that a basic content of what reciprocity requires of us in Confucianism and care ethics cannot be provided. In what remains I will demonstrate how reciprocity might function in a Confucian care ethic as a virtue, motivation, epistemic standard, and political ideal.

Both Confucianism and care ethics agree that caregiving should be generally reciprocated, and they both have ways of determining who ought to be reciprocating what to whom. However, the structure of this virtue is not always made explicit in these traditions. Such content is offered by Lawrence Becker, who, while working within the framework of virtue ethics, provides one of the most detailed theoretical accounts of reciprocity developed outside of social contract theory (Becker 1990). In his book, *Reciprocity*, Becker gives a basic outline for understanding reciprocity as it functions as a virtue, and this outline helps to give substance to reciprocity as a virtue in a Confucian-influenced care ethic (Becker 1990). For Becker, understanding reciprocity as a virtue means that we ought to be disposed, as a matter of moral character, to make reciprocity a moral obligation (74). This may seem to conflict with the claim that reciprocity will stop short of being a strict moral duty in a Confucian care ethic, but this is not the case. Understanding reciprocity as a moral virtue means that caring agents will feel strongly inclined to reciprocate care, and will be encouraged to develop relational reciprocity as a habitual disposition. But this injunction will not be categorically determined, and this disposition will not trump other caring considerations, such as the value of unconditional love or spontaneous gifts.

Becker identifies eight components of reciprocity which can be compressed as six basic guidelines to virtuous reciprocal behavior (74, 89–130):

1. Good received should be returned with good.
2. Evil received should not be returned with evil, but should be resisted.
3. Evil done should be made good.
4. The returns should be made by the one who received the good or committed the evil, and should be fitting and proportional.
5. Returns should be made for goods received, not merely for goods accepted.
6. Reciprocity should be a matter of retrospective moral obligation.

Incorporating Becker's guidelines for reciprocity as a virtue in a Confucian care ethic provides substance for understanding what *li*, or proper behavior, might entail with regard to the return of care, both good and bad. To the extent that care received was good, it recommends that care ought to be returned to others. To the extent that care has been performed badly, or has led to exploitation, it should be resisted, but such harms should not be returned. When care has failed, reparations should be made to those who were negatively affected. Becker's standards further stipulate that care should be typically reciprocated by those who received care, and reparations should be made by those who failed to care, or who cared poorly. As such, Becker's theory provides a basic framework for understanding how a person who exhibits the virtue of caring reciprocity should behave toward others. However, Becker's account of reciprocity as a virtue stops short of explaining why someone might be motivated to reciprocate care, how good and bad care is to be determined and by whom, and how society can be best organized to foster reciprocally caring dispositions.

Here, collaboration between Confucianism and care ethics creates a useful synthesis. As a motivational and epistemic concept, reciprocity appears in both care ethics and Confucianism differently, but a synthesis of their approaches creates a more balanced foundation for distinguishing good and bad forms of care. For Noddings, reciprocity is "vital," both in being motivational, and for contributing to the epistemic assessment of care completion (Noddings 1984, 151). Noddings finds that what care ethics seeks out of reciprocity is not "payment in kind" between caregiver and care-receiver, but an exchange of response that inspires future caregiving, and "the special kind of reciprocity that connotes completion" (151). This reciprocity is "direct response," "happy growth," or "personal delight," and children reciprocate care when they share parents' engrossment and concern, and communicate their own aspirations (74). Genuine reciprocity cannot be demanded or manipulated. Nonetheless, the capacity to complete care involves reciprocal response to the extent that care which cannot be reciprocated is care that is not owed (157).

Noddings' account of reciprocity thus serves two functions. First, reciprocity is understood as a response on the part of the care-receiver that both signifies the successful completion of care, and motivates a caregiver to want to continue giving care. In this reciprocal exchange, Noddings grants epistemic authority for care completion to the care-receiver, such that care-receivers are entitled to be the final judges of whether care was successful, and if they deem not, to make the choice to not reciprocate caring response. Second, Noddings' concept of reciprocity keeps care obligation manageable, in that a caregiver is not obligated to care for another with whom there is no hope of completion or reciprocity of response.

Noddings' claim that the epistemic authority to assess care completion belongs to care-receivers raises problems for a Confucian ethic. This is because Confucius grants this authority to caregivers, or at least limits the extent to which care-receivers can act upon their self-assessment to critique caregivers, or to distance relations with them. In *The Analects*, Confucius recommends remonstrance against superiors when they are acting immorally. However, Confucius also makes clear that in some role relations, such as that between child and parent, remonstrance is to be limited:

> The Master said, "In serving his parents, a son may remonstrate with them, but gently; when he sees that they do not incline to follow his advice, he shows an increased degree of reverence, but does not abandon his purpose; and should they punish him, he does not allow himself to murmur." (Confucius 500 BCE 15: 23)

On the one hand, this advice improves upon Noddings' account of epistemic authority, which is problematic when children are too immature to assess their own best interests. Contrary to Noddings' claim that genuine reciprocity cannot be demanded, this passage requires that children develop their capacity for disciplined responsive reciprocity. On the other hand, Noddings recognizes that it is vital for the care-receiver to be the ultimate judge of care in order to avoid misapplying care. This is a point that likewise recommends that care-receivers develop their capacity for determining what is a proper reciprocal response to the "care" they have received, moving this concept beyond mere "happy growth" to a normative and epistemic phase. But Noddings' view additionally suggests that the Confucian limitation on remonstrance is also in peril of misapplying care, because it favors the virtue of filial piety and respect for parents over the personal integrity of a child/care-receiver. It carries within it a dangerous suggestion that even abuse and neglect is to be met with near-silent respect and honor, although it stops short of requiring total conformity of perspective.

Sin Yee Chan grapples with this dilemma in the aptly titled article "Can *Shu* Be the One Word that Serves as the Guiding Principle of Caring Actions?" (Chan 2000). Chan contends that the concept of *shu* helps to answer the question of whether, when caring for another person, we should go by her perspective or our own in deciding what to do on her behalf. Chan's analysis of *shu* affirms going both with the perspective of the caring agent, and with the perspective of the cared-for, but gives priority to the former. To make this argument, Chan draws from Herbert Fingarette's interpretation of *shu* as "*identifying with another person while remaining her critic*" (Chan 2000, 507, italics in the original; Fingarette 1980). Chan interprets *shu* as involving a kind of reversibility that involves both imagining one's own self in the position of the cared-for, and also empathetically discerning the perspective of the cared-for, as it may differ from one's own (Chan 2000, 509). Chan argues that what it means to "put oneself into another's shoes" is that a caregiver takes into account both objective and subjective features of the cared-for as a unique person, including their circumstances. This carves out space for an autonomous critical reaction on the part of the would-be caregiver. But because a caring person cannot assume that her own perspective is always accurate, "the caring person follows a much more stringent standard . . . when she decides about the actions on the other person's behalf," such that she should have "clear evidence for the wrongness of the other person's perspective if she decides to act contrary to it" (519).

Chan's analysis of Confucian reciprocity as involving critical empathy enhances Noddings' account of caring reciprocity. However, Chan's recommendation to apply a "stringent standard" for determining the wrongness of the cared-for's judgment is hopelessly vulnerable to subjective and self-serving beliefs. It is also vulnerable to the harms associated with paternalism, and overlooks how epistemic authority is a developmental goal and communal process. A better synthesis of care ethics and Confucianism in this regard would adopt an ongoing *reciprocal* and communal epistemic assessment of care completion. Having a reciprocal exchange of critical assessment power gives caregivers an opportunity to independently consider what is really the best interests for the person they seek to care-for, for evolving response from the care-receiver, and in cases where there is dispute, for an ongoing dialectic of communication that involves others outside of the direct care relation. As children grow older, it is more appropriate for them to assume responsibility for the assessment of the care that they received, because as they age children are expected to assume more responsibility for reciprocating care to parents and others. And when care is exchanged between adults, this epistemic assessment should be as autonomously mutual as the situation allows. It may be the nature of caregiving that at some point a would-be caregiver has to decide how best to respond, but the process of care is typically one that extends into the future, allowing for enduring opportunities for reflection, as indicated by Becker's last stipulation that reciprocity is matter of *retrospective* obligation.

This synthesis of Confucian and care ethical reciprocity as an exchange of epistemic privilege is thus superior to a one-sided approach, and is a prerequisite for applying Becker's standards for responding to good and bad care. It enhances the argument that reciprocity is a relational ideal that can be understood as a virtue by offering methodological and epistemological standards for this virtue. However, it does not itself fully reckon with the problem of sex-based care inequality and exploitation. What is additionally needed is broad-based social support of care relations that extends reciprocal obligations for care to businesses, governments, and other social institutions. In the final section I explore how care ethics and Confucianism share a notion of reciprocity as a political ideal, respond to three challenges to this approach, and consider how this ideal will likely manifest differently in the East and West.

Reciprocity as Political Ideal—the Great Community and Caring State

The final point of compatibility in Confucianism and care ethics is how reciprocity as a relational ideal features for both theories as part of a political philosophy of care. In these two traditions, reciprocity emerges both as a quality of the just state and as a principle for generating the obligation to support cooperative caring schemes that provide care well, and in a just manner.[6] Both theories seek to establish a reciprocal exchange of care between the state and its citizens, in the form of social support for the work of care. In Confucianism this ideal political state is called the "Great Community," while in care ethics it has been called the "Caring State."

The political model of the Confucian "Great Community" is described by Julia Po-Wah Lai Tao in her analysis of the differences between Confucianism and feminist care ethics. Tao agrees that there are "deep and important differences" underlying Confucianism and feminism, and finds that Confucianism does better in dealing with strangers than the care ethics of Noddings, where it is more compatible with later versions of care ethics (Tao 2000, 216, 225). Specifically, Tao reports that the Confucianism vision of the "Great Community" is a political philosophy of care characterized by "good faith, friendly relations, caring for others, and the fulfillment of reciprocal obligations" (226). The passage that Tao quotes from Confucius in the *datong* (Great Community) describes this vision more at length:

> When the great Dao prevailed, the world belonged to the general public (tianxia wei gong). They chose the worthy and the capable, were trustworthy in what they said, and cultivated harmony. Therefore, the people did not love only their parents and did not treat only their children as children. Thus, the aged could live out their lives, the grown-ups all had their function, the young could be reared, and the widowed, the lonely, the orphaned, the crippled and the sick all found their care. Men had their roles, and women kept their homes. They hated casting away goods, but not necessarily to keep them for themselves. They hated leaving their strengths unemployed, but not necessarily to employ it themselves. Therefore, scheming had no outlet, and theft, rebellion and robbery did not arise, so that the outer doors were left unlocked. This is called the Great Community (datong). (Tao 2000, 226; Confucius 500 BCE 15: 11, 2: 23)

Tao acknowledges that feminism demands reform of the sexual division of labor described in this passage, but finds it to be otherwise similar to the views of later feminist care ethicists, such as Tronto, who agree with Confucius that a society cannot be morally admirable unless it provides adequate care for all of its members and territories. In the Great Community, care is an emotion that ideally creates concern and loving sentiment between family members, and then emanates outward to motivate care on a larger social scale. Although Tao acknowledges similarities to Tronto's political philosophy of care, Tao concludes that Confucianism

> provides a more positive answer for dealing with strangers than either feminist care ethics or the popular liberal answer... [where] we are perfectly justified to leave moral strangers where we find them on the doorstep of communities, because there is no such moral requirement to extend caring and concern to strangers beyond chosen communities and voluntary relationships. (225)

Tao is correct to question the way in which the responsibilities for care have been privatized and limited in liberal theory, as well as to examine how reciprocity of care might be established between the "sovereign and citizen" prong of the five-fold relations. But she errs when she attributes this same tendency to "feminist care ethics." A feminist care ethic agrees that it is wrong to care exclusively for one's one family, and that a fully adequate principle of reciprocity must include both public and private relations.

Similar arguments for more reciprocal social relations of care, reminiscent of the Confucian "Great Community," have been developed by care ethicists Kittay and Engster (Kittay 1999; Engster 2007). In her book, *Love's Labor*, Kittay calls for an expansion of the concept of reciprocity found in John Rawls's theory of justice, and opens "conceptual space for dependency concerns within social cooperation in a just society" (1999, 106). For Kittay, the concept of reciprocity is rooted in the idea of nested dependencies "linking those who help and those who require help to give aid to those who cannot help themselves" (107). She bases her principle of reciprocity on the concept of a doula—a post-partum nurse who cares for a newly delivered mother so that the mother can in turn care for her child. This arrangement serves as a metaphor for the need to care for caregivers in a socially nested sense. Her principle of doulia states that "just as we have required care to survive and thrive, so we need to provide conditions that allow others—including those who do the work of caring—to receive the care they need to survive and thrive" (107). Later, Kittay uses this principle to establish an ideal of caring reciprocity that creates a broad social responsibility "for enabling dependency relations satisfactory to dependency worker and dependent alike," as well as for "creating social institutions that enable caregivers to do the job of caretaking without becoming disadvantaged in the competition for social benefits" (109).

In his book, *The Heart of Justice*, Engster develops a concept of caring obligation that expands Kittay's political vision via his "principle of consistent dependency" (PCD) (Engster 2007). This principle states:

> Since all human beings depend upon the care of others for our survival, development, and basic functioning, and at least implicitly claim that capable individuals should care for individuals in need when they can do so, we should consistently

> recognize as morally valid the claims that others make upon us for care when they need it, and should endeavor to provide care to them when we are capable of doing so without significant risk to ourselves, seriously compromising our long term functioning, or undermining our ability to care for others. (49)

Unlike Kittay, Engster refrains from categorizing the PCD as a principle of reciprocity, stipulating that the PCD grounds our duty to care for others "not in relations of reciprocity, but in our common human dependency" (50). His reluctance to characterize the PCD as a principle of reciprocity heralds three challenges with understanding reciprocity as a caring political ideal. First, political theory premised on reciprocity may fail to deal adequately with beings incapable of full reciprocity. Second, such models may endorse an overly maternal state. Third, political schemes of caring reciprocity are subject to deep cultural variation. Responding to these objections is necessary in order to fully defend the political philosophy that seems to be recommended by Confucianism and care ethics alike.

The first two of these challenges are raised at length by Martha Nussbaum in her book *Frontiers of Justice* (Nussbaum 2006). Here Nussbaum critiques how reciprocity has functioned in social contract theory to stunt moral relations with those who cannot reciprocate as fully autonomous and rational beings, such as animals, disabled humans, and nations (98, 130). She notes that in basing political theory on the ability to reciprocate and the expectation of mutual advantage, social contract theory gives no justification for caring for those who cannot reciprocate, and misrepresents the basic human condition of dependency. Nussbaum's argument on behalf of her Aristotelian capabilities theory draws heavily from the critiques developed by Kittay and other care ethicists, but Nussbaum is simultaneously critical of care ethics for being overly maternal at the expense of personal liberty. While Nussbaum's denunciation of social contract theory is one that both care ethicists and Confucianists can accept, her critique raises difficulties for the thesis that Confucianism and care ethics possess a promising compatibility in understanding reciprocity as a political ideal.

Specifically, Nussbaum's critique raises the concern that characterizing the obligation to care as a matter of reciprocity implies that individuals who are unable to return care are undeserving of care, and that those who have not received (much, or adequate) care are not obliged to care for others. This problem is evident in Kantian and Rawlsian political theory, where the capacity for forming rational ends and for reciprocating cooperative schemes is a prerequisite for full moral citizenship. It is also evident in Becker's criteria for the virtue of reciprocity, where good returned is based on good given, and returns are made directly by those who have received them. In liberal political theory, the moral worth of those who are unable to reciprocate fully in socially productive schemes is thereby diminished, and their political status curtailed (Nussbaum 2006, 118). Nussbaum writes that such theories handle severe mental impairments and related disabilities as "an afterthought," and that "people with mental impairments are not those for whom and in reciprocity with whom society's basic institutions are structured" (98). Nussbaum argues that the tendency to link citizenship to a capacity for reciprocity, and political motivation to an expectation of mutual advantage, has the effect of characterizing the obligation to meet the needs of those incapable of full reciprocity as an act of private charity, rather than as a matter of political entitlement (123).

If Nussbaum's critique of reciprocity correctly extends also to Confucianism and care ethics, this would speak strongly against understanding any principle of caring exchange as one of reciprocity. However, Kittay's doulia-based principle of reciprocity shows that Nussbaum's first concern is unfounded as applied to these theories. Kittay premises her principle of reciprocity on unequal vulnerability in dependency, unequal powers to respond to others in need, and the primacy of human relations in happiness and well-being (Kittay 1999, 113). She adapts a Marxist-based principle of reciprocity that does not make the ability to reciprocate care a prerequisite for citizenship or care entitlement:

> To each according to his or her need for care; from each according to his or her capacity to care, and such support from social institutions as to make available resources and opportunities to those providing care, so that all will be adequately attended to in relations that are sustaining. (114)

Such a principle establishes that there are reciprocal obligations without entailing that all individuals have an equal obligation to return care in kind. All who need care should receive it, including individuals who are unable to make intentional or equal returns. At the same time, if you are able, you should reciprocate this care to others to a reasonable extent. As Engster's PCD states, those who are able to reciprocate care and do not are morally remiss, unless they can show that doing so would have caused significant moral sacrifice. However, for caring reciprocity to meet Becker's sixth standard of being "fitting and proportional," returns need not always be the product of rational intent, nor returns of the kind that create direct mutual advantage. Although a just scheme of caring reciprocity will be one that is generally advantageous to all, the expectation of mutual advantage is not the sole or primary motivation for such a scheme. This is especially the case when we are speaking of relations with disabled humans, and with animals, who are sometimes capable of reciprocating in morally significant ways, but who are not always as equally capable of creating a rational moral intention to reciprocate care, and who cannot return care in kind. Neither is reciprocity always best understood as a direct return to the one who gave care. When it comes to human families and communities, caring reciprocity to older generations can also involve "paying forward" care to younger or future generations, as well as caring more generally and spontaneously for those whose needs manifest in our lives.

Nussbaum acknowledges that there are understandings of reciprocity that do not duplicate the social contract expectations of rational equality, autonomy, and mutual advantage (Nussbaum 2006, 97). She refers to the capacity for reciprocity exhibited by disabled persons like Sesha, Kittay's daughter, and Jamie, a boy with Down's syndrome (97). Their behavior exemplifies that reciprocity need not only be understood in Rawlsian and Kantian terms (134). Nussbaum states:

> If we consider the lives of people with mental impairments and those who live with them, it seems obvious that their lives involve complex forms of reciprocity... Jamie interacts in a generous way with his family and other children. Sesha hugs those who care for her, dances with joy... and shows appreciation for the care she is given. (133–4)

This sense of reciprocity is similar to Noddings' understanding of reciprocity as responsiveness to care, and with it care ethics and Confucianism can extend moral subjectivity to those who lack the full capacities for rational or intentional reciprocity, but who nonetheless reciprocate care by responding positively to care.

However, Nussbaum raises a second relevant critique to the claim that care ethics is compatible with the Confucian understanding of reciprocity as a political ideal—that such a political philosophy of care is overly maternal. Nussbaum criticizes Kittay's care-based political theory as one that neglects the importance of personal liberty, and that would "provide comprehensive support for need throughout all citizens' lives, as [a]... welfare state—but a welfare state in which liberty is far less important than security or well-being" (217). She faults Kittay for viewing the state as a "universal mother" and for rejecting independence as a major social goal (218). Nussbaum doubts that being "some mother's child" is a sufficient image for being a citizen or that care is a sufficient image for motherhood. She concludes that humans have political needs that extend beyond care—such as the needs for liberty, opportunity, the chance to form life plans, the ability to learn and think for oneself, and the right to form relations that are chosen, not given.

This critique speaks against the collaboration between care ethics and Confucianism because both ethics might be accused of characterizing the state as a universal mother when they endorse a conception of reciprocity that establishes state obligation to support the work of care on every level. In attempting to create a political philosophy of care that adequately supports the work of care, and that eliminates sexist exploitation, both Confucianism and care ethics could make individuals vulnerable to having their individual rights diminished via state surveillance and legislative intervention into personal life. This critique shows that it is naïve to suggest that a state is likely to be "caring" in the same sense that a mother is inclined to "care" for a child, and turns the notion of the Great Community into a hopelessly utopian one. Moreover, rather than overthrowing gender-based assumptions around care, such an approach feminizes politics.

While Nussbaum's concerns are legitimate in pointing out a source of potential tension between the political understanding of reciprocity in Confucianism and care ethics, she fails to appreciate that both care ethics and Confucian ethics can respond to this concern when reciprocity is brought to the fore as a political ideal. This is because both care ethicists and Confucians can argue that the aim of care is in part to cultivate the capacities of individuals, and that the inclusion of reciprocity moves us away from a political model of unconditional love that is associated with maternal care. The injunction to support cooperative schemes of care when one is able does not necessarily inhibit personal liberties, but can enhance them, by making it possible to cultivate the abilities of all, to whatever extent possible. Being "some mother's child" is not meant to exhaust the possible understandings of citizenship, but to enforce a mindfulness of the origins of dependency for all human life, and the pre-necessity of care for the capacity to exercise personal liberties. Personal liberties are not at odds with the vision of the Caring State, and nor is Nussbaum's capabilities theory, because fostering basic capabilities that are individually variable can be understood as one of the central goals of the Great Society or Caring State. Indeed, the capacity to reciprocate care with more deliberative intention and efficacy could be said to be an important capability that might be added to Nussbaum's list.

However, there is no doubt that the precise balance to be struck between personal liberty and state-sanctioned, care-based reciprocity is subject to cultural variation. There are many practical examples of this variation, but one of the most poignant is found in how Confucian and Western societies differ in their approach to providing care for the elderly. Confucianism has a strong expectation that grown children will reciprocate the parental care they received when young by caring for parents as they age. Traditionally, the reciprocal duty to care for one's own aging parents fell most directly to sons, in that daughters were expected to care for the parents of their husband (Lei 2013). While this sex-based expectation is not as common in the West, in both societies the work of care has been subject to traditional sexual divisions of labor, with sons often more expected to provide financial support for aging parents, and daughters often more expected to provide the hands-on work of care. In both societies, market relations have begun to evolve such that women are increasingly participating in the paid workforce, allowing them to share the financial burden of caring for parents, and putting pressure on men to provide more direct care. Additionally, both sexes are moving away from their extended families to gain employment. These trends strain traditional understandings of who is responsible for the care of the aged, and contribute to a more general "crisis of care."

Creating a political philosophy of care capable of responding to this crisis in a non-exploitative way is valuably assisted by a principle of reciprocity that establishes a state obligation to support the work of care. But this principle is likely to be applied differently in China than in Western liberal democracies. One way this difference is evident is in how moving parents to an elder care facility is more likely to be viewed as a failure of filial piety in a Confucian context than in the West. The erosion of traditional Confucian values of filial piety and reciprocal care for aging parents is so offensive to the Chinese that in 2013 the federal government reissued laws requiring children to care for their parents by visiting often and occasionally sending greetings (Da and Zuo 2013). The law is called the "Protection of the Rights and Interests of Elderly People," and has nine ordinances that delineate the duties of children to tend to the "spiritual needs of the elderly." It permits a neglected parent to sue her child for financial and temporal reparations. The law also encourages other social institutions to reciprocate the work of care by giving employees time off so they can make parental visits, although it creates no avenue for the formal enforcement of this recommendation. This type of law reflects a belief that the state plays an important role not only in encouraging the return of care to aging parents, but in enforcing parent–child reciprocity through legislative sanction. This belief gains philosophical support from Ruiping Fan, who characterizes the increased Chinese reliance on Western-style "nursing homes" as a decline in Confucian filial piety that has led to a heightened suicide rate among the elderly, and that could be reversed through a return to Confucian reciprocity (Fan 2007; 2010).

Such a law is a compelling instance of how a government might serve to reinforce a principle of Confucian and caring reciprocity as a political ideal, but it is unlikely to be a strategy that would be acceptable in most Western liberal democracies. A law that penalizes children for neglecting their parents would be seen by most Westerners not only as futile, but also as an intolerable government infringement on personal liberty. It seems to further send the message that the entitlement of being cared for in old age is premised on having had children, which is eroded in the contemporary environment of the "one child only" policy in China, and conflicts with the Western liberal value of reproductive autonomy, as well as the individual right to have one's needs met in old age regardless of whether or not one has had children.

The latter concern can be addressed by re-emphasizing that care for the aged is not the sole responsibility of children, or strictly rooted in an obligation to reciprocate care given. As earlier stated, both Confucianism and care ethics agree that the elderly deserve to receive basic care simply because they need it, and that both the state and the family have distinct roles to play in providing such care. To the extent that a parent–child relationship exists, it supplements whatever state provisions may be offered, and satisfies the psychological and emotional desire of parents to have ongoing relations with their offspring. The legitimacy of this desire is reflected in the Western Christian admonition to "Honor your mother and father," and in the parental reverence shown via holidays like "Mother's Day" and "Father's Day." But the obligation to return care to one's parents is unlikely to be seen in Western liberal democracies as a social injunction strong enough to warrant litigious sanctions on children who neglect this duty. Moreover, in political atmospheres that glorify individual autonomy, and in economic markets where quality elderly care is more often privatized than socialized, the ability to secure private institutional care can be seen as a sign of prestige and privilege, and an opportunity for mutual independence.

Ultimately, it is possible to defend the compatibility of Confucian *shu* and the caring principle of political reciprocity despite these cultural tensions. This is because both moral theories accept that the reciprocal caring obligations are subject to the contextual circumstances of culture, as well as other variables. While some care ethicists, like Kittay, move toward Marxist and socialist models for understanding how care may be best provided and distributed, others like Engster remain open to the creative ways that the private market could also help to meet caring needs and alleviate the disparate burdens of direct care that currently fall to women. In societies characterized by Chinese Confucianism, it may be possible to affirm that the *li* governing what children owe parents is rightly subject to state enforcement, just as it is thought appropriate in the West that the state delineate and enforce obligations that parents have to their children. At the same time, it is possible to affirm that individuals are within their rights to resist government enforcement of filial duties in favor of non-governmental mechanisms for the cultivation of reciprocal inclinations.

But even if we wish to retain the idea that children are expected to reciprocate the care that they received as children to their aging parents, this is not incompatible with creating rites of *li* that govern this expectation more equally between men and women. *Li*, revised to include this goal, could diffuse patriarchal hierarchies in the family and state, and serve to reciprocate care in many directions. Social expectations in family and work can become more reciprocal if girls as well as boys are assured that they will be cared for as much they give care, by not suffering care-based wage gaps and lesser social welfare provisions. Businesses and governments can share in the work of care by supporting these responsibilities via the provision of paid leave and job security for employed adults who take time from work to care for children or parents. In this way, the Confucian "Great Society" and the care ethical PCD both posit a political ideal of reciprocity that can be feminist in its orientation by distributing the burdens of care between men and women more equitably. This approach need not exclude those incapable of full reciprocity, and can disassociate itself from maternalism by reformulating care as a universal human good and responsibility. It can also recognize that the strategies needed to provide care that is both adequate and just will admit to cultural variation, without having to jettison the basic idea that caring reciprocity as a political ideal can contribute to this project.

Conclusion

Ultimately, it is important to acknowledge that the complexity and theoretical autonomy of moral traditions means that Confucianism will always differ from a Western-influenced feminist care ethic in significant ways. However, this does not mean that their collaboration cannot yield mutually beneficial insights. I have argued that a Confucian ideal of reciprocity, when infused with the feminist considerations central to later articulations of care ethics, helps to develop a more adequate political philosophy of care that does not limit care obligation to the private sphere of the family. This concept of reciprocity, found in both Confucianism and care ethics, is best understood as a relational ideal that encompasses being a virtue, caring motivation, epistemic method, and political ideal. As a political ideal, the sense of reciprocity that emerges from a collaborative synthesis between Confucianism and care ethics provides a model for how care might be more equally distributed in society between men and women, as well as others, without requiring that the capacity for reciprocity be prerequisite for being a citizen and moral subject. It also offers a justificatory principle for obligating the provision of care through both private and public relations that eliminate sex-based role expectations and double standards in how care is distributed. Such political strategies admit to cultural variation, as is evident in how the Chinese understanding of reciprocal caring obligation departs from the Western tendency to rely on institutionalized care of the family. However, this does not mean that Confucianists and care ethicists cannot agree on the very basic idea that care ideally admits to give and take on all of these levels, and that individuals and institutions benefitting from the receipt of care are more virtuous to the extent that they attempt to return on these received goods.

Notes

1. I would like to thank the editors of this volume for their insightful feedback on original drafts of this chapter, as well as for the valuable comments I received at two 2014 conferences, the Western Political Science Association Seattle meeting, and "In the Unjust Meantime: A Conference in Honor of Alison Jaggar," at the University of CO-Boulder.
2. The five-fold relations originate from the most central relation of father/son, which gives rise to other key relations, including ruler and citizen, older and younger sibling(s), husband and wife, and older and younger friend. The individual self is exhaustively constituted by these relations, and certain moral duties involving proper observance of norms and rites are associated with each position.
3. The principle is found in the fifteenth book of *The Analects*: "Tsze-kung asked, saying, 'Is there one word which may serve as a rule of practice for all one's life?' The Master said, 'Is not RECIPROCITY such a word? What you do not want done to yourself, do not do to others'" (Confucius 500 BCE, 15: 24).
4. Care ethics and feminist ethics are sometimes treated as if they were synonymously exhaustive of one another, while in other cases they are treated as distinct. To avoid the conflation of moral theories and the subsequent reduction of moral diversity, I recommend a collaborative strategy that situates Confucianism, feminist ethics, and care ethics, such that they serve as supports and correctives to one another, without the need for categorical assimilation (Sander-Staudt 2006). This would allow for numerous collaborations between these *three* theoretical traditions without their oversimplification or conflation. In this way, the collaborative ideal of reciprocity that is developed later for guiding interpersonal relations can also be modeled at the theoretical level.
5. Reciprocity is not typically thought of as an emotion, but acts of reciprocity do seem to generate corollary emotions in humans. Recent studies in infant psychology show that even very young children express disapproval when they witness the return of altruistic acts with acts of selfishness (Schmidt and Sommerville 2011). The authors of this study posit that humans experience innate feelings of approval and disapproval associated with reciprocity or the lack of it, and that these emotions have developed as an evolutionary adaptation in favor of social cooperation.
6. Some care ethicists like Star argue that care ethics differs from Confucianism in eschewing general principles altogether, as opposed to just acknowledging that principles may be suspended or revised. However, I do not agree. Rather, I am more inclined to adopt the position of Virginia Held, who argues that care ethics need not be entirely unprincipled, but is likely to adopt principles differently from other moral and political theories like social contract theory. The principles of justice in care ethics, which I hope to show are inherently reciprocal, exemplify Held's thinking on this point.

References

Becker, Lawrence. 1990. *Reciprocity*. Chicago, IL: University of Chicago Press.

Chan, Sin Yee. 2000. "Can *Shu* Be the One Word that Serves as the Guiding Principle of Caring Actions?" *Philosophy East and West* 50(4): 507–24.

Confucius. 500 BCE. *The Analects of Confucius*, translated by James Legge, 1893. Accessed 20 November 2013 at: <http://www.sacred-texts.com/cfu/conf1.htm>. Adelaide, South Australia: University of Adelaide.

Da and Zuo. 2013. "Chinese Virtue is Now the Law." *New York Times*. 2 July. <http://www.nytimes.com/2013/07/03/world/asia/filial-piety-once-a-virtue-in-china-is-now-the-law.html?>

Engster, Daniel. 2007. *The Heart of Justice: Care Ethics and Political Theory*. New York: Oxford University Press.

Fan, Ruiping. 2007. "Which Care? Whose Responsibility? And Why Family?: A Confucian Account of Long-Term Care for the Elderly." *Journal of Medicine and Philosophy* 32(5): 496–517.

Fan, Ruiping. 2010. *Reconstructionist Confucianism: Rethinking Morality after the West*. New York: Springer.

Fingarette, Herbert. 1980. "Following One Thread of the *Analects*." *Journal of the American Academy of Religion* 47(3): 373–405.

Gilligan, Carol. 1982. *In a Different Voice*. Cambridge, MA: Harvard University Press.

Hamington, Maurice. 2004. *Embodied Care: Jane Addams, Maurice Merleau-Ponty and Feminist Ethics*. Chicago, IL: University of IL Press.

Held, Virginia. 2006. *The Ethics of Care: Personal, Political, Global*. New York: Oxford University Press.

Herr, Ranjoo. 2003. "Is Confucianism Compatible with Care Ethics? A Critique." *Philosophy East and West* 53(4): 471–89.

Herr, Ranjoo. 2012. "Confucian Family for a Feminist Future." *Asian Philosophy* 22(4): 327–46.

Kittay, Eva. 1999. *Love's Labor: Essays on Women, Dependency, and Equality*. New York, NY: Routledge.

Lei, Lei. 2013. "Sons, Daughters and Intergenerational Support." *Sociological Review* 45(3): 26–52.

Li, Chenyang. 1994. The Confucian Concept of *Jen* and the Feminist Ethics of Care: A Comparative Study." *Hypatia* 9(1): 70–89.

Li, Chenyang. 1999. *The Tao Encounters the West*. Albany, NY: State University of New York Press.

Li, Chenyang. 2000. *The Sage and the Second Sex: Confucianism, Ethics and Gender*. Chicago, IL: Open Court Press.

Li, Chenyang. 2002. "Revisiting Confucian Jen Ethics and Feminist Care Ethics: A Reply to Daniel Star and Lijun Yuan." *Hypatia* 17(1): 130–40.

Noddings, Nel. 1984. *Caring: A Feminine Approach to Ethics and Moral Education*. Berkeley, CA: University of California Press.

Nussbaum, Martha. 2006. *Frontiers of Justice: Disability, Nationality, Species Membership*. Cambridge, MA: Harvard University Press.

Sander-Staudt, Maureen. 2006. "The Unhappy Marriage of Care Ethics and Virtue Ethics." *Hypatia* 21(4): 21–40.

Schmidt, M. F. H., and J. A. Sommerville. 2011. "Fairness Expectations and Altruistic Sharing in 15-Month-Old Human Infants." *PLoS ONE* 6(10): e23223. doi: 10.1371/journal.pone.0023223

Star, Daniel. 2002. "Do Confucians Really Care? A Defense of the Distinctiveness of Care Ethics: A Reply to Chenyang Li." *Hypatia* 17(1): 77–106.

Tao, Julia Po-Wah Lai. 2000. "Two Perspectives of Care: Confucian *Ren* and Feminist Care." *Journal of Chinese Philosophy* 27(2): 215–40.

Tronto, Joan. 1994. *Moral Boundaries: A Political Argument for an Ethic of Care*. New York: Routledge.

Wei, Xiao. 2008. "Caring: Confucianism, Feminism, and Christian Ethics." *Contemporary Chinese Thought* 39(2): 32–48.

Yuan, Lijun. 2002. "Ethics of Care and Concept of *Jen*: A Reply to Chenyang Li." *Hypatia* 17(1): 107–29.

Yuan, Lijun. 2005. *Reconceiving Women's Equality in China*. New York: Lexington Books.

12

Practicing care at the margins

Other-mothering as public care

Julie Anne White

Work on the ethics of care has evolved significantly since the publication of Carol Gilligan's *In a Different Voice* (1993). Several of the early associations with the ethic of care positioned care as a private virtue, gendered feminine, and central to mothering practice. Over thirty years of scholarship these associations, particularly the taken-for-granted association between care and mothering, have been compellingly contested. With Daniel Engster (2007) I am interested in revising and rethinking care as a public virtue; with Joan Tronto (1993) I work toward reconceptualizing care as practice central to our democratic commitments. And drawing on the methodological insights of many care theorists from Gilligan forward, I ground my normative approach to developing a model of democratic public care in an analysis of the existing social practices of care.

"Other-mothering," I will argue in this chapter, is a resistant practice with important implications for care ethics. Within the context of neoliberal hegemony—both its cultural and its economic hegemony—the work of care is increasingly commodified; other-mothering as a practice resists any simple reduction of care to property for exchange while also and relatedly challenging taken-for-granted organization of public and private life. In this sense, other-mothering may provide insight into a model of public care that can resist the reduction of democratic logics to market logics.

The move to build a model of public care from any practice of mothering probably rightly invites some suspicion. Yet, neoliberalism has so thoroughly privatized and commodified care that the family may be the lone site of care that is not purchased. "Mothering" as a private practice has ironically become less visible and yet more important in a neoliberal order. Like old liberalism, neoliberalism still needs to create the next generation of workers and citizens, but it tries to do so with an even more minimal investment on the part of the state. As Nancy Folbre (2002) has suggested, in this model, children are more like pets—an individual choice—than like public goods worthy of collective "investment." Because I want to take an approach that recognizes care as a practice that can be organized in ways consistent with democratic practice, such privatization and commodification are troubling. By "privatizing" or locating care in domestic space, neoliberalism risks reinforcing patriarchal divisions of labor between public and private spaces that reproduce the traditional status of financial dependency for women. But alternatively, "privatization," understood as locating care in the market, may do little better at resisting this order; given the exploitive organization of paid care work even in relation to other forms of work in the capitalist economy, paid care workers often remain dependent and vulnerable and are, disproportionately, white women and people of color. In either of these two senses of "privatized" care—domesticated or marketed—the practice is inconsistent with a meaningful democratic equality.

In this chapter I argue that other-mothering as a practice sustained in many African-American communities provides insight into the problems and possibilities for public care. Other-mothering practices 1) challenge taken-for-granted understandings of the "natural" extension of caregiving responsibilities, 2) pluralize our understandings both of care and of vulnerability, and 3) foster a relationship between identifying and meeting proximate and immediate needs and a larger struggle for social transformation (Collins 2000). Such struggles target and address needs as particular while recognizing them as generated within a broader structure marked by systematic inequalities. These aspects of other-mothering productively challenge conventional practices of maintaining public and private, and thus provide more adequate grounding for public care than Virginia Held's mothering or Eva Kittay's doulia model of care practice (Held 1989; Kittay 1999). Because other-mothering is a practice within historically marginal and struggling communities, it is a practice that links care as an intimate practice with care as political struggle. Drawing on the work of Stanlie James (1993), Patricia Hill Collins (2000), and Cheryl Gilkes (1987), I outline the model of care that emerges from other-mothering practices and draw out its implications for a prospective public care.

Care Literature on Gender and Mothering

As a place to begin, I want to offer a brief historiography of work on care that focuses on two early writers on the ethic of care: Carol Gilligan and Virginia

Held. Both Gilligan and Held identified the practice of mothering as central to the ethic of care, albeit for quite different reasons and in quite different ways. I outline the place of mothering in their work, the critiques and responses offered, and then go on to ask whether other-mothering as Collins outlines it might draw on the productive insights around traditional mothering practices while also avoiding what critics saw as a reiteration and a potential defense of traditional gender roles.

In *In a Different Voice*, Gilligan identifies what she sees as an alternative and gendered orientation to moral problem solving. In interviews with adolescent girls reflecting on real-world moral dilemmas, Gilligan consistently found a process of problem solving that she interpreted as focused on "needs" rather than rights, and identified the importance of context with the inadequacy of formalistic and principled approaches. On Gilligan's account, of course, this orientation could be explained in large part by referencing Nancy Chodorow's (1979) psychoanalytic account of gender development to which the role of woman as mother is central. On Chodorow's account, the male ego individuates in response to the mother figure with whom he does not identify. By contrast, girls experience identification with the mother figure on the basis of shared gender and also experience connection to the father figure as love object. Gilligan suggests this account of identity development helps to explain the gendered differences she observes in moral reasoning. Women's reasoning, she argues, reflects a recognition of multiple needs and the centrality of relationship: moral dilemmas are resolved by reference to an ethic of care.

The role of mothering in the development of Virginia Held's normative theory differed in significant ways (1995). For Held, mothering is a valuable practice completely neglected or misunderstood within the dominant traditions of social and political thought. Such traditions derive obligations from contractual models of consent. But, Held argued, these models are inadequate to understanding the nature and implications of mothering responsibilities. Held proposed a revision of the dominant tradition's moral theory in light of this attention to care; for anything as central to the human condition as rearing children should inform the core concepts within our social, moral, and political traditions.

Given these two accounts, we might have anticipated the immediate flurry of scholarly responses that challenged the necessity of any gendered relationship to care at least as a normative rather than a historical or psychoanalytic model. As Held herself adopted the position that either men or women could "mother," many moved to the language of "parenting." And later work by Gilligan and her colleagues suggested that the tighter association between care and gender was increasingly challenged as women took on roles in the professional workforce.

The worry that celebrating the ethic of care meant celebrating a more traditional place and role for women was widespread (Bartky 1990; Okin 1989). Even in some of the early attempts to bring together (wed?) justice to care, there was an almost too convenient reiteration of a gendered division of labor between values appropriate to the domestic and intimate and, alternatively, values appropriate to principled and public relationships (Benhabib 1987; Okin 1996; West 2002). Care then would require, as it always had, a well-bounded domestic sphere, the extension of care would be to biological kin, and care would be rooted in this spatial and familial exclusivity. There were very good reasons, and good feminist reasons in particular, to resist this as a normative model.

The Invisibility of Care

Nancy Folbre's *The Invisible Heart* (2002) explores the way the association of care work with women helps to explain its historical invisibility. She suggests that care as both a value and a practice was made invisible in societies that intellectually and materially privileged the workings of the invisible hand. Because historically so much of the practice of care was non-wage work, and because much of this work was done by women and people of color in contexts where their formal political power was limited or non-existent, there has been little attention to care in either political life or political theory. For the dominant traditions of contract pay little if any attention to how the next generation of "autonomous" citizens and "self-sufficient" workers comes into existence. Gilligan and Held emerge in a space created in feminist political struggle and shift our attention to exactly these sorts of issues.

The progress of neoliberalism complicates these successes. In *The Outsourced Self* (2012), Arlie Hochschild suggests that one of the aspects of a neoliberal society in which all value is ultimately exchange value is that "we may fail to notice the value of things we cannot buy." Hochschild's argument is disturbing because it suggests the difficulty of calling sustained attention to the value of care in a market-driven society. One way in which shifts in the gendered composition of the labor force called attention to care is that they often required the conversion of what had been non-wage labor to wage labor—more often paying for childcare or elder care or emotional care than had historically been the case. These measurable costs essentially converted unrecognized work to recognized work by converting it to the common currency—both materially and metaphorically. Care workers in this market model are typically grossly underpaid and overworked, but now that care is commodified for exchange it becomes visible work.

Yet this practice of commodifying care is also a repackaging in which some aspects of "care" as it was configured in the work of Held and Gilligan are lost. Markets are, for example, designed to make history, context, and particularity irrelevant, and they work on a contractual model of exchange. The care orientations identified by Held and Gilligan identify contextuality and particularity as central and resist contractual models of responsibility. While it seems essential that those who value care take seriously better working conditions for care workers and recognize the ways in which the demands of care work exceed traditional ways of understanding labor, it also seems essential that we recognize the aspects of care which are valuable and which are largely obscured when we convert care work to wage work.

Neoliberalism and the Present Absence of Care

I have suggested that there is much about neoliberalism that troubles a commitment to care. Elsewhere I have focused on liberalism's commitment to a particular understanding of self-hood, one that understands autonomy as economic self-sufficiency and so resists the centrality of relationship as well as pathologizing need as a characteristic of the uniquely vulnerable (White 2000). Responsibility on this account is reduced to earning wages sufficient to meet one's needs in the marketplace. But there is a wide range of human needs that are obscured in such a model. Most fundamentally, the model of the invisible hand treats the identity of the provider of care as irrelevant. Yet, in the face of trauma, not only may I need help, but for intervention of any kind to qualify as "helpful" it may need to be provided by someone I trust. When one is vulnerable it is particularly important that they can trust those to whom they turn, for in the absence of trusting relations, one's sense of vulnerability may be exacerbated rather than remediated. When I say "I need someone to talk to"—it is pretty clear that it is not an anonymous stranger whom I am in need of. Hochschild depicts a society in which we increasingly see even needs like these "professionalized" and care provision as purchasable; we may even have the sense that such care is better exactly because we pay for it and it is therefore clearly valuable.

This is a hazard of a culture so thoroughly shaped by neoliberalism—one typified on Hochschild's account by the practice of outsourcing. But such outsourcing, the commodification of care by anonymous providers, may leave a critical but often implicit aspect of need unmet: the need to be responded to as a particular person with a particular history by someone trustworthy and familiar. Market logics cannot account for the simple fact that, especially when we are needy, not any provider/producer will do. It is often a familiar hand and not the invisible hand that we need.

The metaphor of the invisible hand is meant to capture the beautiful efficiency of exchange between unfamiliars. Neoliberalism promotes the discursive hegemony of such exchange logics. Romand Coles (1997) has argued that these logics in turn depend on a kind of discursive common currency that may create little possibility for the recognition of multiple and incommensurable values. Yet on his account, our democratic commitments in a diverse society require such a recognition of incommensurability. In his commitment to the enduring presence of alterity, his resistance to a politics of the commons that is a politics of assimilation and commensurability, Coles prompts at the very least a careful consideration of what we give up in efforts to commodify care. Democratic commitments so configured require us to resist reducing "care" to its exchange value, for the common currency in which value is determined is itself a mechanism for effacing and undermining plurality.

The struggle to resist a common currency model of care will be an uphill one. This is well captured in Arlie Hochschild's description:

> Over the last century, the world of services has changed greatly. A hundred—or even forty—years ago, human eggs and sperm were not for sale nor were wombs for rent. Online dating companies, nameologists, life coaches, party animators, and paid graveside visitors did not exist, even as ideas. Nor had a language developed that so seamlessly melded village and market—as in "Rent-a-Mom," "Rent-a-Dad," "Rent-a-Grandma," "Rent-a-Friend"—insinuating itself, half joking, half serious into our culture.
>
> These services are only likely to proliferate in a world that undermines community, disparages government, marginalizes nonprofits, and believes in the superiority of what's for sale. (Hochschild 2012, 222)

For feminists to have argued that care work should be paid work was a no-brainer. A central feature of both women's political marginalization and their economic exploitation was unremunerated labor. Yet perhaps it is time also to recognize that there is a loss in the conversion of care to a good or service for purchase. As Hochschild puts it, "the more we apply market language, habits of emotional detachment, and focus on the 'purchase moment' to our most intimate life, the more fragile it becomes" (225).

Hochschild provides a fairly devastating critique of the consequences of the pervasiveness of exchange logics as a way of navigating our relationships. It is a critique that will be particularly recognizable to the white, middle-class, educated consumer. But as Hochschild herself notes, we don't all have the same relationships to things that are for sale. For the kind of "dependence on the market" that Hochschild claims has subtly undermined our intimate life is accessible only to those with the resources to purchase services. Moreover, Alison Wolf has recently argued that there is significant evidence that, while this ability to purchase services has facilitated more gender equality within upper-middle-class marriages, this equality often comes at the expense, even the exacerbation, of gender inequality among the working class (Wolf 2013). Patterns of services purchased by these households tend, Wolf argues, to reinforce historical associations of women service-providers with underpaid care work and male service-providers with better compensated work in fields like home renovation and maintenance. The more equitable division of care work between couples in the upper middle class may be accomplished by commodifying care for purchase, but this very practice of commodification reinforces the association between women, particularly women of color, and underpaid care work. In the domestic context, Wolf has argued that the rise of working professional women, while perhaps fostering greater equality between educated middle-class men and women, has widened the inequality gap between women. In the global context, there are an increasing number of "transnational families"—leaving children in low GDP contexts in mother-away families and providing migrant second mothers to children in higher GDP contexts (Parrenas 2005).

We should thus have concerns about the commodification of care from both the perspective of our democratic commitments and from the perspective of commitments to gender justice in the economy. In what follows I look to practices of "other-mothering" to suggest the possibilities for moving beyond domestic and commodified care and to practices that might ground and foster a commitment to public care. Practices of other-mothering, because they challenge many of our hegemonic cultural assumptions about how care functions, denaturalize these assumptions. I am not making the argument for other-mothering as the alternative model of public care. Rather I suggest that such a model of public care might be grounded in fostering practices that are counter-hegemonic in ways similar to other-mothering.

Other-Mothering and Marginalization

Because access to commodified care is closely associated with race and class privilege, and because communities of color (here I will specifically focus on African-American communities), historically lacked access to traditional sources of power, these communities developed coping mechanisms dependent on non-traditional resources and forms of intervention.

For the purposes of this chapter, I will rely primarily on Patricia Hill Collins description of other-mothering. It is a practice that she links to the specific history of African-Americans in the US context, while also acknowledging cultural contributions to these practices from the African context. These practices were rooted in the recognition that "vesting one person with full responsibility for mothering a child may not be wise or possible. As a result, othermothers, women who assist bloodmothers by sharing mothering responsibilities, traditionally have been central to the institution of Black motherhood" (Collins 2000, 117). This recognition produces social and familial relations that invite more fluid boundaries between biological mothers and other women who care for children. Carol Stack notes in her canonical work, *All Our Kin* (1974), that long-term care or informal adoption of non-kin children was a common response by women in the community when a child was in need. Stack identifies these women-centered networks of community-based childcare as "fictive kin" relationships.

These non-traditional forms have often been portrayed as part of the "crisis in the Black family" or an aspect of a kind of culture of poverty. At best they were read as a merely functional survival strategy. Recently, for example, it has been suggested that other-mothering as a practice is made necessary by high rates of incarceration of young black men. But other-mothering as a practice long precedes this more recent trend in criminal injustice. The separation of black men from their families, of course, dates back to slavery and was sustained during reconstruction as newly freed black men had to move north in an attempt to escape the racism that was pervasive in southern trade unions. Alternative family structures in US black culture have been made necessary by the system of white privilege that undermines the supposedly more natural and tightly bounded nuclear family. While in the hands of Senator Moynihan this story is told as one of dysfunction and cultural pathology, an alternative telling is about racism and community survival. As Stephanie Coontz argues,

> these alternative family forms and gender roles were hardly "pathological" or "disorganized." They were part of a rich extended kin and community life. In nineteenth century Washington, D.C., for example, black working people supported more than one hundred associations, while poor alley residents developed vibrant and cohesive community networks. Studies of many cities in the nineteenth and twentieth centuries reveal that African-American families maintained tighter and more supportive kin ties than did other urban families, taking care of elders, paupers, and orphans within family networks rather than institutionalizing them as frequently as other groups did. (Coontz 1992, 241)

Given the structure of white supremacy, the concern about institutionalization should not be read as a more general resistance to institutions. Rather it is a recognition of the need to construct black care networks as a space apart within that structure. The very insistence on the part of Coontz that these are not "pathological patterns" is made necessary only because of race. For in an age where we find so much in our history to celebrate about earlier forms of "social capital" and civil society, this story is not part of our shared legacy.

Moreover, as Coontz suggests, the dysfunction of the black family is measured by reference to a very particular white, middle-class ideal-type—one that prioritizes the nuclear family as the site of care, that purchases the care that family members themselves can't provide, and that thus sees the intimate and the domestic as tightly bounded. This ideal has a much shorter and demographically limited history than contemporary public policy debate encourages us to recognize: normalizing the tightly bounded nuclear family amounts to sentimentalizing, the "way things never were" according to Coontz. Coontz argues that families have always been in flux and often in crisis; given this, the sentimentalization of the 1950s "Ozzie and Harriet" model confuses what was in fact a novelty with an enduring and natural model of family (1992, 25).

Not only is the traditional nuclear family a nostalgic trap, as Coontz argues, but recognizing it as such may open the way to see practices of other-mothering as not mere functional adaptations for a marginalized community but also practices in many ways more consistent with democratized care. Stanlie James argues, for example: "Not only have forms of other mothering nurtured and sustained African-American communities, but they were also powerful non-traditional resources utilized to intervene creatively in situations or conditions that threatened the survival of the community" (James 1993, 51). Both James and Collins articulate a vision of other-mothering as a practice that emerges within and nurtures a much broader sense of responsibility to the vulnerable. James narrates a story of her grandmother's participation in other-mothering networks. It was because her "grandmother believed that . . . all children must be clothed and educated, [so] if their biological parents could not discharge these obligations, then some other member of the community should accept that responsibility" (James quoted in Collins 2000, 179).

Stanlie James identifies three important consequences of attending to other-mothering. The first consequence is to dispel feelings of impotence through illustrating historical non-traditional patterns of empowerment for black women. Second, through examining the activism of such women as Ella Baker and Daisy Bates (activists and other-mothers) emphasis is placed on the conceptualization of power as a verb as opposed to a noun. Finally, the ability to analyze, critique, and strategize around issues developed through community other-mothering is a critical resource that can and should be creatively utilized to address contemporary needs.

James continues by arguing that knowledge and respect put other-mothers in unique positions to provide analyses and or critiques of conditions or situations that may affect the well-being of their community. "Whenever necessary, she serves as a catalyst in the development and implementation of strategies designed to remedy these harmful conditions." Other-mothers can be key not only in supporting children but also in helping blood-mothers with the material dimensions of caregiving, supporting maternal authority and providing for the voice of that authority in a blood-mother's absence. In confronting racial oppression, maintaining community-based childcare and respecting other-mothers who assume childcare responsibilities can serve a critical function in African-American communities (Collins 2000, 180).

I want to be clear here that, while Collins has linked this practice to patterns of familial practices in Africa (174), my argument does not depend on demonstrating the cultural link. As Stephanie Coontz suggests, "To be sure, many black families have differed from the white middle-class ideal, because their circumstances were different, but these differences have often been exaggerated, and where they have prevailed they have frequently been the sources of strength rather than weakness" (Coontz 1992, 237). Collins argues that in this context, those African-American women who continue community-based childcare challenge a fundamental assumption underlying the capitalist system itself: that children are "private property" and can be disposed of as such. For example, the exclusive parental "right" to discipline children as parents see fit, even if discipline borders on abuse, parallels the widespread assumption that property owners may dispose of their property without consulting members of the larger community. By seeing the larger community as responsible for children and by giving other-mothers and other non-parents "rights" in childrearing, those African-Americans who endorse these values challenge prevailing capitalist property relations.

In all these ways, Collins anticipates the more radical implications of other-mothering. It is a survival strategy for those at the margins for whom the privatization, domestication, and nuclearization of the family is not an option. But it is not just that. Practices of survival at the margins are also the practices that generate and are sustained by alternative normative visions. These are the visions that produce both critique of the privilege of the center and hope for more just alternatives.

Other-Mothering, the Economy, and Exchange Logics

Anne Roschelle, in her work *No More Kin* (1997), argues that while Stack and Collins had perhaps correctly identified other-mothering as a productive coping strategy for those raced and gendered at the socioeconomic margins, in the context of the 1980s and 1990s there has been significantly less evidence of these kinds of social networks. Collins too acknowledges that the socioeconomic environment shifts patterns of dependence on other-mothering. It should not be surprising that, as circumstances changed, so did family structures. For example, desegregation had some significant consequences for traditions of other-mothering:

> In some fundamental ways, moving into the middle class means adopting the values and lifestyles of White middle-class families. While the traditional family

> ideal is not the norm, the relative isolation of such families from others is noteworthy. US middle-class family life is based on privatization—buying a big house so that one need not cooperate with one's neighbors, or even see them. American middle-class families participate in the privatization of everything from schools and health care, to for-fee health clubs and private automobiles. Working-class African-Americans who experience social mobility thus may encounter a distinctly different value system. Not only are woman-centered networks of blood-mothers and other-mothers much more difficult to sustain structurally—class stratified residential and employment patterns mean that middle-class Black women often see working-class and poor Black women only as their employees or clients—such ideas are often anathema to the ethos of achievement. From the security firms that find ways to monitor nannies, to the gated-communities of suburbia, purchasing services appears to be the hallmark of American middle-class existence. In this context, stopping to help others to whom one is not related and doing it for free can be seen as rejecting the basic values of the capitalist market economy. (Collins 2000, 182)

The circumstances of black middle-class families may undercut the historic role of other-mothers, for one's status as middle class is marked by assimilation to both the material and the cultural aspects of neoliberalism.

Similarly, as the socioeconomic conditions of the marginal get even more desperate, Roschelle makes the point that this desperation also undercuts other-mothering practices and social support systems. When this decline converged with the 1996 Welfare Reform Act, the consequences were particularly devastating. For while perhaps not celebrated as functional, much of the 1996 welfare reform assumed that there was something like a fictive kin network/social support system on which AFDC/TANF participants could rely: there would be the non-state safety net at the end of the state's temporary assistance. In the face of this assumption, Roschelle's evidence that these networks are in serious decline is important to consider.

> Although the women in the Flats were economically disadvantaged, perhaps they had the minimal resources necessary to participate in their exchange networks. One could argue that current economic conditions have become so severe that they prevent minority families from participating in their social support networks because these families no longer have any resources to share. (Roschelle 1997, 184)

Roschelle's language for describing the extent of this crisis is itself telling. For while she worries that the continued economic erosion of these communities has left them without anything to exchange, we might note that this is exactly why practices motivated by the gains of exchange are inadequate at the extreme margins.

Care and Democracy

Danielle Allen (2004), in a chapter entitled "Sacrifice, a Democratic Fact," explores the narrative of black families in a quite different context: the 1957 desegregation struggles in Little Rock. Allen contrasts Hannah Arendt's infamous account of desegregation with Ralph Ellison's response. Arendt argued that black parents "in pursuing social advancement, were exploiting their children. 'The girl was obviously asked to be a hero,' Arendt wrote, '[which] is, something neither her absent father nor the equally absent representatives of the NAACP felt called upon to be'" (Arendt quoted in Allen 2004, 25). Allen sees Arendt's analysis as tightly connected to her work in *The Human Condition* (1958), where she affirms a strong distinction between public, private, and social spheres. Parenting is an appropriately private act and for Arendt it marked a failure of citizenship that parents had attempted to achieve desegregation through children rather than direct participation in the public sphere.

Ralph Ellison, Allen notes, sharply disagreed with Arendt's account of Little Rock. Ellison remarked: "I believe that one of the important clues to the meaning of [American Negro] experience lies in the idea, the ideal of sacrifice. Hannah Arendt's failure to grasp the importance of this ideal among Southern Negroes caused her to fly way off into left field in her 'Reflection on Little Rock'" (Ellison quoted in Allen 2004, 27). Allen quotes Ellison's response to Arendt again at greater length:

> She has absolutely no conception of what goes on in the minds of Negro parents when they send their kids through those lines of hostile people. Yet they are aware of the overtones of a rite of initiation which such events actually constitute for the child, a confrontation of the terrors of social life with all the mysteries stripped away. And in the outlook of many of these parents (who wish the problem didn't exist), the child is expected to face the terror and contain his fear and anger precisely because he is a Negro American. Thus he's required to master the inner tensions created by his racial situation, and if he gets hurt—then his is one more sacrifice.

Allen concludes that "Whereas Arendt developed a political theory that might protect children from politics by transforming politics into an epic arena for full-grown warriors only, Ellison has a more tragic vision: rituals to solidify social order inevitably involve children in politics, however much one might wish the case otherwise" (Allen 2004, 28). She goes on to connect Ellison's view to democracy. His view is one rooted in a more "honest account of collective democratic action" that

> begin[s] by acknowledging that communal decisions inevitably benefit some citizens at the expense of others, even when the whole community generally benefits.

> Since democracy claims to secure the good of all citizens, those who benefit less than others from particular political decisions, but nonetheless accede to those decisions, preserve the stability of political institutions. Their sacrifice makes collective democratic action possible. Democracy is not a static end state that achieves the common good by assuring the same benefits to everyone, but rather a political practice by which the diverse negative effects of collective political action, and even of just decisions, can be distributed equally, and constantly redistributed over time, on the basis of consensual interactions. The hard truth of democracy is that some citizens are always giving things up for others. Only vigorous forms of citizenship can give a polity the resources to deal with the inevitable problem of sacrifice. (Allen 2004, 29)

It has become commonplace in the contemporary context to hear that markets can do no wrong and government can do no right. We would do better to recognize that both are the sites of tragic loss. These losses are perhaps more visible in a deliberative democratic setting where losers in any decision-making process continue to be present as co-deliberators—political members with the potential for regret, resentment, and reflective revision as potential responses to loss—than where they are a defeated minority in a politics of winner-takes-all. And over time this visibility may mean reckoning with a very different kind of justice: justice may mean co-deliberators trying to ensure that tragedy equally befalls all.

Care probably requires both an ethic of generosity and one of sacrifice, each of which looks irrational from the perspective of a market model. This is not to say that paid care workers don't often engage in acts of generosity that well exceed their contractual obligations. Of course they do. It is also not to say that care workers don't make incredible sacrifices, often sacrifices of their own intimate relationships, in the course of their work. What it is, however, to say is that when these acts of sacrifice or generosity occur they exceed our ability to recognize them when we work within market models. They remain invisible.

Recognizing these moments of sacrifice and generosity, making them visible, is a critical strategy of resistance to neoliberal hegemony. Such generosities often begin with a very different way of attending to the world, one consistent with a democratic politics of care. A generous attention resists naturalized and privatized notions of responsibility. This resistance cultivates a much broader attention to the needs of others that recognizes both the plurality and specificity of needs; James and Collins argue that in other-mothering this attention is cultivated and works across rather than within the public/private distinction, broadening the resources and strategies for responsiveness. As a consequence, other-mothering widens participation in networks of care but also pluralizes authority within these networks. Other-mothering as a practice nurtures generous attention and responsiveness. It is a practice that resists the vision of autonomy as self-sufficiency that is at the core of neoliberalism.

Moreover, the values associated with this model of care are also values consistent with democratic commitments. For democracy as Allen understands it fails the project of equality when care work becomes commodified and its value is reduced to the value of exchange. Such commodified care is both unevenly distributed and often inadequate. A democratic equality must reckon with the fact that responsiveness to the needs of fellow citizens often requires sacrifice. Like Jane Mansbridge (1983), Danielle Allen's account encourages us to recognize that democracy is marked by moments of loss. Democracy, notes Mansbridge, requires coercion if we are not to "imagine" it as the practice of consensus. There are thus losses. But meaningful democratic equality also requires that we ensure that the losses are not always accumulating for the same constituencies—that the role of "loser" is not fixed. This will require parallel moments of generosity.

Some more recent work on care has tried to resist the idea that care is a "burden." Indeed, it seems clear from much of the ethnographic work on mothering and care work that to view caregiving merely as a burden obscures important dimensions of the practice of care that are experienced as positive by caregivers themselves. But it seems to me that both this argument and the claim that the work of care is chiefly burdensome are often problematically formulated within logics of exchange: the work of care doesn't pay enough but it is "rewarding" in other ways. Or Folbre's argument that "investing" in our children now will reap economic benefits for us all later. Care workers may or may not experience these rewards, and our "investment" may or may not pay off—though there are good economic reasons to be optimistic.

But with respect to our broader democratic values, such approaches to care seem to give over to economic logics in ways that undermine care's ability to serve as a democratic resource. Other-mothering might be construed as a form of friendship; as Arlie Hochschild suggests, "If a friend did you a favor, you weren't obliged to repay it right away, as when we pay for a service. In fact, that might have seemed rude. It would have defeated the purpose of the gift exchange, which ensured long-term bonds" (Hochschild 2012, 6). Ellison, Allen, and Mansbridge are offering accounts of our democratic lives that require relations that are irreducible to "the purchase moment." It should not surprise us that these relationships of friendship and gift-giving are as incompatible with the tradition of economic contract as they were with the traditions of political contract.

It should also not surprise us that these relationships are found in communities most marginalized in a world dominated by contract. But caring relationships, such as other-mothering, associated with social marginality have too readily been turned into a justification for pathologizing communities that encourage permeable boundaries to the family, that extend resources without security, and that make parental authority more public. Community survival may well require such practices. They may be functional. But they may also be "good."

In their work "Use of African-American Family Structures and Functioning to Address the Challenges of European American Post-divorce Families," Crosbie-Burnett and Lewis (1993) argue that not only are the family structures more common in African-American families not dysfunctional. They may be normatively preferable for a society where divorce is more common than not, where what job security that ever existed is evaporating, and mobility is expected:

> strengths of African-American families (AA families) can inform European American post-divorce families (EAPD families), whose ideology and frame of reference is based on the traditional nuclear family, leaving them ill-prepared to cope with the complex family structures and relationships in which they find themselves. The continued welfare of dependent children as their parents change partners and households is probably the most important challenge to post-divorce families. AA families have had to cope with the same challenge. Historically, in African societies strong communal interpersonal networks including extended families existed for the purpose of caring for children. AA families can inform post-divorce family roles and relationships in several ways. The literature on AA families shows that sex roles are more androgynous in these families than in European American families. Both males and females learn and perform what has been traditionally dichotomized as the instrumental and expressive functions. A pedi-focal conceptualization of family may suggest a more appropriate unit of analysis. (243)

There is much that is functional about such a model of family as a site for meeting the immediate needs of parent and child. It is a way of coping. But it need not merely reproduce marginality. It may also be resistant to hegemony. It is functional and transformational simultaneously. Moreover, in the context of public care, the blurring of the boundary between family as kin and communal and interpersonal networks provides a more appropriate context for identifying and addressing needs and more appropriate training for the citizens of a caring democracy.

Conclusion

Drawing on Ellison's concept of "ritual," it is possible to see other-mothering as a kind of "ritual" that is politically appropriate for a diverse democracy like our own. It is a practice that links survival and social transformation. Perhaps the most important aspect of its transformative potential lies in the ways other-mothering cannot be well understood and is thus not easily assimilated to a model of economic rationality, or a logic of exchange. Other-mothering is a practice of maintaining relationships and communities rather than acquiring goods.

Moreover, if parenting is a site for the preparation of democratic citizens, the practice of other-mothering is critical for exactly this reason. Its status as a gift rather than a service is critical to the ways that it resists and restructures the boundaries and authority of care. If citizens are to live in diverse democracies, families that resist the exclusivity of "nuclear" patterns, that resist the conventional property relationship between parent and child, that expose children to a plurality of distinct and respected voices of authority, that model generosity as well as sacrifice not merely within but beyond kin relationships—these are family structures consistent with democratic citizenship.

References

Allen, D. 2004. *Talking to Strangers: Anxieties of Citizenship since Brown v. Board of Education*. Chicago, IL: University of Chicago Press.

Arendt, H. 1958. *The Human Condition*. Chicago, IL: University of Chicago Press.

Bartky, S. L. 1990. *Femininity and Domination: Studies in the Phenomenology of Oppression*. Florence, KY: Psychology Press.

Benhabib, S. 1987. "The Generalized and the Concrete Other: The Kohlberg–Gilligan Controversy and Moral Theory." In *Women and Moral Theory*, edited by E. Feder Kittay and D. T. Meyers, 154–77. Lanham, MD: Rowman and Littlefield.

Chodorow, N. 1979. *The Reproduction of Mothering: Psychoanalysis and the Sociology of Gender*. Berkeley, CA: University of California Press.

Coles, R. 1997. *Rethinking Generosity: Critical Theory and the Politics of Caritas*. Ithaca, NY: Cornell University Press.

Collins, P. H. 2000. *Black Feminist Thought: Knowledge, Consciousness and the Politics of Empowerment*, 2nd ed. New York: Routledge.

Coontz, S. 1992. *The Way We Never Were: American Families and the Nostalgia Trap*. New York: Basic Books.

Crosbie-Burnett, M., and E. A. Lewis. 1993. "Use of African-American Family Structures and Functioning to Address the Challenges of European-American Post-divorce Families." *Family Relations*, Special Issue on Family Diversity, 42(3): 243–8.

Engster, D. 2007. *The Heart of Justice: Care Ethics and Political Theory*. New York: Oxford University Press.

Folbre, N. 2002. *The Invisible Heart: Economics and Family Values*. New York: New Press.

Gilkes, C. T. 1987. "Building in Many Places: Multiple Commitments and Ideologies in Black Women's Community Work." In *Women and the Politics of Empowerment*, edited by A. Bookman and S. Morgen, 53–76. Philadelphia, PA: Temple University Press.

Gilligan, C. 1993. *In a Different Voice: Psychological Theory and Women's Development*. Cambridge, MA: Harvard University Press.

Held, V. 1989. *Rights and Goods: Justifying Social Action*. Chicago, IL: University of Chicago Press.

Held, V. 1995. *Justice and Care: Essential Readings in Feminist Ethics*. Boulder, CO: Westview Press.

Hochschild, A. 2012. *The Outsourced Self: Intimate Life in Market Times*. New York: Metropolitan.

James, S. 1993. "Mothering: A Possible Black Feminist Link to Social Transformation?" In *Theorizing Black Feminisms: The Visionary Pragmatism of Black Women*, edited by S. M. James and A. Busia, 44–54. London: Routledge.

Kittay, E. 1999. *Love's Labor: Essays on Women, Equality and Dependency*. New York: Routledge.

Mansbridrge, J. J. 1983. *Beyond Adversary Democracy*. Chicago, IL: University of Chicago Press.

Okin, S. 1989. *Justice, Gender, and the Family*. New York: Basic Books.

Okin, S. 1996. "Sexual Orientation, Gender, and Families: Dichotomizing Differences." *Hypatia* 11(1): 30–48.

Parrenas, R. S. 2005. *Children of Global Migration: Transnational Families and Gender*. Stanford, CA: Stanford University Press.

Roschelle, A. R. 1997. *No More Kin: Exploring Race, Class, and Gender in Family Networks*. London: Sage.

Stack, C. 1974. *All Our Kin: Strategies for Survival in a Black Community*. New York: Basic Books.

Tronto, J. 1993. *Moral Boundaries: A Political Argument for an Ethic of Care*. New York: Routledge.

West, R. 2002. "The Right to Care." In *The Subject of Care: Feminist Perspectives on Dependency*, edited by E. F. Kittay and E. K. Feder, 88–114. Lanham, MD: Rowman and Littlefield.

White, J. A. 2000. *Democracy, Justice and the Welfare State: Reconstructing Public Care*. University Park, PA: Penn State University Press.

Wolf, A. 2013. *The XX Factor: How the Rise of Working Women Has Created a Far Less Equal World*. New York: Crown.

Part IV

Challenging Dominant Paradigms

13

Care in the state of nature

The biological and evolutionary roots of the disposition to care in human beings

Daniel Engster

Care ethics is often described as a naturalistic philosophy. Following David Hume, many care theorists assert that human beings have an innate disposition to care for others, rooted in natural features of our psychology or biology (see, for example, Noddings 2010; Richards 2013, 19–23; Slote 2010a, 157–8). This naturalistic quality of care ethics represents, by some accounts, one of its distinguishing features (Kittay 2009). Whereas rationalist, and particularly Kantian, moral theories typically attempt to transcend or idealize the psychological, biological, and practical world of human affairs, care ethics gives voice to the natural caring inclinations of human beings who exist within it (Jaggar 2000).[1]

Although care theorists have frequently claimed that an innate sentiment of care exists in human beings, few have provided much (or any) scientific evidence for this claim. Michael Slote (2007, 13–16) and David Richards (2013, 19–23) have identified some evidence for the existence of a natural sentiment to care, but their analyses are very brief. Nel Noddings (2010) argues at length for the innate bases of care but with limited attention to scientific evidence. In this chapter, I provide a more complete exploration of the natural bases of care ethics. Drawing on recent research in evolutionary theory, neurobiology, ethology, and developmental psychology, I argue that human beings have an innate disposition to care for others.

By providing evidence for an innate disposition to care in human beings, this chapter challenges traditional Western ideas about human nature and strengthens the justification for care ethics. At least since the seventeenth century, one of the main stories we have told ourselves about ourselves in the West is that we are by nature selfish and competitive creatures. These stories have influenced not only how we behave and view others but also what we consider to be morally and politically possible. For individuals reared in this tradition, care ethics might seem an attractive but naïve moral and political philosophy. By demonstrating the existence of an innate disposition to care in human beings, however, I upend this perception. While human beings are no doubt in part selfish and competitive, we are also naturally inclined toward care and compassion. Evolutionary biology, neuroscience, and behavioral studies all overwhelmingly support this conclusion. A caring political order is therefore not beyond our reach. Far from being a utopian moral and political theory, care ethics is firmly rooted in human nature.

This chapter also complicates somewhat our understanding of care ethics. Although scientific evidence shows that human beings are naturally disposed to care for one another, it also indicates that our natural caring inclinations tend to be parochial. We tend naturally to care for kin and others in our group but to be indifferent to unrelated strangers or humanity at large. Natural caring sentiments can therefore take us only so far in motivating care for others. Moral argumentation, community building, political institutions, and other acts of human agency are necessary for bridging the gap between our natural caring sentiments and a broad social concern for others.

This chapter finally offers some unique insights into the challenges associated with creating a caring or just political order. Although our innate dispositions to care for one another provide a natural basis for human society, their parochial character can generate significant obstacles to the creation and maintenance of large-scale political communities. Human beings are naturally disposed to care for our own and those with whom we identify but not all others in society. If large-scale political societies are to remain stable over time and function smoothly, states thus need to devote some attention to expanding our natural caring dispositions to encompass diverse others in society. Simply exercising a monopoly over legitimate coercive force is not enough.

Altogether, I outline a counter-narrative in this chapter to traditional state of nature and social contract theories. Human beings never existed in an anarchical state of nature and never needed anything like a social contract to join them together. Even in pre-political times, human beings lived together in groups organized around care. The main challenge of morality and politics is not so much to generate moral concern and political order out of chaos as to expand our natural but parochial dispositions of care to encompass strangers and distant others. Care ethics offers essential insights for achieving this task.

In the first part of this chapter, I define my understanding of a caring disposition and outline the evidence for a natural disposition to care in evolutionary theory, neurobiology, ethology, and developmental psychology. In the second part, I offer a new vision of the state of nature that takes into account human beings' innate disposition to care, and draw out the implications of this new framework for moral and political theory.

A Preliminary Methodological Note

Applying evolutionary, biological, psychological, and other scientific findings to moral and political theory is fraught with perils. Too often in the past, pseudo-scientific evidence has been used to support sexist, racist, and classist moral and political conclusions (Haraway 1991; Hrdy 1999; 2009; Lloyd 1993). It is therefore important to clarify a couple of points about my argument before proceeding. First, my argument is not intended to support, and in fact does not support, any claims about innate differences between men and women or any other human subgroups.[2] Although human sociability and morality may have distant roots in a mammalian maternal instinct (Noddings 2010), and maternal bonding remains today a fruitful area for studying the biochemical processes associated with caring, mothering appears to be—at least among human beings—simply one vivid instantiation of a general caring tendency found among virtually all individuals (the apparent exception being psychopaths). Indeed, most scientific studies have found that women are not any more naturally caring than men, and that men can be every bit as empathic and caring as women under the right circumstances (Batson 2011 57; Jaffe and Hyde 2000).[3] My argument thus steers clear of questionable claims about innate dispositional and behavioral differences based on socially constructed categories (a binary division of human beings into two sexes) and instead defends the more general thesis that human beings (as well as most higher mammals) are innately disposed to care for others.

I should also make clear that I do not mean to make any deterministic claims about human behavior. Genes, neurotransmitters, hormones, and the like can at best predispose or incline us to feel and act in certain ways. When I say that human beings are naturally disposed to care for others, all I mean is that we are "prewired" for certain feelings and actions (Haidt 2012, 130–1). Our upbringing, experiences, worldview, reasoning, and circumstances nonetheless all play important roles in determining the precise nature of our beliefs and actions (Fiske 2010).

Virginia Held (2002) has offered a more general warning about naturalism in ethics. Defining any moral philosophy in naturalistic terms, Held argues, threatens "to subordinate the normative to the natural," mask normative judgments behind scientific claims, and undermine "our ability to make the needed distinction between what we observe and describe and what we normatively commit ourselves to" (2002, 9, 13). While Held's concerns are important, my purpose here is not to naturalize care ethics but only to demonstrate and clarify the natural bases or sentiments underlying it. Caring dispositions as I understand them function to motivate caring behaviors and provide some pre-cognitive, action-guiding intuitions. They provide the basis for what Nel Noddings calls natural caring as distinct from ethical caring (1984, 81–3; 2002, 29–31; 2010, 1–2, 33–8). My argument therefore does not collapse "ought" into "is" or blur the distinction between norms and facts. I aim instead only to identify the innate caring dispositions (the "is") that motivate and form the basis for a moralized understanding of care ethics (the "ought"), demonstrate that care ethics is not a pie-in-the-sky ethic but rooted in natural human dispositions ("ought" implies "can"), and draw out some lessons for care ethics, and moral and political theory more generally, from our innate disposition to care for others.

Caring Dispositions

By caring dispositions, I mean internal impulses, intuitions, and emotions motivating concern for a person's welfare.[4] These internal states may include feelings of sympathy, empathy, compassion, concern, tenderness, sorrow, or distress. While care theorists disagree about which of these sentiments is most important for motiving caring behaviors (Noddings 2002, 13–14; 2010, 12; Slote 2007; 2010b), we need not concern ourselves too much with these debates as long as we are clear about the emotions we are discussing. Caring dispositions involve, on the one hand, more than merely imagining or knowing the internal state of others, matching their neurological responses, or coming to feel as they feel (Batson 2011, 11–19). Feeling another's pain is not in itself a caring disposition unless it also *motivates* a concern to help them. On the other hand, caring dispositions need not be entirely selfless. If one person is sufficiently distressed by the circumstances of another that they feel an urge to help them, then personal distress can also function as a caring disposition. Caring dispositions therefore encompass a broader set of affective motivations than purely altruistic motivations (Batson 2011, 19–23; Tronto 2013, 32).

In saying that caring dispositions motivate concern for others' welfare, I mean they dispose one to show solicitude for their biological, emotional, and developmental needs and well-being. Protecting others from harm or blights is particularly important. A caring disposition may thus be defined as any feeling, intuition, or other internal state that inclines us to help others, or wish to see others helped, by comforting them, protecting them, feeding them, soothing them, or otherwise attending to their needs. Caring dispositions are, of course, only one factor in determining whether or not a person actually cares for others; a person's mood and worldview, the presence or absence of others, his or her sense of efficacy, and other factors all also play a role in caring actions (Fiske 2010, chapter 9; Hamington 2010). A caring disposition is nonetheless at the root of most voluntary caring.

Jonathan Haidt and his colleagues (e.g., Graham et al. 2013) have identified care as one of five innate or prewired foundations of human morality, along with fairness, loyalty, respect for authority, and a concern for sanctity or cleanliness. In support of their moral foundations theory, they have carried out cross-cultural studies demonstrating the presence of care and other fundamental moral values among groups throughout the world. Skeptics have nonetheless argued that a very high evidence bar needs to be met before any disposition or trait can be confidently deemed innate (Churchland 2011, 112–16). Specifically, they have suggested that cross-cultural data need to be supplemented by evidence from evolutionary theory, genetics, neurobiology, and developmental psychology (Suhler and Churchland 2011). In the next three sections, I provide this evidence for an innate disposition to care.[5]

Natural Selection and Care

In earlier times, philosophers regularly appealed to divine design to explain the existence of natural sentiments in human beings, but at least since the nineteenth century, evolutionary theory has become the preferred scholarly discourse for discussing this topic. At first glance, the theory of evolution might not seem a very promising framework for explaining the development of caring dispositions. At least in the popular imagination, natural selection is often thought to mean survival of the fittest, where the fittest are equated with most ruthless, selfish, and brutal individuals ("red in tooth and claw") (Hrdy 1999, 12–15).[6] This is, however, a very simplistic, if not simply wrong, understanding of the theory. Natural selection defines fitness to mean above all the ability to reproduce offspring that survive, reproduce, and propagate one's genes. At least among higher mammals and especially primates and humans, adaptive fitness is therefore very closely bound up with ability to give and receive care (Fuller 1992).

Because the offspring of most mammals are unable to fend for themselves for a long time after birth, they depend heavily on caregivers for their survival and development (Batson 2011, 54). Primate babies, in particular, are all born needing a great deal of care (Hrdy 2009, 227). A baby chimp orphaned in the wild before the age of three will not survive, and even up to age five, losing a mother is considered a life-threatening liability (266–9, 408–9). Human beings require even more care: "All apes mature slowly, but none so slowly as apes belonging to the genus Homo," a group of large-brained hominids with origins stretching back over two million years (Hrdy 1999, 267, 284; 2009, 146). Given the high degree of dependency of mammal and particularly primate infants, researchers have theorized the evolutionary development of attachment behaviors in them (Bowlby 1982; Hrdy 1999, 387–407; Lieberman 2013, 47–50). According to this theory, natural selection favored infants who were prewired to cry, fuss, suckle, cling, and otherwise demand the attention of their caregivers. These adaptations have come down to us today in the well-documented need for attachment among human and primate infants:

> For more than thirty-five million years, primate infants stayed safe by remaining close to their mothers day and night. To lose touch was death. This explains why, even today, separation from a familiar caretaker provokes first unease, then desperation, followed by rage, and finally despair. (Hrdy 1999, 97)

Primate infants who did not cling to their parents or cry when put down were much more likely to be forgotten, trampled, eaten, or killed. Over time, natural selection thus favored infants who were born with a prewired disposition for attachment to their caregivers over those who were not.

Just as natural selection favored infants who fussed, cried, and demanded attention, it similarly favored mammalian parents who were more attentive and caring toward their infants. Mammalian parents who provided better care for their offspring would have greatly enhanced their offspring's chances of surviving, developing into healthy adults, and passing on their genes to the next generation. Inasmuch as the offspring of these more caring parents carried genes that similarly inclined them to care more for their offspring, genes associated with more parental care would have gradually increased in frequency in the population.[7] Conversely, mammalian parents who showed less care and concern for their young would have been less reproductively successful and their genes would have been gradually selected out of the population (Batson 2011, 46). These selection pressures would have been especially prominent among higher mammals with longer developmental periods. Today, there is widespread agreement among evolutionary theorists that the motivation to care for one's offspring was almost certainly an important evolutionary adaptation selected for among higher mammals including primates and human beings (Bell 2001; Dawkins 2006; Hrdy 1999; 2009; Singer 1981; Sober and Wilson 1998). A good deal of evidence (see below) further indicates that parents' disposition to care for their children has an innate genetic basis and can, in fact, be passed on to their offspring (Batson 2011, 46–53; Bartz et al. 2011, 307).

In addition to favoring more caring parents, evolutionary theorists also argue that individuals who showed care and concern for kin and as-if kin (i.e., group members who help to protect, support, and provision one's kin) would have enjoyed an adaptive advantage over those who did not (Dawkins 2006; Hrdy 1999; 2009; Singer 1981). Siblings conceived by the same parents share on average the same percentage of genes with one another (50 percent) as parents share with their children. Grandparents share on average 25 percent of their genes with their grandchildren; uncles and aunts share 25 percent of their genes with their nephews and nieces; half siblings share 25 percent of genes with one another; and so forth. Just as natural selection favored the genes of parents who better cared for their offspring, the theory of kin selection or inclusive fitness suggests that individuals who cared for kin would also have been more successful at propagating their genes than those who did not.[8] In the small, hunter-gatherer groups that early human beings lived in (probably numbering around twenty-five to thirty-five members), care for kin would have effectively meant a generalized caring concern for almost everyone in one's group (Hrdy 2009). Inasmuch as the disposition to care for as-if kin would also have increased the survival and reproduction rates of one's offspring and kin, this, too, would have been adaptively advantageous.[9] Evolutionary theory thus suggests that a general tendency to care for others in one's group was probably selected for among early human beings because of its proclivity to enhance the survival prospects of one's genetic relations who, in turn, would have borne some of these same tendencies.

Although the account of human evolution outlined above supports a more congenial (and I dare say realistic) description of human nature than simplistic "survival of the fittest" accounts, evolutionary theory also identifies some limits to the adaptive advantages of an innate disposition to care. Successfully propagating one's genes through kin selection depends in part on discriminating between group members and outsiders, and showing preference strictly for the former. Any early humans who showed an inclination to care indiscriminately for all others regardless of kin relations would have been at an evolutionary disadvantage for propagating their genes compared to individuals who favored only kin and kin supporters. Over time, a narrower caring concern would therefore have been selected for over a broader one. Evolutionary theorists also point to the selective advantages to being able to distinguish between cooperative members within one's group and freeloaders or non-cooperators. Individuals who were able to discriminate between contributing and non-contributing group members and direct their care only towards the former would have been at an adaptive advantage over individuals who indiscriminately cared for all group members regardless of contribution.

Once our hominid ancestors developed the ability to discriminate between cooperative and uncooperative group members, Christopher Boehm (2012) argues that this capacity very likely further functioned (over the last 50,000 years or so) to select for individuals with more caring or prosocial genes while decreasing the prevalence of genes for in-group aggression, domination, non-cooperation, and free riding. Anti-social, domineering, and exploitative individuals would have most likely been, according to Boehm, banished or killed by early human groups until only more cooperative individuals (or at least individuals who were able to restrain or hide their domineering or exploitative tendencies) would have remained. Over time, social selection therefore may have complemented natural selection to make humans more generally caring toward others in their groups.

Care and Neurobiology

If the motivation to care for others has a genetic basis, as predicted by evolutionary theory, we should find evidence for it in human molecular biology. Genes, after all, do not directly determine behaviors but code for proteins that in combination with other molecules incline us to behave in certain ways. While a full physiological account of how human beings are motivated to care for others exceeds the bounds of this chapter (and current scientific knowledge), a good deal of scientific research points to the central importance of oxytocin and several other hormones and neurotransmitters (vasopressin, dopamine, endogenous opiates, serotonin, prolactin) in this process (Batson 2011, 50–1; Bell 2001; Bartz et al. 2011; Churchland 2011; Taylor 2002). Levels of oxytocin production and uptake are coded for in our genes and passed from parents to children. Variations in the oxytocin receptor gene, in particular, have been associated with sensitive parenting, behavioral and dispositional empathy, and a number of prosocial behaviors (Bartz et al. 2011; Bakermans-Kranenburg and van Ijzendoorn 2008; Israel et al. 2009; Kim et al. 2010; Rodrigues et al. 2009; Tost et al. 2010). When coupled with the arguments from evolutionary theory, this biochemical evidence goes a long way toward demonstrating an innate or natural basis for care in human beings.

Oxytocin is a peptide of nine amino acids that is produced in the hypothalamus and released into the brain and bloodstream (De Dreu et al. 2010, 1408). Generated in especially high amounts among female mammals during labor, oxytocin functions to induce uterine contractions and promote the flow of milk during breastfeeding (Bell 2001, 221). It also inhibits the natural fear response in mammals, increases feelings of relaxation and well-being, and promotes maternal bonding behaviors (Churchland 2011, 33–4; Bell 2001; Broad, Curley, and Keverne 2006; Hrdy 1999, 151–6; Lieberman 2013, 93–4).[10] In fact, the development of oxytocin and the closely related vasopressin some 200 million years ago appears to be one of the key biochemical developments that set early mammals apart from their reptilian ancestors. While most reptilian parents will flee from or kill any of their offspring they may encounter, oxytocin in mammals encourages the desire for closeness and contact necessary for breastfeeding (Bell 2001).

How exactly oxytocin works to stimulate parenting behaviors is not entirely understood, but one account suggests that the release of oxytocin in the brain leads to the release of dopamine and other endogenous opiates, causing mammalian mothers to associate caregiving with decreased fear and anxiety and higher pleasure and contentment (Churchland 2011, 55, 63; Lieberman 2013, 92–4). Whatever the exact chemical mechanisms, a large number of animal studies demonstrate the central role of oxytocin in maternal caregiving. Female sheep who have no concern for lambs will become highly maternal and bond with unrelated lambs when given oxytocin injections (Keverne 1988; Keverne and Kendrick 1990). High levels of oxytocin have further been found to correlate with high levels of maternal behavior in rats, prairie voles, monkeys, and human beings (Churchland 2011, 53; Hrdy 2009, 215). Among human beings, researchers found a strong association between a mother's oxytocin levels and various cognitive and behavioral factors associated with positive mother–infant bonding behaviors (Feldman et al. 2007). Conversely, when an oxytocin antagonist is given to a mother rat or mother sheep, or oxytocin receptors are blocked, the mother will not care for her infants, leading to high rates of infant mortality (Bell 2001, 223; Churchland 2011, 50; Lieberman 2013, 159).

Although oxytocin has been closely linked with maternal caregiving, it is also found in men and along with vasopressin and other hormones and neurotransmitters likewise appears to play an important role in motivating a wide array of prosocial behaviors. Oxytocin has been associated, for example, with the formation and maintenance of mate attachment and long-term partner bonds in human beings and a number of other mammals (Churchland 2011, 46–53, 56–7; Lim and Young 2006; Scheele et al. 2013). Larger numbers of oxytocin receptors in the human brain are further associated with greater empathy, generosity, and other-regarding behaviors (Churchland 2011, 50; De Dreu et al. 2010, 1408). Research has also linked oxytocin with more trusting and cooperative behaviors, higher levels of social motivation and awareness, and longer eye gaze (for reviews, see Bartz et al. 2011; Heinrichs et al. 2009; MacDonald and MacDonald 2010). In laboratory experiments, men who were given doses of oxytocin using a nasal spray and then asked to play a variety of economic strategy games were much more likely to exhibit trusting and cooperative behaviors than men who were not given oxytocin. In one case, while 52 percent in control group were selfish and only 20 percent were cooperative, in the group who inhaled oxytocin only 17 percent were selfish and 58 percent were cooperators (De Dreu et al. 2010). In other experiments, individuals who were given oxytocin were significantly more generous and empathetic to others (Kosfeld et al. 2005; Zak et al. 2007).

Although levels of oxytocin production and uptake are coded for in our genes, they also appear to be mediated by parental care (Churchland 2011, 53; De Dreu et al. 2010, 1411). Rat pups whose mothers produce high levels of oxytocin produce high levels of oxytocin in response to their mother's licking and grooming behaviors. When these female pups mature and have their own litters, they too have high oxytocin levels and are highly caring, and their pups similarly produce high levels of oxytocin (Champagne and Meaney 2001). Similar relations have been found in humans: high levels of oxytocin in mothers correlate with high levels of caring behaviors and high levels of oxytocin in babies (Feldman et al. 2010). Both genetic and environmental factors thus appear to play a role in the transmission of caring dispositions from parents to children.

Consistent with the predictions of evolutionary theory, oxytocin appears to motivate care primarily toward individuals whom we consider trustworthy or members of our in-group (Bartz et al. 2011). While oxytocin correlates with higher in-group benevolence in animals, for example, it has been found to generate feelings of heightened anxiety and aggression toward strangers (Bell 2001, 221; Churchland 2011, 50). Similar effects have been found in human beings. When individuals are given the choice between helping in-group or out-group members in laboratory experiments, individuals who inhaled oxytocin show increased bias toward their in-group (De Dreu et al. 2010; 2011).[11] Carsten De Dreu and his colleagues (De Dreu et al. 2011, 1265) who conducted these experiments conclude in one of their studies that:

> There is no doubt that oxytocin is implicated in the development of trust, empathy, and prosociality, but these tendencies appear limited to individuals belonging to one's in-group. Thus, rather than making humans prosocial, oxytocin functions to strengthen an evolutionary evolved and rather functional tendency to discriminate between in-group and out-group as well as to give members of one's own group preferential treatment. Such ethnocentrism has adaptive value to individuals and their groups but, unfortunately, also paves the way for intergroup bias, conflict, and violence.

Depending on circumstances, and particularly the degree to which members of one group perceive others as potential threats, the very same genetic and physiological adaptations that underlie the motivation to care for others can also give rise to their opposite.

Oxytocin, vasopressin, dopamine, and the like are not the sole physiological bases of caring motivation in human beings. Other physiological features, such as mirror neurons, may also play some role. Yet, the relation between mirror neurons and caring dispositions appears to be at best indirect. Mirroring another's physical or emotional states can lead to any number of feelings or responses. We might turn away or flee from others in distress in order to protect ourselves from unpleasant feelings or even experience glee if we place negative value on their welfare (Batson 2011, 41–2, 61–3). In order for our mirror reflex to give rise to caring motivation, we must also have feelings of caring concern for the person in need—perhaps because we know them or identify with them, associate them with someone we know or care for, or feel some sense of responsibility for them (Bloom 2013, 43–7). Oxytocin, vasopressin, and other hormones and neurotransmitters appear to play vital roles in stimulating these feelings.

Ethology and Behavioral Studies

Thus far, I have argued for an innate or natural basis of caring motivation in human beings based on evolutionary theory and neurobiological research. If the motivation to care is innate in human beings, there should also be behavioral evidence for it; and of course, there is plentiful evidence. Caring behaviors occur all around us all the time among parents and children, friends, partners, co-workers, and sometimes even strangers. Raw acts of selfishness, greed, incivility, and cruelty stand out in our minds and capture so much of our attention because they represent such threats to our lives and well-being and exist in sharp contrast to the general care that forms the background of society. Psychological studies have confirmed the presence of strong dispositions to care for others in most human beings. As noted above, Haidt and his colleagues (Graham et al. 2013) found that individuals from diverse religious and cultural backgrounds across the world endorse caring values. C. Daniel Batson (1991; 2011) and others (Hoffman 2000) have likewise found evidence not just for caring behaviors but also for altruistic behaviors among large percentages of individuals. Since most psychological studies on empathy and altruism have been carried out on adults, there is unfortunately no way to know for sure whether these caring dispositions are rooted in natural impulses, cultural conditioning, social pressures, or other factors.

Where the goal is to demonstrate a natural basis of caring concern in human beings, probably the most compelling behavioral evidence comes from research on primates and human infants.[12] Primates are the nearest genetic relatives of human beings among existing species, with chimpanzees and bonobos sharing over 98 percent of our DNA. Since in primates the prefrontal cortex, which is generally associated with self-control, choice, reasoning, and behavioral adaptability, is smaller relative to body size and less dense in neural pathways than in humans, primate behavior is often thought to provide some insight into the innate, physiological tendencies underlying human behavior.

A broad body of research supports the existence of caring dispositions in primates (De Waal 2006; 2009; Hrdy 1999; 2009). Virtually all female primates, for example, show an innate attraction and responsiveness to infants (Hrdy 2009, 217, 229). In most primates, males likewise provide special protection for their (presumed) offspring (Hrdy 1999, 215–16; 2009, 158–61). In many species of monkeys—albeit not most apes—males even engage in extensive direct care for the young, with some males carrying babies for as much as 90 percent of the time (Hrdy 2009, 88–9, 160–1). As Hrdy writes (1999, 209), "If the circumstances are conducive, almost any primate male can be induced to behave in a nurturing way."[13]

There is also extensive anecdotal and experimental evidence for a more general caring concern among primates (De Waal 2009; Langergraber et al. 2007). Male and female chimpanzees regularly groom one another, support one another, and share food—usually keeping track of who has previously done them a good turn and reciprocating in kind (De Waal 1997; Gomes et al. 2009; Koyama et al. 2006; Melis et al. 2008). In experiments, chimps have been shown to help other chimps and humans without expectation of a reward (Greene 2013, 38–9; Warneken and Tomasello 2006; Warneken et al. 2007; Warneken and Tomasello 2009). When given a choice between rewarding themselves only or also rewarding another monkey, capuchin monkeys and marmosets overwhelmingly choose to reward the other (De Waal 2009, 112–13, 193; Hrdy 2009, 96–8; Lakshminarayanan and Santos 2008). Alternatively, hungry rhesus monkeys will refrain from pulling a lever to get food if doing so gives another monkey a painful electric shock (Bloom 2013, 48). Primate care nevertheless tends to be directed mostly toward kin and reciprocating group members. In the experiments mentioned above, chimps will usually only pull a rope that delivers food to themselves and another chimp if the other chimp is kin or an ally. If the other chimp has no significant relationship to them, most chimps are indifferent to them (Hrdy 2009, 35–6; Jensen et al. 2006; Silk et al. 2005). In the experiment on capuchin monkeys described above, the probability that the monkey would benefit others likewise varies depending on the closeness of their relational ties (De Waal 2009, 113, 194).

If primates provide one source for discerning our natural inclinations, human infants are another. Newborns lack a number of capacities necessary for the full expression of care and empathy, including physical mobility, strength, and the ability to differentiate self from others clearly. Nonetheless, the capacity for rudimentary care and empathy are evident almost from birth. "Right from the first days of life," Sarah Hrdy writes, "every healthy human being is avidly monitoring those nearby, learning to recognize, interpret, and even imitate their expressions" (Hrdy 2009, 7, 115–16). Newborns cry in response to the cries of other babies and mimic the facial expressions of adults. Even if these behaviors fall short of caring concern, they at least provide evidence that newborns respond to the cues of others and, in the case of crying, are distressed by vocalizations of distress (Bloom 2013, 47–8; Eisenberg et al. 2003; Hoffman 1981, 64–6). As noted above, newborns further enter the world with a need for attachment and undergo physiological changes (related to oxytocin production and receptors) depending on the level and quality of care provided to them. This, too, suggests the presence of a prewired disposition for caring behaviors in them.

By the time they are three to six months old, babies are able to distinguish helping from hindering puppets in short skits and overwhelmingly prefer helping puppets over the hindering ones (Bloom 2013, 7, 27–8; Greene 2013, 46–7). By 12 to 18 months old, children will pat and stroke others in distress, share resources with others, provide helpful information to others in need, and help others to achieve their goals (Hoffman 2000, chapter 3; Warneken and Tomasello 2006; 2009). Felix Warneken and Michael Tomasello (2009, 397), who have carried out studies on helping behaviors in both human infants and chimpanzees, observe: "The early ontogenetic emergence of spontaneous helping in young children and its presence in our nearest primate relatives, suggest that helping others with their instrumental goals somehow comes naturally to humans, not exclusively through cultural transmission or explicit teaching." We are, according to this research, born with an innate disposition to care. Yet, human babies, too, are highly parochial. They quickly develop a preference for individuals who look and speak like their primary caregivers. They prefer to accept toys from native over non-native language speakers, and even react favorably to individuals who treat similar others well and dissimilar others poorly (Bloom 2013, 105, 111; Greene 2013, 50; Hamlin et al. 2013).

Drawing together the insights from evolutionary theory, neurobiology, and behavioral studies, we may conclude that "the circuitry for caring" is innate in human beings and probably underlies a good part of our moral behavior (Churchland 2011, 8, 71, *passim*). "We may assume," Frans De Waal writes (2006, 24), "that empathy first evolved in the context of parental care, which is obligatory in mammals," and then expanded to encompass concern for kin and other group members. The naturally motivated caring of parent for child "may provide a biological substrate for all intrinsic valuing of another's welfare" (Batson 2011, 46). It may very well be the case, in other words, that "morality originates in the neurobiology of attachment and bonding" (Churchland 2011, 71). And yet our natural disposition to care for others appears to be limited. It evolved to incline us to care for kin and others who support our survival and the survival of our offspring, but leaves us for the most part indifferent to the welfare of those outside our group. In some cases, it can even give rise to aggression and violence, particularly when we feel threatened by others.

Care in the State of Nature

Whatever else this brief survey of evolutionary theory, neurobiology, and behavioral psychology may suggest, it certainly upends traditional views of human beings in the state of nature. Hobbesian, Lockean, and Rousseauean accounts of state of nature are, as Frans De Waal notes, leftovers "from pre-Darwinian days, based on a totally erroneous image of our species" (De Waal 2009, 21). Although there can be little doubt that human beings are in part self-interested creatures (prone to acts of self-promotion and sometimes violence), we are also clearly disposed to care for others (which can also generate conflict and violence). The disposition to care is not the only or perhaps even the predominant sentiment in us, but it is an important one. Any theory of politics or morality that ignores this sentiment will be misleading in important ways.

Care theorists (Held 1993, 195) have long criticized state of nature stories for ignoring the importance of care. Even if we were to incorporate care into the state of nature, there are still reasons to be skeptical about these accounts of human behavior. Whatever human beings' innate dispositions may be, their expression depends in large part on environmental circumstances. Thus, in any state of nature scenario, a great deal depends on whether one imagines nature to be a place of scarcity or plenty, or high or low population density. These concerns can be avoided in part if, instead of imagining the state of nature in wholly philosophical terms, we base it on the probable living conditions of *Homo sapiens* in the years prior to the development of the first agricultural settlements roughly 12,000 years ago. The individuals who lived in these hunting and gathering—or foraging—communities were anatomically and genetically identical to modern humans, but had not yet moved into settled political communities (Boehm 2012, 82). Hence they provide some insight into human behaviors in the real pre-civil state of nature. By imagining human life in this pre-civil state of nature, we can develop an alternative account of human nature to replace the misguided theories of Hobbes, Locke, and Rousseau.

Prior to the Neolithic era, human beings probably lived in small, multi-family groups consisting of about twenty-five to thirty-five members.[14] Care and loyalty to individuals within these groups was probably high, but most individuals were likely indifferent to most outsiders. Because human population densities tended to be low, contact between groups was probably infrequent (Hrdy 2009, 18–19, 29). There is no clear evidence of widespread warfare among human groups prior to the Neolithic Age, but group warfare may have taken place depending on circumstances (Boehm 2012, 77; Hrdy 2009, 19–20; see, however Choi and Bowles 2007). Small skirmishes and occasional raids seem more likely (Boehm 1999, 221–3).[15] Alternatively, some groups may have forged loose alliances with one another based on cross-group kin membership and rudimentary exchange relations (Hrdy 2009, 26).

Early human groups in the pre-civil state of nature were also likely egalitarian (Boehm 1999; 2012, 9–10, 69, 82, 95–6, *passim*). As much as some individuals may wish to rule over others, nearly all human beings appear to have a natural revulsion (perhaps rooted in basic survival instincts) against being dominated. Thus, in most existing hunter-gatherer human groups, counter-dominant coalitions regularly form to shame, banish, punish, and sometimes kill bullies, free-riders, and other anti-social types who try to dominate or take advantage of others in the group.

The status of women in the prehistoric state of nature probably varied between groups, but in general was probably relatively high (Boehm 1999, 4–9; Boehm 2012, 80; Hrdy 1999; 2009; Wood and Eagly 2002).[16] Women would have played a central role in the economies of these early groups, as either hunters or foragers (Boehm 2012, 137; Hrdy 2009, 147). They would likewise have been actively involved in the politics of these groups, engaging in the shaming and punishing of bullies and freeloaders. Perhaps most importantly, many of these groups may have had a matrilocal basis. Until recently, it was generally assumed that men tended to stay put in early human groups and trade sisters and daughters between groups. This received wisdom, however, ignores the centrality of care to human existence. Women who remained with kin to have and raise their children, Hrdy argues (2009, chapter 8), would have enjoyed significant advantages from an evolutionary perspective over those who did not. They would have received much more support during pregnancy and childbirth and would have been able to trust other group members (kin) to help them care for their infants. This, in turn, would have greatly increased the survival chances of both mothers and children and allowed women to reproduce much more frequently than, say, other ape mothers who cared exclusively for their young. The matrilocal thesis helps to explain a number of developments in humans' evolutionary history that are otherwise mysterious: why humans were able to reproduce so much faster than other apes after our near extinction 70,000 years ago, why human mothers are so much more willing than other ape mothers to allow other individuals to hold and care for their infants, and why humans developed such more advanced social and cooperative capacities than other apes (Hrdy 2009, 101–2, 279–80, chapters 3 and 8).

Closely related to this last point, early humans almost surely depended on alloparents (i.e., individuals other than the biological parents) to help raise their children (2009, chapter 5; see also Diamond 2012, 186–90). The nutritional and other demands of life in hunter-forager groups would have made it difficult for individual parents to meet their own needs and those of their children by themselves—particularly parents with very young children.

Alloparenting, by contrast, would have greatly increased the survival chances of children and allowed adult women to have babies more frequently. A brief survey of caretaking practices across traditional hunting and gathering peoples—the closest proxies for Pleistocene hominids—confirms the nearly universal prevalence of alloparenting (Hrdy 2009, 73–9). "Around the world, wherever traditional ways of life persist... " Hrdy writes (77–8), "shared care is the rule." Researchers have also found that fathers play on average a much greater role in the care of children in hunter-gatherer societies than in any other (agricultural, pastoral, industrial) social form (Diamond 2012, 187; Hrdy 2009, 126–32, 161–2).

I do not mean to romanticize human life in the prehistoric state of nature. Everyday subsistence was no doubt very hard. Occasional acts of violence—probably mostly aimed against bullies and freeloaders—would have occurred within groups, and occasional skirmishes or raids probably occurred between groups. This description of human life in a pre-civil state of nature nonetheless does provide an important corrective to the theories of Hobbes, Locke, and Rousseau. Indeed, taking care seriously in the state of nature changes everything.

First, the state of nature certainly was not a war of all against all. Most individuals would have had a great deal of difficulty surviving outside their groups, and children in particular would not have survived without kin networks (Hrdy 2009, 18–19). Even if warfare was more frequent than indicated above, it still would have been between groups and not individuals. Second, human beings did not naturally live in traditional patriarchal families, as Locke supposed, or follow any universal moral law of the sort he imagined. The "typical or natural Pleistocene family" was "kin-based" and "very, very flexible," with ambiguity probably surrounding the paternity of many children (Hrdy 2009, 166).[17] Alloparenting, or community care, would have been the norm. While care and compassion would have been strong within groups, it would have been weak toward humanity at large. Moreover, self-policing within groups would have been fairly efficient. Third, the historical state of nature bears very little resemblance to Rousseau's vision of human beings as solitary and self-sufficient creatures. Even though Rousseau recognized pity as an innate human characteristic, he greatly underestimated the degree to which we are naturally disposed to care for our children and kin and form communities around them.

The above description of human life in the pre-civil state of nature further challenges some of the basic premises of social contract theory. Contrary to the views of classical liberal theorists, human beings already lived in relatively orderly groups with fairly effective self-policing practices in the state of nature of the late Pleistocene. In moving to larger, more settled agricultural civilizations, the main moral and political problem was not so much to forge morality and order out of chaos as to encourage individuals who already existed in families and groups to care for others beyond their kin and tribes. The main motivation for this move was almost certainly to improve opportunities for care by securing more regular food sources. Whether we look at the challenges faced by the early Greek polis—immortalized in dramas such as Aeschylus' *Oresteia* and Sophocles' *Antigone*—the formation of states in early modern Europe, the consolidation of the United States into a nation, or the consequences of state failure in contemporary Rwanda, we nevertheless find the same problem continually reoccurring. In all cases, the central moral and political challenge involves melding groups together and getting individuals to care about others beyond their self-identified in-groups (families, tribes, ethnic groups, religious groups). The collapse of domestic sovereignty and return to the state of nature leads not so much to anarchy as to group conflict and sometimes genocide.

Here, then, we come to the importance of care ethics as a moral and political theory. Care ethics is the moral and political theory par excellence for studying what it means to care for others—on an individual, family, social, and international level—and exploring how a caring concern can be fostered across diverse individuals and groups. Care theorists have, in fact, outlined a number of strategies for extending our natural caring dispositions to unknown others. Noddings (2005; 2010) has written extensively about the importance of a caring education for cultivating and training our natural caring dispositions and directing us toward broader ethical ends (see also Engster 2007, chapter 5). Held, Kittay, Tronto, and other care theorists have further outlined a variety of proposals for developing political institutions and social policies that support and facilitate care (Engster 2007; Held 2006; Kittay 1999; Noddings 2002; Tronto 1993, 2013). The construction of fair and reliable social, economic, and political institutions appears particularly important for fostering more caring relations among strangers. As Patricia Churchland (2011, 65) observes, "Trust can be expanded beyond the circle of kin and familiar folks if the institutional arrangements can be counted on to assure a reasonable level of trustworthiness of participants, known and unknown." When states establish fair governing institutions and generous social welfare policies, individuals tend to show more trust for other members of society and appear more willing to extend caring concern to them (Rothstein and Uslaner 2005). Corrupt political institutions and patronage, by contrast, tend to reinforce parochial caring sentiments.

Despite the important contributions that care theorists have made to the question of how our caring sentiments can be cultivated and expanded, more work needs to be done on this topic. Although care theorists have long acknowledged the challenge of parochialism to care ethics, for example, this problem is perhaps deeper than they have estimated (e.g., Noddings

2010, 188–9).[18] If our most basic innate dispositions to care are parochial, then parochialism cannot be simply dismissed as a corruption of care. There is nothing natural about caring for strangers and distant others. These sentiments need to be cultivated and maintained and their value explained.

Care theorists nonetheless at least appear to be on the right track. Human beings are by nature caring and relational. Starting out from the assumption of isolated individuals in a disorderly state of nature is not very helpful in thinking about the most basic political problems. States are generally not tasked with the challenge of creating moral concern and order out of nothing, but instead with coaxing individuals to extend some measure of the care they already feel toward family and friends to unknown others. In this alternative, caring vision of politics, creating institutions that establish connections and breed trust among strangers is every bit as important for achieving stability and order as setting up coercive political institutions and enforcing laws.

While traditional state of nature and social contract theories generally left out care, I have attempted to demonstrate its centrality to society and politics. Human society very likely originally arose out of relations of care, and feelings of trust and care continue to play an important role in sustaining political stability and order. The central political problem is not so much binding isolated individuals together in society as surmounting parochial loyalties and promoting empathy across groups. Care is not then below or outside politics, as is so commonly assumed, but intimately tied up with the most basic political question: how can order be established and maintained?

Conclusion

Human beings are not the narrowly self-interested, solitary creatures of traditional social contract theories. We are all born (with only rare exceptions) with a natural disposition to care for others. This disposition is quite sensitive to environmental factors and is most fully activated only in highly caring environments, but it is nevertheless written into our genes and biochemistry. The origins of this natural disposition to care are speculative, but there are good reasons for thinking it initially developed out of a very basic mammalian (or near-mammalian) adaptation to care for offspring, and eventually expanded in social mammals to encompass care for kin and other supportive group members (as-if kin). By the time our hominid ancestors had developed into recognizable human beings, they inhabited a state of nature that was already social and contained a great deal of care within groups (e.g., alloparenting). Life was no doubt brutish and short for these early humans, but it was not solitary or even necessarily nasty. Early humans lived in societies organized around care. While moral and political theorists would be foolish to ignore the selfish and egotistical drives within human beings, they would be just as foolish to ignore our innate dispositions to care. Human beings are naturally caring creatures. Much of the strife and suspicion that exists between peoples appears to arise, in fact, not from egoistic tendencies but rather from the parochial nature of our caring dispositions. Recognizing this fact does not necessarily make it any easier to reduce mistrust or conflict, but it does offer a ray of hope. The roots of a more caring world already exist within us. The main political task for those committed to realizing this world is to identify the institutions, policies, and practices that will enable our natural caring dispositions to expand and grow.

Notes

1. I wish to thank Maxine Eichner, Maurice Hamington, Willie Hale, Adam Johnson, and Julia Barbosa Landois for reading and providing valuable comments on earlier drafts of this chapter.
2. My argument is in this respect very different from Noddings' argument in *The Maternal Factor* (2010), which asserts a number of innate differences between men and women.
3. Batson notes that there nonetheless may be innate gender differences that moderate the experience of empathy. "There is some evidence that women are, in general, more emotional than men, or at least are more emotionally expressive" (2010, 57). Even if it were true that women are naturally more caring than men, of course, no moral or social conclusions would follow from this fact. What is natural is not always right or desirable.
4. Caring dispositions can also motivate care for oneself (Churchland 2011, 27–31), but my central concern here will be care for others.
5. I am skeptical about the innate roots of some of Haidt's other moral foundations, such as sanctity. Others, such as fairness and loyalty, are closely related to, and perhaps even rooted in, the innate disposition to care.
6. In a 2007 opinion piece in the *New York Times*, David Brooks wrote, "From the content of our genes, the nature of our neurons and the lessons of evolutionary biology, it has become clear that nature is filled with competition and conflicts of interest."
7. By genes here, I mean a cluster of chromosomal material (Dawkins 2006, 28–32). The relation between genes and behavior is not one-to-one but many-to-many. It takes many genes working together to create an inclination toward any complex behavior, and many genes have multiple effects (Churchland 2011, 97–103).
8. Theories of kin selection and inclusive fitness generally assert a sharp distinction between genetic relations (kin) and other group members, and assert that natural selection would have favored individuals who helped only the former. This

obviously presents problems in explaining the development of a more generalized disposition to care for all group members. If, however, as-if kin played an important role in caring for, provisioning, and protecting one's kin, a selective advantage would have developed for individuals who included them in their ambit of caring concern. There still would have remained an advantage for individuals who showed some preference toward kin, but extending some concern to other group members who supported one's kin (as-if kin) would have also been more advantageous than not doing so. For a discussion of these and other points, see Boehm (2012, especially chapter 3).

9. Although most evolutionary theorists argue that natural selection takes place primarily or exclusively at the individual or genetic level, a few argue that group selection is necessary to explain at least in part the increased frequency of caring dispositions in humans (Nowak et al. 2010; Sober and Wilson 1998; Wilson and Wilson 2008). I do not take a position on this debate, but generally assume (without denying the possibility of some group selection) that individual-level selection was the stronger force in human evolution.
10. Preliminary research also suggests that oxytocin is implicated in human beings' innate responsiveness to infants and readiness to bond with adoptive and other children (Churchland 2011, 33–4; Hrdy 2009, 213–15).
11. Importantly, all experiments included only male subjects. It is thus unknown whether oxytocin triggers what De Dreu et al. dub the "tend and defend" response in women.
12. Graham et al. (2013, 112) note, "The case for innateness grows much stronger when a behavior or ability is found in non-human primates (particularly chimpanzees and bonobos) and when it can be shown to emerge in young children before they have been exposed to relevant teaching or reinforcement."
13. Hrdy makes a similar point about maternal care. Mother love is, by her account, natural, but varies depending on circumstances and may sometimes even give rise to a decision to abandon a newborn (Hrdy 1999, 315–17, 376, 378).
14. This account of life in the late Paleolithic is based on Boehm (1999; 2012) and Hrdy (1999; 2009), and to a lesser extent Diamond (2012). Boehm and Hrdy provide much more detailed descriptions of human life in late Paleolithic times, while Diamond describes life in contemporary traditional societies which tend to be larger, more settled, and in more continuous contact with other human societies than the hunter-forager groups that existed prior to the Neolithic Era.
15. As Hrdy (2009, 28) notes, however, "once local conditions promote the emergence of warlike societies, that way of life (as well as the genes of those who excel at it) will spread."
16. Men's greater upper-body strength and speed made them more efficient agricultural workers than women. At the same time, the increased food supply increased the number of living offspring, placing greater demands on women for nursing. Over time, these "small differences" became "much magnified" (Hrdy 1999, 211–13).
17. Many traditional groups believe that fetuses are a composite product of several different men with whom the mother had sexual relations. All these "fathers" typically cooperate in rearing "their" children (Hrdy 1999, 246–7).

18. Noddings, in particular, paints natural caring in a fairly rosy light and characterizes parochialism as exogenous to it.

References

Bakermans-Kranenburg, Marian, and Marinus van Ijzendoorn. 2008. "Oxytocin Receptor (OXTR) and Serotonin Transporter (5-HTT) Genes Associated with Observed Parenting." *Social Cognitive and Affective Neuroscience* 3(2): 128–34.

Bartz, Jennifer, Jamil Zaki, Niall Bolger, and Kevin Ochsner. 2011. "Social Effects of Oxytocin in Humans: Context and Person Matter." *Trends in Cognitive Science* 15(7): 301–9.

Batson, C. Daniel. 1991. *The Altruism Question: Toward a Social-Psychological Answer.* Hillsdale, NJ: Lawrence Erlbaum Associates.

Batson, C. Daniel. 2011. *Altruism in Humans.* Oxford: Oxford University Press.

Bell, David. 2001. "Evolution of Parental Caregiving." *Personality and Social Psychology Review* 5(3): 216–29.

Bloom, Paul. 2013. *Just Babies: The Origins of Good and Evil.* New York: Crown.

Boehm, Christopher. 1999. *Hierarchy in the Forest: The Evolution of Egalitarian Behavior.* Cambridge, MA: Harvard University Press.

Boehm, Christopher. 2012. *Moral Origins: The Evolution of Virtue, Altruism, and Shame.* New York: Basic Books.

Bowlby, John. 1982. *Attachment and Loss*, Vol. 1: *Attachment*, 2nd ed. New York: Basic Books.

Broad, K. D., J. P Curley, and E. B. Keverne. 2006. "Mother–Infant Bonding and the Evolution of Mammalian Social Relationships." *Philosophical Transactions of the Royal Society B.* 361(1476): 2199–214.

Brooks, David. 2007. "Human Nature Redux." *New York Times*, 17 February 2007.

Champagne, Frances, and Michael Meaney. 2001. "Like Mother, Like Daughter: Evidence for Non-genomic Transmission of Parental Behavior and Stress Responsivity." *Progress in Brain Research* (133): 287–302.

Choi, Jung-Kyoo, and Samuel Bowles. 2007. "The Coevolution of Parochial Altruism and War." *Science* 318(5850): 636–40.

Churchland, Patricia. 2011. *Braintrust: What Neuroscience Tells Us about Morality.* Princeton, NJ: Princeton University Press.

Dawkins, Richard. 2006. *The Selfish Gene*, 30th anniversary ed. Oxford: Oxford University Press.

De Dreu, Carsten, Lindred Greer, Michel Handgraaf, Shaul Shalvi, Gerben Van Kleef, Matthijs Baas, Femke Ten Velden, Eric Van Dijk, and Sander Feith. 2010. "The Neuropeptide Oxytocin Regulates Parochial Altruism in Intergroup Conflict among Humans." *Science* 328 (11 June): 1408–11.

De Dreu, Carsten, Lindred Greer, Gerben Van Kleef, Shaul Shalvi, and Michel Handgraaf. 2011. "Oxytocin Promotes Human Ethnocentrism." *Proceedings of the National Academy of Sciences* 108(4): 1262–6.

De Waal, Frans. 1997. "The Chimpanzee's Service Economy: Food for Grooming." *Evolution of Human Behavior* (18): 375–86.

De Waal, Frans. 2006. *Primates and Philosophers: How Morality Evolved*. Princeton, NJ: Princeton University Press.

De Waal, Frans. 2009. *The Age of Empathy: Nature's Lessons for a Kinder Society*. New York: Three Rivers Press.

Diamond, Jared. 2012. *The World Until Yesterday: What Can We Learn from Traditional Societies?* New York: Penguin.

Eisenberg, N., S. Losoya, and T. Spinrad. 2003. "Affect and Prosocial Responding." In *Handbook of Affective Sciences*, edited by R. J. Davidson, K. R. Scherer, and H. H. Goldsmith, 787–803. Oxford: Oxford University Press.

Engster, Daniel. 2007. *The Heart of Justice: Care Ethics and Political Theory*, Oxford: Oxford University Press.

Feldman, Ruth, Ilanit Gordon, and Orna Zagoory-Sharon. 2010. "The Cross-Generation Transmission of Oxytocin in Humans." *Hormones and Behavior* 58(4): 669–76.

Feldman, Ruth, Aron Weller, Orna Zagoory-Sharon, and Ari Levine. 2007. "Evidence for a Neuroendocrinological Foundation of Human Affiliation: Plasma Oxytocin Levels across Pregnancy and the Postpartum Period Predict Mother–Infant Bonding." *Psychological Science* 24(11): 965–70.

Fiske, Susan. 2010. *Social Beings: Core Motives in Social Psychology*, 2nd ed. Hoboken, NJ: Wiley and Sons.

Fuller, Robert. 1992. *Ecology of Care: An Interdisciplinary Analysis of the Self and Moral Obligation*. Louisville, KY: Westminster/John Knox Press.

Gomes, Cristina, Roger Mundry, and Christophe Boesch. 2009. "Long-Term Reciprocation of Grooming in Wild West African Chimpanzees." *Proceedings of the Royal Society B* (276): 699–706.

Graham, Jesse, Jonathan Haidt, Sena Koleva, Matt Motyl, Ravi Iyer, Sean Wojcik, and Peter Ditto. 2013. "Moral Foundations Theory: The Pragmatic Validity of Moral Pluralism." *Advances in Experimental Social Psychology* (47): 55–130.

Greene, Joshua. 2013. *Moral Tribes: Emotion, Reason, and the Gap between Us and Them*. New York: Penguin.

Haidt, Jonathan. 2012. *The Righteous Mind: Why Good People are Divided by Politics and Religion*. New York: Pantheon Books.

Hamington, Maurice. 2010. "The Will to Care: Performance, Expectation, and Imagination." *Hypatia* 25(3): 675–95.

Hamlin, J. Kiley, Neha Mahajan, Zoe Liberman, and Karen Wynn. 2013. "Not Like Me = Bad: Infants Prefer Those Who Harm Dissimilar Others." *Psychological Science* 24(4): 589–94.

Haraway, Donna. 1991. *Simians, Cyborgs, and Women: The Reinvention of Nature*. New York: Routledge.

Heinrichs, Markus, Bernadette von Dawans, and Gregor Domes. 2009. "Oxytocin, Vasopressin, and Human Social Behavior." *Frontiers in Endocrinology* 30(4): 548–57.

Held, Virginia. 1993. *Feminist Morality: Transforming Culture, Society, and Politics*. Chicago, IL: University of Chicago Press.

Held, Virginia. 2002. "Moral Subjects: The Natural and the Normative." *Proceedings and Addresses of the American Philosophical Association* 76(2): 7–24.

Held, Virginia. 2006. *The Ethics of Care: Personal, Political, and Global*. Oxford: Oxford University Press.

Hoffman, Martin. 1981. "Is Altruism Part of Human Nature?" *Journal of Personality and Social Psychology* 40(1): 121–37.

Hoffman, Martin. 2000. *Empathy and Moral Development: Implications for Caring and Justice*. Cambridge: Cambridge University Press.

Hrdy, Sarah Blaffer. 1999. *Mother Nature: Maternal Instincts and How they Shape the Human Species*. New York: Ballantine.

Hrdy, Sarah. 2009. *Mothers and Others: The Evolutionary Origins of Mutual Understanding*. Cambridge, MA: Belknap Press.

Israel, Salomon, Elad Lerer, Idan Shalev, Florina Uzefovsky, Mathias Riebold, Efrat Laiba, Rachel Bachner-Melman, Anat Maril, Gary Bornstein, Ariel Knafo, and Richard Ebstein. 2009. "The Oxytocin Receptor (OXTR) Contributes to Prosocial Fund Allocations in the Dictator Game and the Social Value Orientations Task." *PLoS ONE* 4(5): e5535.

Jaffe, Sara, and Janet Shibley Hyde. 2000. "Gender Differences in Moral Orientation: A Meta-analysis." *Psychological Bulletin* 126(5): 703–26.

Jaggar, Alison. 2000. "Ethics Naturalized: Feminism's Contribution to Moral Epistemology." Metaphilosophy 31(5): 452–68.

Jensen, Keith, Brian Hare, Josep Call, and Michael Tomasello. 2006. "What's In It for Me? Self-regard Precludes Altruism and Spite in Chimpanzees." *Proceedings of the Royal Society B* 273(1589): 1013–21.

Keverne, Eric. 1988. "Central Mechanisms Underlying the Neural and Neuroendocrine Determinants of Maternal Behavior." *Psychoneuroendocrinology* 13(1–2): 127–41.

Keverne, Eric, and K. M. Kendrick. 1990. "Neurochemical Changes Accompanying Parturition and Their Significance for Maternal Behavior." In *Mammalian Parenting: Biochemical, Neurobiological and Behavioral Determinants*, edited by N. A. Krasnegor and R. S. Bridges, 281–304. Oxford: Oxford University Press.

Kim, Heejung, David Sherman, Joni Sasaki, Jun Xu, Thai Chu, Chorong Ryu, Eunkook Suh, Kelsey Graham, and Shelley Taylor. 2010. "Culture, Distress, and Oxytocin Receptor Polymorphism (OXTR) Interact to Influence Emotional Support Seeking." *Proceedings of the National Academy of Sciences of the United States of America* 107(36): 15717–21.

Kittay, Eva. 1999. *Love's Labor: Essays On Women, Equality, and Dependency*. New York: Routledge.

Kittay, Eva Feder. 2009. "The Ethics of Philosophizing: Ideal theory and the Exclusion of People with Severe Cognitive Disabilities." In *Feminist Ethics and Social and Political Philosophy: Theorizing the Non-ideal*, edited by L. Tessman, 121–46. New York: Springer.

Kosfeld, M., M. Heinrichs, P. J. Zak, U. Fischbacher, and E. Fehr. 2005. "Oxytocin Increases Trust in Humans." *Nature* 435(7042), 673–6.

Koyama, N., C. Caws, and F. Aureli. 2006. "Interchange of Grooming and Agonistic Support in Chimpanzees." *International Journal of Primatology* (72): 1293–309.

Lakshminarayanan, V. R., and L. R. Santos. 2008. "Capuchin Monkeys are Sensitive to Others' Welfare." *Current Biology* 18(21): R999–1000.

Langergraber, K. E., J. C. Mitani, and L. Vigilant. 2007. "The Limited Impact of Kinship on Cooperation in Wild Chimpanzees." *Proceedings of the National Academy of Sciences* 104: 7786–90.

Lieberman, Matthew. 2013. *Social: Why Our Brains are Wired to Connect*. Oxford: Oxford University Press.

Lim, Miranda, and Larry Young. 2006. "Neuropeptidergic Regulation of Affiliative Behavior and Social Bonding in Animals." *Hormones and Behavior* 50(5): 506–17.

Lloyd, Elisabeth. 1993. "Pre-theoretical Assumptions in Evolutionary Explanations of Female Sexuality." *Philosophical Studies* 69(2/3): 139–53.

MacDonald, Kai, and Tina Marie MacDonald. 2010. "The Peptide that Binds: A Systematic Review of Oxytocin and its Prosocial Effects in Humans." *Harvard Review of Psychiatry* 18(1): 1–21.

Melis, Alicia, Brian Hare, and Michael Tomasello. 2008. "Do Chimpanzees Reciprocate Received Favours"? *Animal Behavior* (76): 951–62.

Noddings, Nel. 1984. *Caring: A Feminine Approach to Ethics and Moral Education*, Berkeley, CA: University of California Press.

Noddings, Nel. 2002. *Starting at Home: Caring and Social Policy*, Berkeley, CA: University of California Press.

Noddings, Nel. 2005. *The Challenge to Care in Schools: An Alternative Approach to Education*, 2nd ed. New York: Teachers College Press.

Noddings, Nel. 2010. *The Maternal Factor: Two Paths to Morality*, Berkeley, CA: University of California Press.

Nowak, Martin, Corina Tarnita, and Edward Wilson. 2010. "The Evolution of Eusociality." *Nature: International Weekly Journal of Science*, 466(7310): 1057–62.

Richards, David. 2013. *Resisting Injustice and the Feminist Ethics of Care in the Age of Obama*. New York: Routledge.

Rodrigues, Sarina, Laura Saslow, Natalia Garcia, Oliver John, and Dacher Keltner. 2009. "Oxytocin Receptor Genetic Variation Relates to Empathy and Stress Reactivity in Humans." *Proceedings of the National Academy of Sciences* 106(50): 21437–41.

Rothstein, Bo, and Eric Uslaner. 2005. "All for All: Equality, Corruption, and Social Trust." *World Politics* 58(October): 41–71.

Scheele, Dirk, Andrea Wille, Keith Kendrick, Birgit Stoffel-Wagner, Benjamin Becker, Onur Güntürkün, Wolfgang Maier, and René Hurlemann. 2013. "Oxytocin Enhances Brain Reward System Responses in Men Viewing the Face of their Female Partner." *Proceedings of the National Academy of Sciences of the United States of America*. Published online before print 25 November 2013, doi: 10.1073/pnas.1314190110.

Silk, Joan, Sarah Brosnan, Jennifer Vonk, Joseph Henrich, Daniel Povinelli, Amanda Richardson, Susan Lambeth, Jenny Mascaro, and Steven Schapiro. 2005. "Chimpanzees are Indifferent to the Welfare of Unrelated Group Members." *Nature* 437(7063): 1357–9.

Singer, Peter. 1981. *The Expanding Circle: Ethics and Sociobiology*. New York: Farrar, Straus, and Giroux.

Slote, Michael. 2007. *The Ethics of Care and Empathy*. New York: Routledge.

Slote, Michael. 2010a. *Essays on the History of Ethics*. Oxford: Oxford University Press.

Slote, Michael. 2010b. *Moral Sentimentalism*. Oxford: Oxford University Press.

Sober, Elliott, and David Wilson. 1998. *Unto Others: The Evolution and Psychology of Unselfish Behavior*. Cambridge, MA: Harvard University Press.

Suhler, Christopher, and Patricia Churchland. 2011. "Can Innate, Modular 'Foundations' Explain Morality? Challenges for Haidt's Moral Foundations Theory." *Journal of Cognitive Neuroscience* 23(9): 2103–16.

Taylor, Shelley. 2002. *The Tending Instinct: How Nurturing is Essential to Who We Are and How We Live*. New York: Holt.

Tost, Heike, Bhaskar Kolachana, Shabnam Hakimi, Herve Lemaitre, Beth Verchinski, Venkata Mattay, Daniel Weinberger, and Andreas Meyer-Lindenberg. 2010. "A Common Allele in the Oxytocin Receptor Gene (OXTR) Impacts Prosocial Temperament and Human Hypothalamic-Limbic Structure and Function." *Proceedings of the National Academy of Sciences* 107(31): 13936–41.

Tronto, Joan. 1993. *Moral Boundaries: A Political Argument for an Ethic of Care*. New York: Routledge.

Tronto, Joan. 2013. *Caring Democracy: Markets, Equality, Justice*. New York: New York University Press.

Warneken, F., B. Hare, A. Melis, D. Hanus, and M. Tomasello. 2007. "Spontaneous Altruism by Chimpanzees and Young Children." *PLoS Biology* (5): 1414–20.

Warneken, Felix, and Michael Tomasello. 2006. "Altruistic Helping in Human Infants and Young Chimpanzees." *Science* 311(5765): 1301–3.

Warneken, Felix, and Michael Tomasello. 2009. "Varieties of Altruism in Children and Chimpanzees." *Trends in Cognitive Sciences* 13(9): 397–402.

Wilson, David, and Edward O. Wilson. 2008. "Evolution 'for the Good of the Group'." *American Scientist* 96(September–October): 380–9.

Wood, Wendy, and Alice Eagly. 2002. "A Cross-Cultural Analysis of the Behavior of Women and Men: Implications for the Origins of Sex Differences." *Psychological Bulletin* 128(5): 699–727.

Zak, Paul, Angela Stanton, and Sheila Ahmadi. 2007. "Oxytocin Increases Generosity in Humans." *PLOS One 2* (11): 1–5.

14

Theories of care as a challenge to Weberian paradigms in social science

Joan C. Tronto

Comparing Social Theories

Theorists of care began with the quotidian concerns of meeting daily human needs and insisted that such concerns were central to revaluing and reorganizing social life. In this regard, theories of care stand in stark contrast to other social and political theories, which presume the importance of economic concerns of creating resources and political concerns of distributing resources, rather than starting from the endpoint of lived daily lives. The concerns of care are far removed from the centers of power and social change in standard sociological theories; consider, for example, Talcott Parsons' place for such activities as a subset of "latent functions" (Parsons 1949). Indeed, while every society needs to determine ways to care for people, most political and social theories presume that what happens in the realms of care is beneath the concerns of politics (Aristotle 1981), or only one last problem to be addressed by relatively wealthy states. Among classical liberals and neoliberals, the presumption is that care happens in a sphere removed from the state, in the "private" realm. Marxists have seen "reproduction" as the obverse of "production," but, with the exception of feminist Marxists, they have prioritized the forms of power and domination that operate in the realm of "production." Outside of Marxist social science, these structures of power and domination are often taken as background conditions and the work of social scientists is to observe actors working within and against such structures. Substantively, then, care theorists change our perspective when they ask: what happens when we put care, rather than production, distribution, and the maintenance of its systems of power, at the center of social life?

In addition to this substantive change, this chapter argues, focusing on care also transforms the ways in which we might want to think about the nature of social scientific inquiry itself. Following Max Weber, the central task of social science is to look at intended action as the root of what is interesting to study in social life. Through understanding the meaningfulness of action for agents, and the consequences of such actions, social scientists construct their views of reality. Thus, much hinges on the meaning of action from the standpoint of social actors (*Verstehen*). Where social scientists make a contribution to understanding the world more broadly, then, is in revealing and thinking about the *unintended consequences* of such social action.

At a deep level, the standpoint of care results in a challenge to such types of "realist" social theories that follow this Weberian model of sociology. For Weber, intentional human action has (often tragic) unintended consequences and the goal of the social theorist is to explicate and mitigate against these consequences. Part and parcel of this account of social action is a limit to responsibility such that responsibility only fits with foreseeable and intended consequences. Responsibility is thus narrowed: actors have intentions and act to achieve their ends. "Social problems" devolve to others to address. As an illustration of this point, I explore Ulrich Beck's risk society as such a social theory. Risks, which are unintended consequences, are viewed as the great disrupter of contemporary life and the cause of a "second modernity." I raise several criticisms of risk society theory. In the end, I suggest that the danger of a social theory that concentrates on unintended consequences is that it never requires a return to a broader understanding of a problem's context. It seems to close off any views of social forms of responsibility per se. In contrast, I shall argue, intrinsic to the approach of care is a challenge to this approach to social science itself.[1]

The Role of Social Theory

The feminist revolutions of the past century profoundly changed relationships between men and women in their daily lives and material conditions. Not only personal relationships changed. As women began to enter the public world that men had largely made by and for themselves, women began to ask as well about the deeply masculinized assumptions that they had built into that world, and about the ideas and values that had concerned women and others so marginalized. Care was among the essential human values that often inhabited greater standing on the margins of modern capitalist society than closer to its center. Women and men in marginalized groups did and continue to do a disproportionate amount of the caring work in society, both the nurturing forms of care and the "dirty work" of care (see Duffy 2011; Roberts 1997; Glenn 2010). In *Moral Boundaries*, I argued that the world would look very different if we placed care closer to the center of values. In subsequent work, I and many other feminist theorists have begun to explore what this different perspective sees and what it offers as an alternative account of the world (see, *inter alia*, Brugère 2011; Clement 1996; Collins 1990; Engster 2005; 2007; Folbre 1994; 2001; Gilligan 1993; Groenhout 2004; Hamington 2004; Hankivsky 2004; 2006; Kittay 1999; Kittay and Feder 2002; Nedelsky 2011; Pettersen 2008; Robinson 2011; Ruddick 1995; Verkerk 2001; Williams 1999; 2001; Williams and Gavanas 2008; Williams 2010). And yet, despite the fact that this adds up to a social theory that offers a profound alternative, few outside of the feminist and other academic communities (especially in the United States) have paid much attention to this radically different perspective.

In one of the first great works in care theory, Sara Ruddick prescribed the task that informs the argument of this chapter:

> for those who are not already committed to the values of caring labor, a case must be made for the moral and epistemological superiority of the kind of thinking to which it gives rise. This requires specific oppositional comparisons between particular concepts and values of caring labor and their counterparts in dominant, abstractly masculine ways of knowing.... These specific comparisons will reveal incrementally the superiority of the rationality of care to the abstract masculine ways of knowing that dominate our lives. (Ruddick 1995, 136)

Rather than trying to demonstrate the widespread quality of the Weberian approach, I focus on one prominent contemporary theory of social science that reflects this view. The language of "risk society" and the argument that a new form of risk has created a second phase of modernity came into existence in the mid-1980s and gained ground throughout the 1990s. "Risk society" from the outset purported to be about some big questions: modernity, postmodernity, knowledge and science, and the changing nature of (European?) society. Seemingly an objective account of society's changes, the "risk society" theory, especially as propounded by Ulrich Beck in Germany and Anthony Giddens in the UK (and, in a different form, by François Ewald in France), fits the classic model of a middle-level social scientific theory, discussing the "unintended consequences" of social action from a "God's eye" space above society, its normative implications assumed but neither explicitly stated nor explicitly defended. (For several important critiques of such a view, see Tronto 1993; Walker 2007.) Risk society describes a problem and then presumes that its solution lies elsewhere, in other forms of political mediation borrowed, for example, from Habermasian deliberation. But it does not, being an objective social science, address these concerns. The claim made here is that in offering this shape to the problem, humans are already left bereft of solutions to address it.

Before leaving this general account of what a theory can and should do, though, there is one more important issue to raise. When theorists write political and social theories, they reflect their own starting places in the world. They cannot avoid doing so. While some thinkers also make claims that their views represent a perspective that goes beyond their own position, and, indeed, can lay claim to being universally applicable at some time or place, few social theorists will any longer grant such a claim. As long ago as Max Weber, sociologists have recognized that the starting point from which a thinker sees the world will influence, at the very least, the significance she assigns to the facts and patterns that are seen in the world (Shils 1986). But it is interesting how rarely this fact affects the way mainstream, "Northern" social theorists conduct their research or present their views.[2]

In a recent book that sets this problem in a global context, Raewyn Connell argues that, at its founding in the late nineteenth century, sociology's main concern was "global difference": that is, the "difference between the civilisation of the metropole and other cultures whose main feature was their primitiveness" (2007, 7). Connell challenges contemporary social theories of globalization as well, pointing out that virtually all of the theories of globalization produced in the global North involve a "scaling up" of theories that were originally created to describe their own societies to encompass the entire globe, rather than thinking more systematically about world relationships (60).[3] Connell's accusations are serious ones, and suggest to us the ultimate criteria by which we should evaluate social theories: can they extend from their starting observations without doing violence to the social facts in other settings? Can they accommodate the insights of others within their framework? Do they invite inclusion, or suggest that an exclusive worldview is the appropriate place for social theory?

By these criteria, theories of social life that begin and end with "our" lives should raise questions about their general applicability, even if they do help us to understand "our" lives better. But rarely do social theorists in the global North raise these questions on their own about the nature of their social theories, what they purport to say about the world as a whole, and hence, about their reliability as social and political theory.

Indeed, from the standpoint of Weberian social science of intended action-unintended consequence, we might be able to forgive Western social science for its incapacity to see its own limits. From the standpoint of intentional action, it is difficult to argue that it is anyone's fault that the social science frameworks adopted from Western social settings reproduce themselves and discover that the rest of the world is inadequate. But if we change the theoretical frame, and say that theories are also responsible for the misdirection they produce, and that the good intentions of their creators are no grounds for dismissing the harms they produce, we will come to quite another conclusion. So the stakes in this kind of investigation are high indeed.

I shall proceed, then, in this order. I shall begin by describing Beck's risk society and offering a critique of it. I shall then turn to theories of care, and argue that both substantively, and as a way to understand the nature of social scientific practice, care is a more promising possibility.

Risk

As a social theory, "risk society" claims to describe something new: that is, a new phase in modernity. While risk itself is not new, "What has changed is the *nature* of risk." Indeed, Jane Franklin insists, "We have all become acutely aware of how it feels to live in risk society. It seems as though there is no way to negotiate the risks that now present themselves to us: global warming, BSE, the E-coli virus are beyond our control" (Franklin 1998, 1).

What makes this new risk different? Leading thinkers of risk society claim that what makes contemporary risk so different is that it arrives "after nature" and "after tradition," to use Anthony Giddens' language. These new risks no longer match with standard accounts of assigning value and blame. "Risks that were calculable under industrial society become incalculable and unpredictable in the risk society. Compared to the possibilities of adjudging blame and causality in classical modernity, the world risk society possesses no such certainties or guarantees" (Beck 1998, 16). For François Ewald, whose approach is somewhat different from, but parallel to, that of Giddens and Ulrich, new risks move beyond the nineteenth-century assignment of responsibility and beyond the twentieth-century solution of distributing risk through "solidarity." The new risks pose too great a threat, Ewald argues, and have now transformed us into a society based on a "philosophy of precaution" and a "politics of prevention" (Ewald 1993; 2002).

For Ulrich Beck (who as the first theorist of "risk society" will be the focus of this analysis), much is at stake in making the claim that this is a risk society. He sees it as the viable alternative explanation to those who believe that Western societies have entered a period of the "post-modern;" in contrast, argues Beck, this moment is a second moment, a "reflexive" moment, of modernity (Beck et al. 2003). For Beck, this moment is post-industrial and post-class. It is characterized by new sets of concerns. As Beck wrote:

> The driving force in the class society can be summarized in the phrase: I am hungry! The movement set in motion by the risk society, on the other hand, is expressed in the statement, I am afraid! The commonality of anxiety takes the place of the commonality of need. (Beck 1992, 49)

Jane Franklin had said that people now know how it "feels" to live in risk society; though feeling hunger and feeling anxiety are not, perhaps, the same thing. This subjective experience of being afraid, though, is not simply a psychological problem for Beck. In risk society, people also feel that they are out of control: "The subject can no longer be conceived of as master of its surroundings with prescribed boundaries" (Beck et al. 2003, 25). For Beck, the consequences of this anxiety-producing recognition of risk could not be more profound. It transforms not only calculations of insurance and other typical risk management devices, but the entirety of social and political institutions. Beck believes that to live in a "reflexive modernity" does not imply that "people today lead a more conscious life." Instead, "reflexive" signifies not "an increase of mastery and consciousness, but a heightened awareness that mastery is impossible." It is this disenchantment and dissolution of "its own taken-for-granted premises" that "leads to the undermining of every aspect of the nation-state: the welfare state; the power of the legal system; the national economy; the corporatist systems that connected one with the other; and the parliamentary democracy that governed the whole" (2003, 3).

Beck sees these problems as emerging from a "mismatch" between the hazards produced by "late industrial society" and the "rules, institutions, and capacities" to control them. There has been, Beck argues, "organized irresponsibility" around addressing these questions (1998, 18). In the end, Beck argues, we need a more robust account of the ways in which "nobody" and "everybody" will become the "*political subject*" of risk society. New institutions and forms of citizen engagement are necessary to move forward; "the utopia of a responsible modernity, a vision of society in which the consequences of technological development and economic change are debated before the key decisions are taken. The burden of proof regarding future risks and hazards and current environment degradation would lie with the perpetrators rather than the injured party." Such a "*second Enlightenment,*" Beck argues, will realize the opportunities, and not succumb to the despair, that this second modernity requires (1998, 21).

Beck's argument about risk society thus purports to describe the problems of contemporary life. His writing is widely read; the questions of risk society and second modernity are considered in numerous books and whole issues of sociological journals. Risk society is an extension of the classical Weberian approach: it describes the unintended consequences of deliberate and intentional action. Where to begin a critique of this approach? As Marxist scholars often observe, to transform unintended consequences into a reified process (such as "rationalization" or "globalization") over which humans can no longer exercise control mystifies and distorts possibilities for action (Marcuse 1971). From a feminist perspective,[4] Beck's description of the ills of modern life and his analysis of their origins are suspect for different reasons that nonetheless revolve around the kinds of masculinist assumptions built into the intended action/unintended consequence model of social theory.[5] Let me raise three main criticisms feminists might raise against the description of the present moment as risk society: the limited human subjects whom Beck includes within his theoretical frame, Beck's failure to identify properly the political agents who have made these "second modernization" processes possible and problematic, and Beck's continuing concern with values of mastery and control as the defining human condition. Taken together, these points demonstrate that Beck's account of risk society remains highly masculinist as well. After examining this feminist critique, we will then be in a good position to see the difference between risk and care.

First, let us consider Beck's limited sense of the human subjects whom he includes in his account of modern society. When Ulrich Beck says "we," whom does he mean?[6] Some scholars have argued that he means "Germans" (Dingwall 1999). Even if we expand this point, though, his description that "anxiety" has replaced hunger means that he is not speaking about the poor. Perhaps he primarily means people already living in "modernity": that is, in Europe. But the problem with that account is that he also claims that there is a world risk society, and that his analysis is global. When Beck writes, for example, that we used to seek risk for a thrill, he is writing about the lives of certain kinds of people. The lives of the poor and marginalized are much more risky and they do not find such risks thrilling (Fineman 2008). Women are told that they are in constant danger of sexual violence. Young black men are killed in Florida and juries find that the shooters were just following an imperative to "stand your ground." Beck is writing about and for people who have achieved a certain degree of control over their material conditions, but that, sadly, does not describe everyone.

Second, Beck offers an account of what is moving us from the old to the new modernity that is remarkably sanitized of actual political actors. For Beck, the changes that are occurring are a result of the incapacity of "science" and "technology" to grasp the risks that they are imposing upon us. But Beck's language ignores the places from which "science" and "technology" have an impetus to move forward. Insofar as he is unwilling to name capitalism as a key source of the processes that lead to the "speedup" of science and technology, it is difficult to take his view as complete. After all, BCE is caused by feeding cows with a commercial food that contains BCE-infected portions of the nervous systems of other cows. Within traditional farming, who would ever have conceived of such a practice as a good idea? But pushed by a desire for greater profits, the imperative to eke every drop of use out of animals turned domestic animals into cannibals.

Beck sometimes reveals an understanding of this point; he acknowledges that "this deeply politicizing meaning of the risk society argument can be used not only by environmentalists but also by global capital, and more effectively too" (1998, 11–12). But this is a very weak recognition of the role that global capital plays in this process.

Instead, Beck begins to refer to risk in the passive voice: "We no longer choose to take risks, we have them thrust upon us" (1998, 12). But this is a strange notion: who is doing the thrusting? Beck does not want to name the drive for capitalist profits as the cause of these increased risks; instead, he suggests that, "Given that risks are no longer attributable to external agency," we are in a state of "organized irresponsibility" (1998, 15).

Similarly, Beck writes as if the interest of people in the welfare state has just dried up because it is no longer of interest to them. But Beck ignores the fact that the hard-won rights of workers to healthcare, pensions, and unemployment protection were a result of political struggles. Now that the political economy has shifted and workers are no longer so strong, these protections for them have eroded. But the change is not because the world is more risky, it is because political elites now claim that the cost of protection has grown too high and workers have lost the ability to insist that these costs can and should be paid.

What Beck perceives, instead, is that the political activism is the *consequence* of risk society rather than something else. He believes that the social dislocation that people experience are the "side-effects" (Beck et al. 2003) of the other problems that he has identified, and that these side-effects produce a "politicization." Beck fails to note that all of these concerns about safety, risk, about how people live their lives, have *always* been politicized; it is just that now the expression of these political consequences is not contained in the state and in the competition for state power. When working-class political parties actually represented a radical alternative that supported working-class political aims, the state put in place social institutions that created solidaristic solutions to what Beck might call "risk." Beck's gloss on Ewald's *L'Etat Providence* is, in this respect, revealing. Beck writes:

> To me, [Ewald's] theory represents a basic shift in the interpretation of the welfare state. While the majority of social scientists have sought to explain the origins and construction of the welfare state in terms of class interests, the maintenance of social order or the enhancement of national productivity and military power, this argument understands the provision of services (health care), the creation of insurance schemes (pensions and unemployment insurance) and the regulation of the economy and the environment in terms of the creation of security. (2003, 20)

What Beck fails to notice, though, is that even if Ewald is correct to say that the creation of the welfare state created security, this does not erase the actual history: people acted politically to push the state to provide for all of their security. The kind of political activity that Beck sees is more a kind of symptom, a kind of static excitement, than an effective response to risk society.

The third problem in Beck's work is his ongoing description of the problem as a lack of mastery and control. What does mastery and control mean? How much should we be able to control? Beck seems to think that scientists should be able to control the effects of their work. This has never been the case. But at the present moment, according to those who describe society as a risk society, these preoccupations have displaced other ways to think about social problems. In the words of Barbara Hudson, "'Risk society' analyses of contemporary life suggest that risk has become a central, generalized preoccupation, to the extent that it is configuring contemporary institutions and contemporary consciousness" (2003, 43).

The seriousness of this sense of a loss of control emerges when we think about what those who still are hoping for mastery do in the face of such unease. Hudson (2003, 59) argues that it signals a shift from risk management to risk control:

> Risk management is an acceptance of risk, a pooling of risk amongst people who see themselves as a group of some sort; risk control is a refusal of risk, it is the response to risks posed by people we do not associate ourselves with.

In this way, she contends, "The values of the unsafe society displace those of the unequal society" (43).

As society moves toward a larger concern with trying to protect the "safety" of those with whom one identifies, it is easy to see the ways in which risk society quickly supports an agenda of wars on terror, on demonizing the other.

One interesting feature of this risk society argument is to note how gendered it is. This is not about men and women, but it is about masculinity and femininity. What characterizes masculine roles in society is that they are tied to protection (Stiehm 1982; Young 2003). Risk society creates an image of the world as "risky," which then requires an understanding of the social world as dangerous and of the human task as protection and management. Risk society thus operates in a masculine metaphorical universe. In a way, then, the argument of "risk society" is an attempt to reassert masculine centrality in a world that looks controlled by "feminine" processes such as increasing comfort and intimacy.[7]

At the same time, the new understanding of risk in risk society is a way to reassert a kind of chastened masculinity. This is the new—to use Weber's phrase—"stigma of our human dignity" (Roth 1978, xxxiii). There is a kind of male heroism, recasting individual and collective threats and lives. It is interesting to see how little Beck mentions gender, and how little credence he gives to new social movements. After feminists criticized his work for ignoring the different place of men and women in the workforce, and how the changes in the workforce have affected men and women differently, he responded by writing a book with his wife that repeats a frequent ploy. In arguing that the chaos in love is "normal," Beck follows a well-trodden path of describing the lives of women, and their concerns, as somehow "outside" of history. Risk has changed modernity, but women and their concerns remain stuck in their old-fashioned, timeless, concerns (Beck and Beck-Gernsheim 1995).

It is intriguing that at the same time that risk society accomplishes this task of reasserting the desirability of masculine control of the outcome of action, it also throws other forms of risk back on to women as individuals. What this represents, above all, is an incapacity to think clearly about responsibility. Beck seems to think that scientists once upon a time had control over their research: "Scientists are becoming lay persons. They do not know what will happen before they begin their research," but now they have lost that control and "there is no one responsible" (1998, 14). If no one is responsible, then things are out of control.

Beck's hope is that somehow citizens will regain trust, through institutions in civil society and through a broadened sphere of political activity, in science and technology. More communication, more opportunities for deliberation, and greater transparency will provide the democratic tools by which citizens will be able to reimpose greater controls in the spheres of science, technology, and environment. Ewald is more optimistic in thinking that the kinds of political processes that exist in the moment of "solidarity" persist, and will assist, in the control of "providence." But the evidence of the past thirty years does not support the view of greater and more meaningful citizen involvement. Instead, the "democratic deficit" has grown.

In short, then, Beck's account of risk society portrays a view of modernity that is nostalgic for a world in which the excesses of capitalism did not present themselves so harshly to men of his standing. As others have gained political power, as Europe has ceased to be the center, as men have lost control, it is not surprising that so many social theorists have found the world to be a place of risk. But the ways in which they describe these risks are more a reflection of their own anxieties than a useful way to think about how people might move forward to offer the world greater protection. To describe the present world as one of "organized irresponsibility" begs the obvious question: how might people, politically, go about reassigning responsibilities in such a way that the "new risks" are controlled? Beck suggests that it is impossible to do so. But why?

Care as an Alternative

Around the same time that Ewald began to write about the "providential society" and Beck began to posit the "risk society," feminist scholars who had been rethinking traditional feminine values associated with caring began to make broader claims for the political value of caring (Ruddick 1989; 1995; Tronto 1987; 1993; Collins 1989; 1990). Among the key questions raised by these early feminist texts is: what are the political values that are associated with women's place in society? Patricia Hill Collins, looking at the experience of African-American women, noted that a "care ethic" emerged as black women tried to support and defend their families in a hostile society. Sara Ruddick posited the philosophical richness of the practices of "maternal thinking" and argued that a "politics of peace" followed from taking seriously mothers' desires to preserve their children. Tronto's early work expanded practices of care to the entire world. As Berenice Fisher and Tronto wrote:

> On the most general level, we suggest that caring be viewed as *a species activity that includes everything that we do to maintain, continue, and repair our 'world' so that we can live in it as well as possible.* That world includes our bodies, our selves, and our environment, all of which we seek to interweave in a complex, life-sustaining web. (Fisher and Tronto 1990, 40)

Care has always been, and will always be, a part of human life. For the most part, and throughout most of human history, though, care has been left to women and to others who are marginalized: servants, slaves, lower-class and lower-caste people, many of whom are marked as "other" by race or religion or language, or by their very work as caregivers. Social scientists have rarely paid much attention to care, and indeed to the changes in how care is organized. As feminists and scholars of slavery, servancy, and the working class have begun to look more closely at care, though, a history of care that parallels the development of what Giddens calls "the affective sphere" could be written, separating out, throughout the nineteenth and twentieth centuries, some forms of "nurturing" care and making them more professional, while leaving "the dirty work" still to women and men from the lower classes and from racial and other minority groups (Duffy 2011).

Care is not simply a sentiment or disposition, and it is not simply a set of actions. It is a complex set of practices, which range from very intimate ones, such as "maternal thinking" (Ruddick 1989/1995) to extremely broad practices, such as devising public systems of education (Noddings 2005). In 1990, Fisher and Tronto proposed four phases of care, and Tronto later added a fifth phase and five moral dimensions of these phases (Tronto 1993, 126–37; 2013). Care processes are complex; they require caring about, caring for, caregiving, care receiving, and caring with. They also require the refinement of many moral qualities, including attentiveness, deep reflection on responsibility, competence in caregiving, and responsiveness both to care receivers and to the process and effectiveness of care itself. Finally, caring with requires the qualities of solidarity and trust.

Understood in this broadest way, and as a practice among people as they "care with" each other to distribute responsibilities for care in their society, this is obviously also a way to describe and to think about political power. But this is a different way to think about power than thinking about it as a form of mastery and control. From the standpoint of care, humans are different and the nature of their action is different.

In the first place, care is *relational* and assumes that people, other beings, and the environment are interdependent (see, among others, Groenhout 2004; Koggel 1998; 2006a; 2006b; Robinson 1999; 2008; 2011; Nedelsky 2011). The care worldview is not about "bodies in motion" that collide, or about unforeseen consequences of such collisions. Instead, care presumes that people become autonomous and capable of acting on their own through a complex process of growth, in which they are both interdependent and transformed as they live. They can be more or less attentive to the effects they have on others and the world, though care approaches err on the side of being more, rather than less, attentive. Assigning responsibility is a collective act, not an abstract or scientific or legal endeavor.

Second, rather than thinking of deliberate action to change the world as the most important way to see society, care theories posit that, in addition to creation, care activities (such as repair, maintenance, and continuity) are equally central to human life and activity. And here, all humans are at once both recipients and givers of care. While the typical images of care are that those who are able-bodied and adult give care to children, the elderly, and the infirm, it is also the case that all able-bodied adults receive care from others, and from themselves, every day. Children as young as ten months old imitate the activity of feeding; they try to feed their caregivers and they open their mouths as the spoon nears the other person's mouth (Bråten 2003). Children describe their activities as caring for parents (Mullin 2005). People are both givers and receivers of care all the time, though their capacities and needs shift for each person throughout life. At any moment in a society, there are those who are the neediest and those who are the most capable of helping themselves and others. This shifting in needs and capacities for care are an important way to think about how our human lives change through time.

But there is another consequence for social theory that comes from the slipperiness of caring and being cared for, the changes and particularities of care from historical, cultural, material, and even psychological conditions. Care theory does not posit that care is perfect, or that it even attains the status of achieving the purpose for which it has been undertaken, which is part of the mastery and control implicit in the intended action model of social life. Instead, there are dangers to the inadequacy of care contained within the practice itself. The most serious of these are paternalism (when caregivers presume that their understanding of caring needs is superior to those of the cared-for) and parochialism (when caregivers presume that they can set the limits to how far their circle of care must extend). Both of these dangers are great: they result in domination, abuse of power, and conversely, neglect. But rather than presuming that these are unintended consequences, and therefore something for someone else to clean up, theories of care presume that these problems are intrinsic to the care process itself. Thus, care theory leads logically to a broader and more democratic perspective, including the cared-for's accounts of needs. From the standpoint of care, it is never appropriate simply to say, "That was not intended" as a defense against a careless act.

At first glance, focusing on care rather than on risk may seem simply to be looking at the same issue from a different standpoint. And, scholars such as Beck may argue, the separation of science and technology allows greater precision in describing human action. Indeed, both social theories seem to end in the same place, in calling for greater involvement on the part of citizens and other democratic political actors. Does it change anything if the language of responsibility is used instead of the language of risk? In fact, to look at the issues raised by Beck and others in thinking about risk society from the standpoint of care changes profoundly how to think about "risk."

Viewing the World of Risk from the Standpoint of Care

From the standpoint of a society that was organized around the goal of caring well, "risk" would look very different. Care posits a different kind of social science.

In contrast to such social theories, care has a different ontology, a different epistemology, and a different account of social theory. As ontology, care posits that human vulnerability is key in understanding who and what humans are. This is not to deny the importance of autonomous and willful activity, but such autonomy is an achievement, not a starting point. Humans are vulnerable and needy not only at some points in their lives, but throughout their lives, though with varying degrees of vulnerability and depending upon their abilities and status (including their status as members of oppressed groups).

Care posits the centrality of starting from relationship, and looking at the ways in which needs are met in common. This epistemological starting point finds inadequate the assumption that individuals pursue social ends and produce external, unintended consequences. Instead, care consists of messy feedback loops and overlapping forms of responsibility, and requires the consideration of multiple perspectives (those of the cared-for and many caregivers at many levels). Care does not leave unintended consequences outside of its own process. Indeed, care theorists have identified two likely kinds of outcomes that must always be monitored: the dangers that care will become parochial (too local and concerned only with others in near proximity) and that care will become too paternalistic (i.e., that the views of caregivers will predominate over the views of those who need care). Because these problems are considered within the framework itself, not as unintended or remote consequences, the theory requires that participants within care processes, if they care well, consider them.

This more holistic form of social theorizing can be focused in on more narrow practices of care, or broadened out to include "everything we do to continue, maintain, and repair our world so that we may live in it as well as possible" (which is how Fisher and Tronto originally define care). Such a social theory may not provide immediate answers to the problems it uncovers, but it does help to clarify why feminist care theorists find their approach more generative of solutions than one that views the problem as one of "unintended consequences."

First, insofar as a care perspective starts from human vulnerability, the notion that risk was somehow once contained but is now more rampant looks quite different. Risk was not formerly a rare, thrill-seeking activity; all humans are vulnerable, though not equally so and not all at the same time. This is not to say that new forms of risk are not grave. But as Ewald explains, using the doctrine of precaution, we might be able to limit them. The problem, of course, is that we need to recognize where these dangers come from in the first place. Beck emphasizes the ways in which scientists cannot know the dangers of the risks to which their work exposes us. But feminist scholars have observed frequently the ways in which scientists couch their own work so that they can engage in a kind of "privileged irresponsibility," of not knowing the consequences of their actions. A classic feminist study of this sort is Carol Cohn's (1987) investigation of defense intellectuals and the ways in which they avoid speaking about death. Beck seems to believe that nothing can stop this kind of scientific advance whose consequences cannot be known. But as Herbert Marcuse argued about Weber's own sense of uncontrollable consequences of actions, insofar as humans create the conditions of processes of rationalization, they can also, if they understand them differently, control the consequences (Marcuse 1971). Is it possible to have scientific pluralism that is also responsible? Answering this question depends upon setting the boundaries of such responsibility. That they are now very wide is true. Yet there does not seem to be any reason why talking about their breadth should be impossible, as Beck seems to suggest.

Indeed, though, if we look more closely at the nature of risk, perhaps it is better captured by the feminist care category of vulnerability. Ruddick made this important point: "Children are vulnerable creatures and as such elicit either aggression or care" (1995, 166). This point is worth close attention. From the standpoint of mastery and control, both aggression and care are dangerous prospects; perhaps this is why vulnerability is so threatening in risk society. Aggression is likely to be harmful, care might be infantilizing. If risk makes one vulnerable, then, there are important reasons to try to avoid it.

Iris Marion Young (2003) argued that in the current security state, one effect of "masculinist protection" was to infantilize citizens and make them afraid. Yet Young's admonition to citizens that they should act in a more adult manner does not help to explain how they might do so. If people are legitimately afraid of the aggressive acts of others, it is difficult for them not to be frozen from acting. If people need care and sense that they are not getting it, they may react by lashing out at others whom they perceive as a threat and as the reasons why they are not receiving this care (Hage 2003). Beck describes the existence of new forms of risk as the cause of "side-effects" that include a loss of trust. But from the feminist standpoint, Beck has the problem backwards. What causes the sense of greater risk is the absence of trust. To be part of a society in which one feels that everyone is "caring with" one another to identify and address collective problems creates the conditions for recognizing and dealing more honestly with these dangers. From the standpoint of care, rather than leave these "risks" outside to be dealt with after the fact, the purposes of political life would be reshaped so that concerns about living well and coping with such "risks" were on the political agenda. It becomes possible to deal with the risky consequences of action only once people are no longer "afraid" (or "hungry"). Thus, with a caring approach it is easier to see the democratic possibilities of broader involvement, even as that involvement requires the more difficult tasks of thinking carefully about responsibilities.

One more important point emerges from Ruddick's view that vulnerability invites either aggression or care. While caring for the vulnerable does not exclude the possibility of aggression, it does lead to this question: are the two responses exclusive? That is, can caring make people less vulnerable to aggression? It seems that the answer to this question is complicated. If caring meets the needs that made people vulnerable in the first place, then it will presumably also eliminate the grounds for aggression. But to answer in this way does not resolve the issue; rather, it reveals another problem with the account of risk society. Caring requires a robust account of needs and social, political, and intellectual processes for recognizing the nature of needs. Risk society starts from the presumption that society does not discuss needs, but suffers the consequences of others acting in accordance with their own views of their rights. In a care society, some rebalancing of needs and rights would be a part of the ongoing political discussion. It would not necessitate that all rights be surrendered, but it would make it less necessary to maintain mastery and control over the self, society, and the world.

In this way, care goes beyond even the feminist critique to suggest that we need to rebalance the ways in which "risk" is conceived in the short run and the long run. As the feminist economist Nancy Folbre has observed, focusing on the economic needs of the short term is in keeping with market thinking, but produces long-term costs. So, too, risk society presumes that there is no way to control the production of risks, only their consequences. Care requires that politics goes beyond the short run to include the long-run provision of care. In that way, it is more likely to exercise a principle like Ewald's "precaution," and to be able to curb some excessive risks.

The final advantage of a caring approach takes us back to one of the opening concerns of this text. Insofar as we need to be able to recognize that theorizing starts from specific social locations, the breadth of the concern of care is an advantage. Care is not the entirety of human existence, but it is a large part of human existence and it involves humans in a variety of essential activities. But while the needs for human care, at the most general level, are universal, the ways in which caring needs will be met are highly specific to the caring practices of particular societies, groups, and individuals. Questions about the justice of forms of care, whether the needs of everyone are actually being met, form the basis for making social judgments. Southern theories may not now begin from or end with care, but asking them to do so does not do violence to them, or ignore them. It does require, though, attentiveness to the experiences of people everywhere in the world. That humans around the globe have different capacities to care for themselves and their world is also true. Addressing these imbalances will require a great deal of thought and action. It should shape our future intellectual agendas.

Risk presumes that people live in a dangerous and untrustworthy world, in large part because it is out of their individual control. This is a world filled with fear, with scholars like Beck hoping for a transition to something with greater safety. When the loss of control that only existed previously for rather well-to-do men is mourned, not everyone will feel the poignancy of this loss. Care presumes that people live in a world in which they cope all the time with vulnerability and need, yet somehow also manage to live with joy. The injustices of the unequal burdens of care are urgent social problems. These real injustices, and not the loss of a false sense of mastery and control, are the right problems for social theorists to address.

Notes

1. This chapter is largely based upon some previous work, though I have sharpened and updated the arguments made here. This is the first time these ideas appear in English (see Tronto 2012).

2. Scholars of feminist and critical race theory seem to be exceptional in admitting that their starting place influences their results.
3. She continues: "This scaling-up was structured by a prior concern—to avoid the main existing theories that understood power on a world scale as worldwide domination. This is quite logical, as the concept of abstract linkage is not compatible with the experience of being colonised. The sociological discourse of globalisation, as it emerged in the early 1990s, explicitly distanced itself from theories of imperialism and neocolonialism, and had at best an embarrassed relationship with world-systems analysis. There was a widespread refusal, in the literature based on a concept of abstract linkage, of any analysis that *named the metropole* as the centre of power, as the agent of cultural domination, or as the site of accumulation. Writers such as Bauman and Beck could certainly *recognise* differences between the global rich and the global poor, but the concept of globalisation gave them no coherent way of *explaining* these differences."
4. There have been relatively few feminist critiques of Beck. I have found especially useful Hudson (2003) and Beer (1992).
5. Bologh (1990) remains an important account of the masculinist elements of Weber's work.
6. For a different feminist argument about "who counts," written from a justice perspective, see Fraser (2009). I will discuss the issue of different feminist approaches later.
7. Studying masculinity and the ways it shapes the lives of women and men is a key part of what gender studies now requires. One important American form of masculinity, for example, abandoning families and problems and going on the road, is only partly forestalled in a risk society. This would be an interesting question for future investigation, but beyond the scope of this project. On this form of masculinity, which Michael Kimmel called "fantasies of escape" (1996, 36), see Faludi (1999) and Kimmel (1996).

References

Aristotle. 1981. *The Politics*. New York: Penguin.

Beck, U. 1992. *Risk Society: Towards a New Modernity*. London: Sage.

Beck, U. 1998. "Politics of Risk Society." In *The Politics of Risk Society*, edited by J. Franklin, 9–22. Cambridge: Polity.

Beck, U., and E. Beck-Gernsheim. 1995. *The Normal Chaos of Love*. Cambridge: Polity.

Beck, U., W. Bonss, and C. Lau. 2003. "The Theory of Reflexive Modernization." *Theory, Culture and Society* 20: 1–33.

Beer, U. 1992. "Das Geschlechterverhältnis in der 'Risikogesellschaft'". *Feministische Studien* 10: 99–105.

Bologh, R. W. 1990. *Love or Greatness: Max Weber and Masculine Thinking—A Feminist Inquiry*. London/Boston, MA: Unwin Hyman.

Bråten, S. 2003. "Participant Perception of Others' Acts: Virtual Otherness in Infants and Adults." *Culture and Psychology* 9: 261–76.

Brugère, F. 2011. *L'Ethique du "Care."* Paris: Presses Universitaire de France.
Clement, G. 1996. *Care, Autonomy, and Justice: Feminism and the Ethic of Care.* Boulder, CO: Westview Press.
Cohn, C. 1987. "Sex and Death in the Rational World of Defense Intellectuals." *Signs* 12: 687–718.
Collins, P. H. 1989. "The Social Construction of Black Feminist Thought." *Signs* 14: 745–73.
Collins, P. H. 1990. *Black Feminist Thought.* New York: Routledge.
Connell, R. 2007. *Southern Theory.* Malden, MA: Polity.
Dingwall, R. 1999. "'Risk Society': The Cult of Theory and the Millennium?" *Social Policy and Administration* 33: 474–91.
Duffy, M. 2011. *Making Care Count: A Century of Gender, Race, and Paid Care Work.* New Brunswick, NJ: Rutgers University Press.
Engster, D. 2005. "Rethinking Care Theory: The Practice of Caring and the Obligation to Care." *Hypatia* 20: 50–74.
Engster, D. 2007. *The Heart of Justice: Care Ethics and Political Theory.* New York: Oxford.
Ewald, F. 1993. "Two Infinities of Risk." In *The Politics of Everyday Fear,* edited by B. Massumi, 221–8. Minneapolis, MN: University of Minnesota Press.
Ewald, F. 2002. "The Return of Descartes' Malicious Devil: An Outline of a Philosophy of Precaution." In *Embracing Risk: The Changing Culture of Insurance and Responsibility,* edited by T. Baker and J. Simon, 273–301. Chicago, IL: University of Chicago Press.
Faludi, S. 1999. *Stiffed: The Betrayal of the American Man.* New York: Harper Collins.
Fineman, M. A. 2008. "The Vulnerable Subject: Anchoring Equality in the Human Condition." *Yale Journal of Law and Feminism* 20: 1–24.
Fisher, B., and J. C. Tronto. 1990. "Toward a Feminist Theory of Caring." In *Circles of Care,* edited by E. Abel and M. Nelson, 36–54. Albany, NY: State University of New York Press.
Folbre, N. 1994. *Who Pays for the Kids? Gender and the Structure of Constraint.* London/New York: Routledge.
Folbre, N. 2001. *The Invisible Heart: Economics and Family Values.* New York: New Press.
Franklin, J. 1998. "Introduction." In *The Politics of Risk Society,* edited by J. Franklin, 1–8. Cambridge: Polity.
Fraser, N. 2009. "Who Counts? Dilemmas of Justice in a Postwestphalian World." *Antipode* 41: 281–97.
Gilligan, C. 1993. *In a Different Voice: Psychological Theory and Women's Development.* Cambridge, MA: Harvard University Press.
Glenn, E. N. 2010. *Forced to Care: Coercion and Caregiving in America.* Cambridge, MA: Harvard University Press.
Groenhout, R. E. 2004. *Connected Lives: Human Nature and an Ethics of Care.* Lanham, MD: Rowman and Littlefield.
Hage, G. 2003. *Against Paranoid Nationalism.* Annandale, NSW: Pluto Press Australia.
Hamington, M. 2004. *Embodied Care: Jane Addams, Maurice Merleau-Ponty, and Feminist Ethics.* Urbana, IL: University of Illinois Press.
Hankivsky, O. 2004. *Social Policy and the Ethic of Care.* Vancouver: University of British Columbia Press.

Hankivsky, O. 2006. "Imagining Ethical Globalization: The Contributions of a Care Ethic." *Journal of Global Ethics* 2: 91–110.

Hudson, B. 2003. *Justice in the Risk Society*. Thousand Oaks, CA: Sage.

Kimmel, M. S. 1996. *Manhood in America: A Cultural History*. New York: Free Press.

Kittay, E. F. 1999. *Love's Labor: Essays on Women, Equality and Dependency*. New York: Routledge.

Kittay, E. F., and E. K. Feder. 2002. *The Subject of Care: Feminist Perspectives on Dependency*. Lanham, MD: Rowman and Littlefield.

Koggel, C. M. 1998. *Perspectives on Equality: Constructing a Relational Theory*. Lanham, MD: Rowman and Littlefield.

Koggel, C. M. 2006a. "Global Inequalities and Relational Ethics." Paper delivered at the Annual Meeting of the American Political Science Association, Philadelphia, PA.

Koggel, C. M. 2006b. *Moral Issues in Global Perspective: Human Diversity and Equality*, 2nd ed. Toronto: Broadview.

Marcuse, H. 1971. "Industrialization and Capitalism." In *Max Weber and Sociology Today*, edited by O. Stammer, 133–51. New York: Harper and Row.

Mullin, A. 2005. "Trust, Social Norms, and Motherhood." *Journal of Social Philosophy* 36: 316–30.

Nedelsky, J. 2011. *Law's Relations*. New York: Oxford University Press.

Noddings, N. 2005. *The Challenge to Care in Schools: An Alternative Approach to Education*. New York: Teachers College Press.

Parsons, T. 1949. *The Structure of Social Action*. New York: Free Press.

Pettersen, T. 2008. *Comprehending Care: Problems and Possibilities in the Ethics of Care*. Lanham, MD: Lexington Books.

Roberts, D. 1997. "Spiritual and Menial Housework." *Yale Journal of Law and Feminist* 9: 51–80.

Robinson, F. 1999. *Globalizing Care: Ethics, Feminist Theory, and International Relations*. Boulder, CO: Westview Press.

Robinson, F. 2008. "The Importance of Care in the Theory and Practice of Human Security." *Journal of International Political Theory* 4: 167–88.

Robinson, F. 2011. *The Ethics of Care and Global Politics*. Philadelphia, PA: Temple University Press.

Roth, G. 1978. "Introduction." In *Economy and Society*, edited by M. Weber, xxxiii–cviii. Berkeley, CA: University of California Press.

Ruddick, S. 1989. *Maternal Thinking: Toward a Politics of Peace*. Boston, MA: Beacon Press.

Ruddick, S. 1995. *Maternal Thinking: Toward a Politics of Peace*. Boston, MA: Beacon Press.

Shils, E. 1986. *Max Weber: Methodology of the Social Sciences*. New York: Free Press.

Stiehm, J. H. 1982. "The Protected, the Protector, the Defender." *Women Studies International Forum* 5: 367–76.

Tronto, J. 1987. "Beyond Gender Difference to a Theory of Care." *Signs: Journal of Women in Culture and Society* 12: 644–63.

Tronto, J. C. 1993. *Moral Boundaries: A Political Argument for an Ethic of Care*. New York: Routledge.

Tronto, J. C. 2012. *Le Risque ou le "care"?* Paris: Presses Universitaires de France.

Tronto, J. C. 2013. *Caring Democracy: Markets, Equality and Justice*. New York: New York University Press.

Verkerk, M. 2001. "The Care Perspective and Autonomy." *Medicine, Health Care and Philosophy* 4: 289–94.

Walker, M. U. 2007. *Moral Understandings: A Feminist Study in Ethics*. New York: Oxford University Press.

Williams, F. 1999. "Good-Enough Principles for Welfare." *Journal of Social Policy* 28: 667–88.

Williams, F. 2001. "In and Beyond New Labour: Towards a New Political Ethics of Care." *Critical Social Policy* 21: 467.

Williams, F., and A. Gavanas. 2008. "The Intersection of Childcare Regimes and Migration Regimes: A Three-Country Study." In *Migration and Domestic Work: A European Perspective on a Global Theme*, edited by H. Lutz, 13–28. Aldershot, UK: Ashgate.

Williams, J. 2010. *Reshaping the Work–Family Debate: Why Men and Class Matter*. Cambridge, MA: Harvard University Press.

Young, I. M. 2003. "The Logic of Masculinist Protection: Reflections on the Current Security State." *Signs: Journal of Women in Culture and Society* 29: 1–25.

15

Politics is not a game

The radical potential of care

Maurice Hamington

Care is irrepressible. It is like the weed that grows through the cracks of a city sidewalk. If the human will to care exists, even repressive circumstances cannot stop it. The genocidal intent of the Holocaust certainly represents the antithesis of a caring context. In the early 1940s, the Nazis implemented the Final Solution, a plan to kill all the Jews of Europe and North Africa. The Nazis controlled France at this time and, as in the rest of occupied Europe, Jews were rounded up and sent to concentration camps. In defiance of the Nazis and the Vichy government, members of a small community in south-central France, Le Chambon-sur-Lignon, decided to assist and care for the fugitive Jews. Led by André Trocmé and Edouard Theis, the people of Le Chambon saved between 3,000 and 5,000 Jews from almost-certain death during the German occupation of France. Located near an SS Division, the Chambonnais hid refugees, fed and generally cared for them, moved them to the countryside when there were raids and inspections, and provided many with falsified papers to aid in their escape. These otherwise ordinary townspeople acted benevolently despite great personal risk. Several Chambonnais were ultimately discovered and killed because of their subterfuge, including Trocmé's cousin, Daniel.

Philosopher Philip Hallie who chronicled the events of Le Chambon during World War II struggles to find a clear ethical explanation for the moral heroism of the townspeople. Despite not having the lens of care theory available to him, Hallie does, however, recognize that simply applying traditional Western moral theory to the action of the Chambonnais is unsatisfying: "The study of ethics must not be afflicted with ecological impoverishment. It must not be a way of trying, by a use of abstract, traditional terms, to cast a fitful light within the inward worlds of men's souls... It must concern itself with the *story* of what individuals do in the context of the story of their times" (1994, 280). Here, Hallie decries abstraction and notes the ethical significance of particularism. Pertinent to the discussion of care theory that follows, Hallie locates the moral import of what the Chambonnais accomplished in terms of caring political action. What they did defied notions of moral calculation or what ethical principles could compel an individual to do. Hallie describes the care that the Chambonnais exhibited as much more than a disposition of empathy: "the Chambonnais cared about what had happened, and cared enough not only to feel pain at the suffering of the victims but also enough to make inferences about future events. They cared enough to think and plan" (106). Ultimately, they took action. Ethics was not a game to the people of Le Chambon, governed by rules of consequence maximization or moral command. It was a human connection to someone in need characterized by empathy, imagination, and action. The choices they made were not only morally significant; they influenced their sense of self-identity and their understanding of the circumstances.[1]

The story of the people of Le Chambon reinforces that caring is simultaneously deeply personal, relational, and political. Although care is resilient, shining through humanity's darkest hours, it is not an autonomous force. Care is a human response to our mutual interdependency (Hankivsky 2004, 34) that requires fostering to flourish and grow (Tronto 2013, 8). During the Holocaust, millions of Jews died and many more suffered because of failures to care—powerful divisive and dehumanizing narratives squelched empathy, imagination, and caring actions on a large scale. Caring is so basic to human development and the survival of human civilizations (Rifkin 2009) that the resource potential to care is present even when suppressed. Yet, ultimately, humans must choose to act. Caring is always a choice. Sometimes it is easy to care, as with family and friends, but in other instances the time and effort needed to care for unfamiliar others is daunting. If we assent to the notion that caring is a worthwhile moral ideal (Noddings 2010, 79) then it is reasonable to interrogate social systems and their philosophies for the extent to which they foment caring and furthermore pursue means of creating the most robust communities of caring possible.

This chapter explores two claims about care. First, care transforms the "game" of political ethics. The political nature of care is not equated with contemporary characteristics of ethics but rather endeavors to reconnect the personal and public spheres in ways that alter our relationship to both. The second claim explored in this chapter is that care is much more than an alternative theory of ethics. In this manner, I agree with the trajectory of care associated with Noddings (2002, 60), and to a lesser extent Bowden (1997, 12–15), that care ethics cannot be captured by principles. Although not antithetical to principles as guides, reducing care to absolute and abstract principles forces a robust theory into a traditional Western paradigm of ethics that limits the scope and liminality of care. I think Noddings is right to be skeptical about principles and I want to outline a performative theory of care that goes even further in a non-principled direction with regard to care. I contend that *care is a performative theory of being* that has implications for identity and epistemology as well as ethics and politics. As such, care has a postmodern character (but not a purely deconstructive one) with the radical potential to reframe how we think about morality. In the conclusion, I address what a performative theory of care might mean for a political approach to widen the circle of care for unfamiliar others.[2]

Care Transforms Political and Ethical Games of Normativity

> Politics, education, and even war are now described in the metaphorical language of gaming, with "war games" preparing high-tech militaries for conflicts that increasingly resemble video games. Do we control this metaphor, or does it control us? (Rigney 2001, 141)

Care theory has the potential to transform how politics and ethics are understood. In philosophy, care ethics does not easily fit into the framework of traditional Western moral theory, resulting in struggles over categories, terms, and ultimately, acceptance. In political theory, care challenges dominant liberal assumptions regarding autonomy and egoistic motivation. One such challenge is in regard to the notion of politics defined as an abstract moral structure governing human participation. In other words, the reality of care means that politics is more than a game. Contemporary Western politics often focuses more on winning elections, and thus the race to accumulate and maintain power, than on responsive governance, which facilitates the flourishing and growth of a populace. The notion that politics is a game to be won or lost is sometimes explicit in calculated decisions to garner popularity, and other times gamesmanship is implicit in the actions and thought processes of those involved. As one recent study of political rhetoric in the media describes, "the framing of politics as a strategic game is characterized by a focus on questions related to who is winning and losing, the performances of politicians and parties, and on campaign strategies and tactics" (Aalberg et al. 2011, 162). Although, in my estimation, care is not altruism, it is "other-directed" in such a way that structures politics as a means to care for citizens rather than a game of power. Care centers on the relationship with particular others and the expressed needs of those others in such a way that resists gaming. In this section, I discuss the politics-as-game metaphor as well as the ethics-as-game metaphor and how care challenges these metaphors in a manner that suggests a different way of thinking about normativity.

The notion that "life is a game" is what Raymond Gozzi Jr. refers to as a master metaphor, "one that organizes a whole field of minimetaphors around it" (1990, 291). Game metaphors pervade politics and much of our academic and theoretical thinking as well (Ching 1993, 44). Metaphors are powerful and indispensible vehicles of human understanding. Identifying, analyzing, and sometimes challenging operant metaphors, such as game metaphors, is not merely linguistically interesting; it is a means for understanding our very structures of knowledge (Lakoff and Johnson 1980).

Epistemologically, metaphors allow us to find the similarities between something that is known and something that is unknown, so as to assist us to better understand the latter. When Marcus Aurelius tells us that time is a river that flows between events, a comparison concerning something familiar and tangible (river) is employed to help us better comprehend an idea that is abstract and elusive (time). The metaphorical understanding need not be consciously attended to in order to impact our behavior. I don't have to explicitly acknowledge that time is actually a river for me to make this part of my worldview. Thus, I may think about time as moving in a single direction and irreversible like a river. However, metaphors, as powerful as they are, are only partially explanatory. Metaphors are never definitions. As philosopher J. J. C. Smart suggests, "It is clear, then, that we cannot talk about time as a river, about the flow of time, of our advance through time, or of the irreversibility of time without being in great danger of falling into absurdity" (1949, 485). Time is not water: one cannot skip rocks across time, or be refreshed by taking a drink of time. I have referred to the phenomenon of eliding the difference between metaphor and definition as the "metaphoric fallacy" (Hamington 2009). This fallacy is not a criticism of metaphor but rather a concern about a slippage in human understanding. In many cases, such sloppy thinking is inconsequential. However, there are certain deep or master metaphors for which the confusion between equivalence and analogy can result in substantial moral fallout. One such metaphor is the idea that politics is a game.

One of the challenges of using metaphors is that there can be substantial differences in how one wishes to employ the intended analogy. To effectively communicate using the metaphor, "Joe is a snake," depends upon similar understanding of the term "snake." If there is a general agreement that snakes imply elusiveness, then the comparison can provide useful insight. However, if someone comes from a culture that reveres snakes as resourceful creatures while another person has been acculturated to think of snakes as the source of evil in the world, the claim that "Joe is a snake" loses its ability to convey shared meaning between them. Accordingly, the idea that politics is a game will only be useful to the point that there are shared understandings of how "game" is understood. Although there is the risk of missing some of the variation in understandings of what "game" means to people, some common characteristics of games include: a controlled and finite environment, compartmentalized and truncated morality, trivialized stakes, and the privileging of adversarial relationships.

Games are closed systems that generally have finite temporal and spatial dimensions. They have rules that define the parameters of the activities associated with the game. These rules represent the primary ethical content of games, such that rule breaking is wrong and sometimes the subject of penalization. Games usually have limited or no stakes at all and are engaged in for the pleasure of the activity or for the joy of winning. Games imply contest and thus they privilege competition and the value of victory. Given contemporary emphasis on winning, treating something like a game is often construed as an emphasis on the outcome over and against authentic participation, such as found in the complaint, "Is love just a game to you?" Ultimately, games are morally neutral human activities, yet to declare that an activity is being treated like a game frequently has a pejorative connotation regarding seriousness, depth of involvement, or fixation on victory.

Certainly, political activity has game-like elements. To the extent that the political goal is to garner the requisite influence in order to achieve a desired outcome, then politics can be viewed by some as a type of game. Strategy and tactics are then methods for achieving advantage in the game. The problem resides in the extent to which people engage in the metaphoric fallacy. *Although political activity has elements that are similar to games, it is not a game.* Ideally, politics should address the public negotiation of serviceable government. As such, politics has many elements that are the antithesis of games. For example, as a major structure of social life, politics is open-ended and often entails momentous consequences. Recent threats by US political parties to shut down the federal government in order to gain advantage may appear to have game-like qualities as characterized by brinkmanship, but there are significant implications for the real lives of people when the government shuts down.

Furthermore, the morality of games is often simplistic in the avoidance of breaking rules. Accordingly, those engaged in political activity sometimes seem to seek this or that technicality to justify a decision, or they engage in a form of eisegesis in the backward interpreting of actions (such as when claiming to be on the right side of a "just war" argument after making the decision for other reasons). Such game-playing behavior sometimes may be morally motivated but it hardly reflects a method designed to support deep ethical deliberation. No matter how much we desire it, political activity is anything but simplistic, and thus hardly a game, given the myriad variables it must navigate.

Care, of course, has political elements to it. In order to influence social theory to promote the growth and flourishing of a society, power must be used to effect the imagination and will of a citizenry that such caring is the best use of time and resources. However, the pursuit of a caring society might involve leadership that does not act in a manner that is always politically expedient to the game. Evelyn Nakano Glenn describes the definition of a good society as "those who cannot care for themselves are cared for; that those who can care for themselves can trust that, should they become dependent, they will be cared for; and that people will be supported in their efforts to care for those they care about" (2000, 84). Pursuing issues such as wealth redistribution, same-sex marriage, and greater social safety net protections, for example, may not be comfortable routes to political gamesmanship when these issues are unpopular with powerful constituencies, but they do represent care for vulnerable or oppressed members of society. This is not to say that caring politics must be naïvely ideological. However, care entails a commitment to be responsive to expressed needs that asks leaders to govern by more than popularity polls or special interest donations. Authentic caring is not a game but rather a meaningful and effective response to needs.

An important corollary to the concern over the notion that politics is a game is the implicit metaphor that ethics is a game. Traditional notions of normativity lend themselves to the truncated morality of games. For example, the idea that a set of finite principles or rules can govern our ethical behavior is an ancient and pervasive idea, yet a problematic one. Rules lend themselves to game playing. Rules interject an abstract external evaluative system to human interaction and are therefore never organic or emergent but always imposed. For example, the very serviceable rule that one should not lie appears very clear but opens the potential for "gaming." One can question what they "can get away with," such as a lie of omission rather than commission. Or one can speculate whether it is acceptable to commit a "white" lie, but this begs the question of what constitutes the dividing line between a white lie and a bald-faced lie. When ethics is merely a set of rules intended to adjudicate acts, then ethics can be turned into a game in a pejorative sense.

Nor is care a simple utilitarian calculation of good and harm—another type of game that can devalue respect for individuals. Although care has elements of consequentialism to it, care centers on the ongoing relationship. As Noddings contends, "moral problems should not be reduced to mathematical dilemmas" (2010, 21). Care theory offers an antidote to the external imposition of the game-like ethics in engaging political morality by reframing ethics around relationships. In other words, the question is not whether a lie is right or wrong as an absolute truth, but rather how lying impacts ongoing relationships. Because authentic caring involves the particulars of those involved in a given context, it resists gaming and offers an emergent form of normativity.

Normative guidance for care emerges out of the specific context of those involved rather than a utilitarian calculus or a deontological duty. However, that guidance is tenuous and marked by deliberation, thus offering more of a trajectory than a rule.

Accordingly, care theory offers a radical departure in thinking about morality that does not fit well within Western concepts of normativity. The tenuous normativity of care comes from a different perspective. The traditional ethics game has a predetermined notion of normativity abstracted from the context of the individuals involved: rules or calculations of actions. This abstraction is supported in the name of objectivity and fairness. Care entails a more organic approach to normativity. Fiona Robinson recognizes this when she describes the naturalized epistemology that underpins care as "*not fully normative* in the strong sense, it still retains normativity" (2011, 27). In a stronger critique, Margaret Urban Walker asks, "I have come to wonder, or rather to worry about, why it is so important to know whether 'we' are right and 'they' are wrong, *tout* court" (1998, 13).

Rather than eschew normativity altogether, care theory offers a context-driven emergent trajectory of moral standards. The moral response (caring) is found within the relationships and the individuals involved. In this manner, care transcends the objectivity/subjectivity dualism. Care is not subjective, in that any response cannot simply be labeled as caring in the manner that care theorists have described. Care is also not objective, in that a single best caring response cannot be predetermined given the complexity of context. Rather, care involves the time and attention to the other, the care receiver, prior to any course of action. A game with unyielding external moral rules is anathema to caring. It is not that caring entails anarchism. Principles can offer guidance—milestones of conversation, and symbols for values held—but they cannot be a substitute for the hard work of caring. Similarly, calculations of aggregate pleasure and pain can also be a useful guide but do not replace the challenge of contextual-driven caring. Care is much more than a game of normative adjudication. In the next section, I will suggest that care is an aesthetic activity of self-and-other development that builds identity and knowledge.

A Political Performative Theory of Care

> Performance describes a genuine act of creation . . . (Fischer-Lichte 2008, 36)
>
> Ethics turns on intelligibility, reconciliation, and beauty. (Caputo 1993, 11)

As the intellectual work on care theory matures and spreads to a variety of disciplines, it is clear that care is not just a privatized relational endeavor. It is also a moral ideal that can enrich social and political morality beyond the game-like behavior that underlies traditional political discourse. In this section, I suggest that care is more than an ethical theory. I offer a performative approach to care that entails a theory of being enmeshed with a theory of knowing. Specifically, I want to claim that caring identity consists of performative acts. As such, *care is a political embodied performance, every iteration of which has the potential to contribute to our dynamic sense of moral identity, adds to our disruptive knowledge of the other, and supports the notion that ethical understanding is a mind–body activity that is ripe for autopoetic development.*[3] What I mean by "disruptive knowledge" is the kind of information about the other that is compelling and disrupts our lives to the point of motivating emotion and action. If care is indeed performative, then a holistic mind–body approach is needed if we are going to foster greater care in our society. Thus understanding care is tied to attending to physicality, bodily comportment, and proximity as well as cognitive consideration of morality. In the previous section I contended that care theory suggests a different approach to normativity. In this section, I focus on the role of care in identity formation through the notion of care as performance.

Care-as-performance is a testament to the idea that, without an aesthetic understanding of the ethical, morality suffers from the danger of becoming a rational decision science. The work of John Dewey is instructive for this approach to care. Dewey's philosophy elided the strict boundary between means and ends, and posited a notion of moral deliberation that he described as dramatic rehearsal appropriate to a performative understanding of care. Dewey defined moral deliberation as "a dramatic rehearsal (in imagination) of various competing lines of action" (1988, 132). Such dramatic rehearsals are context-driven scenario explorations. Furthermore, Dewey had an expansive understanding of aesthetics that makes it more accessible to everyday human experience and connects it to morality. Dewey sought to recover "the continuity of esthetic [*sic*] experience with normal processes of living" (1980, 10).

Given a Deweyan framework, performative care is not about making art but about being artful. In other words, a performative theory of care does not suggest that caregivers are artists in the sense of having exceptional genius or in terms of end products, but it does suggest that caregivers are artists in terms of being aesthetically attuned to the bodies, actions, and relations of themselves and others. Among other things, thinking about care as performative suggests that it is an imaginative aesthetic experience. In a similar way, Dewey wants to revitalize the connection between morality and aesthetics. He not only claims that "imagination is the chief instrument of the good" but that "art is more moral than moralities" (1980, 348). Imagination has been an underexplored aspect of care theory (Hamington 2004, 61–88), yet it is a crucial component of empathy and our self-understanding of our role in providing care. Everyday performances of care are not on stage, yet they are witnessed, and if attended to and reinforced as habits, they can become part of our moral narrative.

Framing care as performance also captures the embodied, relational, and active nature of care. Accordingly, Eva Feder Kittay describes the body as "the place of care" (Kittay 2013). Caring is particularist: experienced individually and through one's body. Quintessentially anti-Cartesian, instead of distrusting the senses, a performative approach assumes that care is embodied. Care-as-performance therefore posits honing the physical skills of caring for better attunement to our particularized reality, resulting in knowledge creation, identity formation, and moral relations in a manner akin to Richard Shusterman's notion of somaesthetics (Shusterman 2008). Shusterman describes somaesthetics as "a framework to promote and integrate the diverse range of theorizing, empirical research, and meliorative practical disciplines concerned with bodily perception, performance, and presentation" (2012, 7).

Although Shusterman is not a care theorist, he is trying to make philosophy more holistic in terms of integrating mind and body in service of human well-being—an approach consistent with a performative theory of care. Given its relational ontology, a performative approach to care gestures toward a robust political analysis, resulting in explorations of who we are, and what we know about one another, intertwined with our inquiry into how we should respond to need. This is much different from the standard ethical discourse of dichotomous evaluations of what is right and wrong. The latter discussion, the focus of traditional ethics, is much easier than a comprehensive discussion of identity and epistemology. The work of care is indeed challenging.

Furthermore, care is marked by action and animated by need. Although in popular conversation the phrase "I care" is pervasively employed, such as in the statement, "I care about the environment," the morally praiseworthy aspect of care theory is *actions* integrated with a disposition of openness and responsiveness to the other. As Virginia Held describes, "care is surely a form of labor, but it is also much more" (2006, 36). It is in the doing that care becomes actualized and experienced, but the actions are intertwined with an other-directed disposition. Caring consists of a series of actions, some large and explicit actions and some small and subtle actions, that inform the quality of a relationship, thus making it caring. Actions that bring care into a relationship can be described as performances.

Fifty years ago, the British philosopher of language, J. L. Austin employed the term "performative" to distinguish sentences that describe from those which actually bring about the phenomenon for which they refer, such as in the proclamation "I do" in a wedding ritual (1962, 6). Judith Butler applied the notion of performative speech acts to corporeal existence to argue that gender identity is not a pre-existing ontological or biological category, but is brought about through performance. Extending Simone de Beauvoir's notion that a woman is not born but becomes a woman, Butler describes that "gender is no way a stable identity or locus of agency from which various speech acts proceed; rather, it is an identity tenuously constituted in time—an identity instituted through a *stylized repetition of acts*" (Butler 1988, 519). For Butler, these performances of gender are neither entirely freely chosen nor entirely the products of social forces.

I argue that one's *moral identity* is also constituted through a stylized repetition of acts.[4] Whether I think of myself as a caring person, and what type of caring person, is instantiated through iterations of actions within the context of my relationships. This identity is inherently political as I negotiate the social forces and disciplines that seek to constrain behavior. Ultimately, a moral identity is performed. This claim is consistent with what some theorists have described as the ontological turn in philosophy. Charles Taylor, for example, describes a moral ontology whereby morality is part of human efforts at defining self-identity (1989, 5–9). The notion of effort is important because "identity" is not posited here as a static or natural understanding. Allison Weir offers a framework similar to a performative theory of care when she describes humanity's quest for freedom as striving to diminish fixed identities. Humans are ontologically dynamic because of our capacity to be transformed through our relations. Weir suggests, "Our practices of self-creation both presuppose and create new connections, new identifications; and as our connections change so do our truths" (2013, 33). There is a hint of existentialism in Weir's claims about freedom and self-creation but without a radical sense of individualism and isolation. Weir also foreshadows the epistemological dimension of care.

A phenomenology of care reveals how caring performances are embedded in relationship and entangled in identity formation, knowledge creation, political negotiation, and of course ethical action. Noddings describes a three-part phenomenology of care behavior that I wish to flesh out and expand (Noddings 2002, 19). In the *first* stage, one becomes aware of the need of another. In the *second* stage, an act of care takes place—a caring performance. In the *third* stage, the care receiver acknowledges the care (with exceptions for those who are incapable of acknowledgement), closing the relational loop.

We might describe stage 1 as an awareness and empathy stage, where knowledge acquisition is entangled with imaginative, emotional, and empathetic understanding. I cannot care about that for which I have no knowledge; however, although knowledge is a necessary condition of care, it is not a sufficient condition. An empathetic or emotional connection must be present regarding the need of others that will move me to contemplate action, and I must perceive that my caring actions can be effective in making a difference on behalf of the other (Hamington 2010). I might read an account of a tragic event that leaves a family in Pakistan in need of money for food. Nevertheless, if I am a subsistence college student in North America, my empathy may not motivate action, as I do not perceive that I have the wherewithal to make a difference. In such circumstances, no caring performances (described as stage 2) take place. The actor must believe that they can effectively care or they may not act, even if they have a caring disposition.

Note that I take exception to one aspect of Noddings' first stage in terms of awareness of need. A performative approach to care need not be only reactive. One can give care without a clear present need. In other words, care can be proactive. A caregiver can anticipate needs or identify needs that the one cared-for does not recognize as a need or simply act out of caring for the individual without any real expressed need. Nevertheless, even pre-emptive caring requires awareness and knowledge of the context of the one cared-for.

The notion of caring as an action is nothing new, as many theorists have associated care with labor and practices (Bubeck 1995; Engster 2007; Fineman 2004; Held 1993; Noddings 2002; Robinson 1999; Ruddick 1989; Sevenhuijsen 1998; Tronto 1993; White 2000). A performative approach is consistent with practice-based theories but emphasizes the public and therefore political nature of care. When attended to, the caring performance creates new knowledge about caring that can influence future acts. Because caring involves a responsive act on behalf of the other, it always exists in an autopoetic feedback loop. Every action results in a response that is a moment of learning about care. So if I am responding to the pain of another who has just experienced a racist act, my first action will elicit a response (stage 3) that may result in a second action on my part and so forth.

If I am attentive, my efforts at caring actions are opportunities for learning that can refine my response and perhaps help me in future responses. In addition, the caring act also takes place in a social and political milieu that is negotiated. We bump up against norms of behavior. A skilled carer has developed the habits and abilities to be open to the possibility of a caring action. Caring entails openness to the possibility of personal disruption, risk, and emotional involvement—in other words, an action that some people are not skilled in doing or assiduously avoid. Accordingly, caring performances are also a form of inquiry.

Caring involves positive actions done in the context of attunement to the other that inform growth, learning, and adjustment. For example, one might discover that a homeless individual on the street needs food and one might share their leftover lunch with them. This performance of care is morally praiseworthy to a point. However, such caring performances lay the groundwork for potential further inquiry. One might learn that sharing lunch does not materially alter this person's situation beyond the short term, but that one has it within their power to make a significant difference in their life. Thus, caring has the potential to beget more caring. One might learn from further inquiry that policy changes could help the homeless person they have gotten to know and others like her or him. Additional performances of care are made possible.

Every conversation or encounter will not necessarily lead to caring actions, but they have the potential to. Rich interpersonal interactions marked by care provide important knowledge bases for political action. A high-profile example occurred in 2013 when Ohio Senator Rob Portman changed his position on same-sex marriage after his son came out as gay (Portman). In the lead-up to his change of heart, Portman did not likely have any new compelling statistical or scientific knowledge, but he did have the disruptive knowledge that stems from a caring relationship (Portman 2013).

Stage 3 of a caring phenomenology can be described as part of an autopoetic feedback loop in the ongoing trajectory of care. As Noddings describes, "In care ethics, our obligation rarely ends with a justified decision or act. Life goes on after the decision, and we must tend to the relations we have established" (2010, 82). This is another way in which care ethics is different from traditional normative approaches to ethics: primacy is given to relationships over individual acts. As political animals, humans engage in self-creation as theatre: a performance intended to ingratiate others and garner power. Similarly, a performative theory of care has an element of self-creation—not as a pejorative performance intended as superficial show for others, but rather as a self-styling that integrates politics, ethics, and ontology. German performance theorist Erika Fischer-Lichte describes the transformative power of performance as emerging from its autopoetic potential. *Autopoiesis* describes regenerative systems that transcend subject/object dichotomies by being both producer and that which is produced in a process of self-creation. Accordingly, caring performances are autopoetic in that acts of care that characterize the relationship also contribute to the identity of the participants.

A number of theorists have explored aspects of autopoiesis that are helpful in providing insight into care theory. Late in his career Foucault made a fascinating turn to exploring ethics in light of ontology through what he described as "technologies of the self," one of these being "care for the self." Foucault describes that "the most certain of all philosophical problems is the problem of the present time and of what we are in this very moment" (1982, 785). Specifically, Foucault describes the "care for the self" as a self-cultivation that is the foundation for ethics and the basis for political engagement (Bernauer and Rasmussen 1987, 5–7). Although no one will characterize Foucault as a feminist care ethicist, his insights into the care of the self have relevance to an expansive theory of care as embodied and performative. For

Foucault, philosophy should support self-discovery. The autopoetic nature of care-as-performance is exhibited in the manner in which caring defies being captured in traditional categories of philosophical functionality. Entangled in the ethical dimension of caring performances are identity formation, epistemology, and aesthetics. Caring and knowledge production are inseparable and mutually motivating. Knowledge acquisition is a prerequisite of care and inquiry is often driven by care (Dalmiya 2002). As mentioned earlier, I cannot care about that for which I do not know. On the other hand, when I care about someone, I am driven to learn more about them. Furthermore, the efficacy of care requires information or suffers from the possibility of being misguided or poorly offered.

Every performance of care implicitly or explicitly contributes to one's identity as a carer—an internal autopoetic corollary to external autopoiesis. Because the performances are public, they leave physical and perceptual imprints on others and ourselves. The frequency and quality of care performances inform self-identity as well as socially inscribed identity. One method of describing this sense of identity formation is through an open-ended notion of habit instantiated in the body, as described in the work of Dewey. For Dewey, "Habit means special sensitiveness or accessibility to certain classes of stimuli, standing predilections and aversions, rather than bare recurrence of specific acts. It means will" (1988, 32). The association of habit and will is counterintuitive, but for Dewey, muscle memory works in conjunction with mental processes to allow caring performances to evolve and grow. Why are some people referred to as caring? Because their actions reinforce this identity and to some extent they have accepted or internalized caring as part of who they are. Human beings are not machines, so a particular caring action does not guarantee subsequent caring actions or habits, but it opens up a potential for reflection and assimilation. A performative approach to care is not mutually exclusive to the inductive approach favored by Slote (2010, 18–22) but it does emphasize the active and engaged element of caring behavior.

These caring performances of body and will are political in their implications for influence. Performative theory, as Butler has developed it, lies at the nexus between autonomy and social construction. Fischer-Lichte describes the artist/performer as "a subject engaged in a continuous process of determining and being determined" (2008, 164). Accordingly, our performances are often dictated by political norms and practices, but we can resist social forces, as in Butler's analysis of drag performances as subverting gender identity (1990, 186–9). Similarly, care performances are in part informed or limited by social norms, but individuals can choose to transgress social expectations. Transgressions—caring more than we ought to—can seep into our identity and become easier with repetition. Such transgressions of the norms of care might be referred to as supererogatory care.

Of course, what constitutes supererogatory acts is a relative concept. Someone who takes the risk to stop to help someone in distress at the side of a country road might decide to do it again if they perceive they effectively administered care (as well as cared-for themselves). Without explicit affirmation, that person might think of themselves as "someone who stops to help strangers." Note that a performative notion of identity formation is always relational. Human identity as a function of relationship is consistent with feminist ontological notions of human beings as "second persons" (Baier 1985, 84; Code 1991, 85) As second persons, we cannot speak of identity outside of the existence of others. Our dynamic identity is cognitively and physically a relational construct (Gallagher 2005). Consequently, the autopoetic feedback loop in our relationships and transactions with others creates and recreates our self-concept in both subtle and profound ways.

The performative theory of care described above is a complex integration of philosophical categories, but that level of intricacy matches the human condition. Identity, epistemology, and morality are vast areas for intellectual exploration, but they are also concurrently manifested in embodied human beings who are interconnected through their caring relationships.

Expanding the Circle of Care

> Once the detailed theoretical discussions [about ethical theories] get under way, far too often the radical potential of care ethics dwindles as the goal becomes one of replacing a masculinist moral theory with a feminist one instead of appreciating the weakness of the entire traditional ethical enterprise. (Bailey 2012, 185)

The contemporary enthusiasm for care among political theorists portends an exciting infusion of relational and contextual concern into political theory and analysis. However, I suggest that if we don't recognize the significant paradigm shift that care represents, there is a danger of limiting the potential of care to radically alter the moral and political landscape. In viewing care as performative, I have endeavored to emphasize how caring has transformative implications for ontology and epistemology as well as morality. Care transcends the dualisms of body and mind, self and other, will and social construction, personal and political. When I care, it is an act of will, a choice, but always a choice mediated by my relational self in a social/political context. In this section, I suggest that political thinking about care should emphasize expanding rich interpersonal experiences with diverse others to expand the capacity of care over policies of responsibility or compliance.

One of the implications of existentially tying care to identity is that robust forms of care cannot be authentically mandated or, perhaps more precisely, cannot be comprehensively mandated. A significant element of care is organic and comes from individual choice in response to circumstances. The psychological dimension of caring cannot be ignored. Accordingly, the language of "duties" "responsibilities," and "rights" to care is inadequate in guaranteeing that care is offered with adequate depth and quality, just as laws against racist activity do not guarantee that racism will not occur. Legalistic approaches are positive steps and have important symbolic value, but they do not equate with holistic interpersonal commitment. At times, such mandates can even foster resistance to authentic care when hearts are not changed. Abstract and external normative approaches can lead to the game playing described earlier. If I have been assigned a responsibility to care, it raises the specter of my relationship to the limitations of that caring—where does my responsibility end?

A performative theory of care makes it clear that one cannot simply replace traditional moral language by the language of care. Even as care has postmodern elements, it is a reconstructive theory rather than a deconstructive one. Care offers an empowering method for understanding how identity is wrapped up in knowledge acquisition and morality without falling into the modernist trap of fixed and universal classifications. However, unlike postmodern theory, care claims a tangible moral ideal. A performative theory of care represents a paradigm shift for philosophical ethics in its integration of ontology, epistemology, and ethics. It suggests a reconstructive approach to human be-ing, including a moral identity that acknowledges liminality, relationality, and uncertainty, while simultaneously providing a framework and trajectory for meaning and action rather than nihilism or subjectivism.

Perhaps the most significant question in care theory is a political one: how do we expand the circle of care? How do we lift the social norms for caring and foster care for those unfamiliar to ourselves, transcending social categories and stereotypes? Given contemporary systems of communication, the availability of information on those who need care is ubiquitous. Duties and principles may help as significant markers of social commitment, but the real radical political potential of care is internalizing caring as a moral ideal that informs our self as well as our relationships.

If we take the suggestions of this chapter seriously that care has epistemological and personal aesthetic qualities as well, then expanding the circle of care requires the kind of "world traveling" suggested many years ago by Maria Lugones (1987). Lugones advocated moving past arrogant perception by humbly listening to and spending time with others to build an understanding, not by erasing difference but by earnestly learning about and inhabiting that difference to the best of our ability. This requires rich and often proximal experiences. Lugones writes, "We are fully dependent on each other for the possibility of being understood and with this understanding we are not intelligible, we do not make sense, we are not solid, visible, integrated, we are lacking. So travelling to each other's 'worlds' would enable us to *be* through *loving* each other" (1987, 8). Lugones uses the language of love rather than care, but the implications are similar: knowing and care are intertwined. Accordingly, a more inclusive politics of caring cannot ignore what we know and who we are.

Barbara Thayer-Bacon frames what Lugones is driving at in terms of a new way to think about connected knowledge. Rather than viewing care as a subjective and touchy-feely emotion, Thayer-Bacon claims that it is the basis for a more robust notion of critical thinking: "Connected knowing is based on an epistemology that emphasizes truth as something that emerges through care" (2000, 79). For Thayer-Bacon, care represents habituated performances of listening for the purpose of sympathetic understanding. She explains:

> We must care in order for us to be willing to reason from others' points of view and in order for us to have the sensitivity to hear their voices (for we know now they must tell us their points of view, that we cannot assume to know them any other way). Caring is an effort to attempt to believe others, in order to be sure we understand, before we move to critiquing the others' views. The effort to believe in order to understand causes us to be willing to suspend our own views and be open to others. What we care about is what we choose to attend to, what we choose to be engrossed with and be receptive to. If we do not care about others we will not listen to their voices, and we will not be able to enlarge our thinking. (Thayer-Bacon 2000, 106)

What Thayer-Bacon and Lugones point to is how care can serve as a reconstructive theory of being. Rather than an overarching and closed metanarrative, care offers a malleable integration of morality, knowledge, and identity consistent with the notion that it includes "everything that we do to maintain, continue, and repair our 'world' so that we can live in it as well as possible" (Fisher and Tronto 1990, 40). What I mean by "reconstructive" here is that care can accommodate the deconstructive analysis of postmodernism which challenges categorical thinking that can separate self from others, identity from morality, subject from object, etc. However, rather than concluding in a deconstructed state, care provides an organizing trajectory around attentive/responsive living.

World traveling and adopting care as a moral ideal can be interpreted as requiring a more assertive effort at learning about others in order to build the resources to care in a process that transforms who we are and what we know—for example, talking to strangers in more than superficial ways or venturing to comprehend cultures, religions, and lives lived much differently than our own. The arts and humanities can be of great assistance in this regard, but so too must be rich experiences of one another. How often does one's political disposition toward the contemporary issues of same-sex marriage, homelessness, and undocumented immigration turn on, or is it transformed by, direct knowledge of someone identified by these circumstances?

The suggestion here is that the performance of care does not begin and end with a particular act of kindness. There must be a dramatic rehearsal, a habituation of going out and learning about others in varied, humble, open, and meaningful ways—world traveling—so that our hearts and minds are prepared for caring in our cosmopolitan world. Social policies and education systems that foment caring opportunities and reflection upon care may move what might be considered supererogatory acts of care according to existing social norms to mainstream or ordinary acts of care. Understood as performative, care requires a vastly different method for teaching ethics that is much more experiential and engaged, and attuned to the body as well as one another, than is currently the standard (Hamington 2012). If one accepts the premise that care is indeed performative and embodied, then teaching ethics would engage cognitive, emotional, and physical aspects of caring, not just learning and understanding normative structures.

The people of the town of Le Chambon not only did not think of their helping as part of an ethical game or equation; they did not think much of it as moral heroism at all. Magda Trocmé, as quoted by Philip Hallie, queried:

> How can you call us "good"? We were doing what had to be done. Who else could help them? And what has all this to do with goodness? Things had to be done, that's all, and we happened to be there to do them. You must understand that it was the most natural thing in the world to help these people. (Hallie 1994, 20–1)

The members of this community were not particularly religious or well educated, but they had enlarged their moral inclusiveness for care such that they did not perceive it as moral exceptionalism. In her contemporary study of heroes of compassion during the Holocaust, Kristen Renwick Monroe corroborates Hallie's findings and concludes that identity is the linchpin of exceptional moral activity:

> The rescuers' sense of who they were, and how they saw themselves in relation to others, so limited the range of actions the rescuers perceived as available that they literally did not believe they had any other choice than to help Jews. Identity played such a critical role in shaping their treatment of others that their extraordinary actions seemed matter-of-fact, unremarkable, and unnoteworthy to the rescuers themselves. (2004, 188)

Renwick Monroe makes it clear that moral rules are not adequate to motivate ethical action on behalf of unknown others, but one's moral identity is. She claims that identity has the power to "shape our most basic political acts, including our treatment of others. How we see ourselves, and how we see others in relation to ourselves, has profound implications for our behavior. This often works in subtle and unconscious ways" (2004, 257). Renwick Monroe does not use an explicit care theory lens of analysis, but she supports the relational ontological claim embedded in a performative theory of care and the notion that care is a reconstructive theory of being. We cannot disentangle moral and political actions from considering who we are and what we know.

Our contemporary political journey to widening the circle of caring inclusion is likely to take a different path from that of the people of Le Chambon. Perhaps we can eschew the gaming of politics and ethics for intentional life choices that provide rich appreciation of the diverse contexts of others, and ultimately ourselves, in body, mind, and action.

Notes

1. Oliner and Oliner studied the rescuers of Jews during the Nazi occupation of Europe and concluded that empathy and concern for other others is "the most common way" in which rescuers apprehended moral claims which lead to their actions (1988, 258).
2. I would like to thank Dan Engster for his very helpful comments on my chapter as well as Michael Slote and all those who participated in the care ethics mini conference at the 2014 Western Political Science Association annual meeting in Seattle, Washington.
3. I am using the notion of autopoiesis here to conceptualize humans as recursive and regenerative systems dynamically reflecting both continuity and ongoing self-creation.
4. In addressing the notion of moral identity, it appears that I am characterizing care theory as a type of virtue ethic. Indeed, care has a great deal in common with virtue theory in terms of de-emphasizing the significance of individual acts. However, I agree with Noddings (2010, 125–37), who recognizes the similarities with virtue ethics but finds care to focus more on the relationship than on individuals. Although Michael Slote (2007) has done a great deal of work to bridge the gap, virtue theory does not challenge liberal notions of isolated individualism in the way that care theory does. Care does not neatly fit into the established categories of moral theories, although it holds much in common with many of them.

References

Aalberg, Toril, Jesper Strömbäck, and Claes H. de Vreese. 2011. "The Framing of Politics as Strategy and Game: A Review of Concepts, Operationalizations and Key Findings." *Journalism* 13(2):162–78.

Austin, J. L. 1962. *How To Do Things with Words*. Cambridge, MA: Harvard University Press.

Baier, Annette. 1985. *Postures of the Mind: Essays on Mind and Morals*. Minneapolis, MN: University of Minnesota Press.

Bailey, Cathryn. 2012. "The Revolutionary Fact of Compassion: William James, Buddhism, and the Feminist Ethics of Care." In *Contemporary Feminist Pragmatism*, edited by Maurice Hamington and Celia Bardwell-Jones, 184–99. New York: Routledge.

Bernauer, James, and David Rasmussen (eds.). 1987. *The Final Foucault*. Cambridge, MA: MIT Press.

Bowden, Peta.1997. *Caring: Gender Sensitive Ethics*. New York: Routledge.

Bubeck, Diemut. 1995. *Care, Gender, and Justice*. New York: Oxford University Press.

Butler, Judith. 1988. "Performative Acts and Gender Constitution: An Essay in Phenomenology and Feminist Theory." *Theatre Journal* 40(4): 519–31.

Butler, Judith. 1990. *Gender Trouble: Feminism and the Subversion of Identity*. New York: Routledge.

Caputo, John. 1993. *Against Ethics: Contributions to a Poetics of Obligation with Constant Reference to Deconstruction*. Bloomington, IN: Indiana University Press.

Ching, Marvin K. L. 1993. "Games and Play: Pervasive Metaphors in American Life." *Metaphor and Symbolic Activity* 8(1): 43–65.

Code, Lorraine. 1991. *What Can She Know? Feminist Theory and the Construction of Knowledge*. New York: Cornell University Press.

Dalmiya, Vrinda. 2002. "Why Should a Knower Care?" *Hypatia* 17(1): 34–52.

Dewey, John. 1980 [1934]. *Art as Experience*. New York: Perigee.

Dewey, John. 1988 [1922]. *Human Nature and Conduct: An Introduction to Social Psychology*. Carbondale, IL: Southern Illinois University Press.

Engster, Daniel. 2007. *The Heart of Justice: Care Ethics and Political Theory*. New York: Oxford University Press.

Fineman, Martha. 2004. *The Autonomy Myth: A Theory of Dependency*. New York: New Press.

Fischer-Lichte, Erika. 2008. *The Transformative power of Performance*, translated by Saskya Iris Jain. New York: Routledge.

Fisher, Berenice, and Joan C. Tronto. 1990. "Toward a Feminist Theory of Caring." In *Circles of Care*, edited by E. K. Abel and M. Nelson, 35–62. Albany, NY: State University of New York Press.

Foucault, Michel. 1982. "The Subject and Power." *Critical Inquiry* 8(4): 777–95.

Gallagher, Shaun. 2005. *How the Body Shapes the Mind*. New York: Oxford.

Glenn, Evelyn Nakano. 2000. "Creating a Caring Society." *Contemporary Sociology* 29(1): 84–94.

Gozzi, Raymond, Jr. 1990. "Is Life a Game? Notes on a Master Metaphor." *ETC: A Review of General Semantics* 47(3): 291–3.

Hallie, Philip. 1994. *Lest Innocent Blood Be Shed: The Story of the Village of Le Chambon and How Goodness Happened There*. New York: Harper Perennial.

Hamington, Maurice. 2004. *Embodied Care: Jane Addams, Maurice Merleau-Ponty and Feminist Ethics*. Urbana, IL: University of Illinois Press.

Hamington, Maurice. 2009. "Business is not a Game: The Metaphoric Fallacy." *Journal of Business Ethics* 86(4): 473–84.

Hamington, Maurice. 2010. "The Will to Care: Performance, Expectation, and Imagination." *Hypatia* 25(3): 675–95.

Hamington, Maurice. 2012. "A Performative Approach to Teaching Care Ethics: A Case Study." *Feminist Teacher* 23(1): 31–49.

Hankivsky, Olena. 2004. *Social Policy and the Ethic of Care*. Vancouver: UBC Press.

Held, Virginia. 1993. *Feminist Morality: Transforming Culture, Society, and Politics*. Chicago, IL: University of Chicago Press.

Held, Virginia. 2006. *The Ethics of Care: Personal, Political, and Global*. New York: Oxford University Press.

Kittay, Eva Feder. 2013. "The Body as the Place of Care." In *Exploring the Works of Edward S. Casey: Giving Voice to Place, Memory, and Imagination*, edited by Azucena Cruz-Pierre and Donald A. Landes, 205–14. New York: Bloomsbury.

Lakoff, George, and Mark Johnson. 1980. *Metaphors We Live By*. Chicago, IL: University of Chicago Press.

Lugones, Maria. 1987. "Playfulness, 'World'-Traveling, and Loving Perception." *Hypatia* 2(2): 3–19.

Noddings, Nel. 2002. *Starting at Home: Caring and Social Policy*. Berkeley, CA: University of California Press.

Noddings, Nel. 2010. *The Maternal Factor: Two Paths to Morality*. Berkeley, CA: University of California Press.

Oliner, Samuel P., and Pearl M. Oliner. 1988. *The Altruistic Personality: Rescuers of Jews in Nazi Europe*. New York: Free Press.

Portman, Rob. 2013. "Gay Couples also Deserve Chance to Get Married." *Columbus Dispatch*, 15 March. <http://www.dispatch.com/content/stories/editorials/2013/03/15/gay-couples-also-deserve-chance-to-get-married.html>

Renwick Monroe, Kristen. 2004. *The Hand of Compassion: Portraits of Moral Choice during the Holocaust*. Princeton, NJ: Princeton University Press.

Rifkin, Jeremy. 2009. *The Empathetic Civilization: The Race to Global Consciousness in a World in Crisis*. New York: Tarcher.

Rigney, David. 2001. *The Metaphorical Society: An Invitation to Social Theory*. Lanham, MD: Rowman and Littlefield.

Robinson, Fiona. 1999. *Globalizing Care: Ethics, Feminist Theory, and International Relations*. Boulder, CO: Westview Press.

Robinson, Fiona. 2011. *The Ethics of Care: A Feminist Approach to Human Security*. Philadelphia, PA: Temple University Press.

Ruddick, Sara. 1989. *Maternal Thinking: Toward a Politics of Peace*. New York: Ballantine.

Sevenhuijsen, Selma. 1998. *Citizenship and the Ethics of Care: Feminist Considerations on Justice, Morality, and Politics*. New York: Routledge.

Shusterman, Richard. 2008. *Body Consciousness: A Philosophy of Mindfulness and Somaesthetics*. New York: Cambridge University Press.

Shusterman, Richard. 2012. *Thinking through the Body: Essays in Somaesthetics*. New York: Cambridge University Press.

Slote, Michael. 2007. *The Ethics of Care and Empathy*. New York: Routledge.

Slote, Michael. 2010. *Moral Sentimentalism*. New York: Oxford University Press.

Smart, J. J. C. 1949. "The River of Time." *Mind* 58(232): 483–94.

Taylor, Charles. 1989. *Sources of the Self: The Making of Modern Identity*. Cambridge, MA: Harvard University Press.

Thayer-Bacon, Barbara J. 2000. *Transforming Critical Thinking: Thinking Constructively*. New York: Teachers College Press.

Tronto, Joan C. 1993. *Moral Boundaries: A Political Argument for an Ethic of Care*. New York: Routledge.

Tronto, Joan C. 2013. *Caring Democracy: Markets, Equality, and Justice*. New York: New York University Press.

Walker, Margaret Urban. 1998. *Moral Understandings: A Feminist Study in Ethics*. New York: Routledge.

Weir, Allison. 2013. *Identities and Freedom: Feminist Theory between Power and Connection*. New York: Oxford.

White, Julie. 2000. *Democracy, Justice and the Welfare State: Reconstructing Public Care*. University Park, PA: Pennsylvania State University Press.

16

Care ethics, political theory, and the future of feminism

Fiona Robinson

In her essay "Feminism Unbound: Revolution, Mourning, Politics," Wendy Brown considers what feminism might be "beyond sex and gender" (2005, 98). "What does it mean," she asks, "for feminist scholars to be working in a time after revolution, after the loss of belief in the possibility and viability of a radical overthrow of existing social relations?" (99). These questions are representative of a wider unease regarding the current state and future direction of feminist theory and practice. From the rise of the term "post-feminism," to analyses of the "aftermath of feminism" (McRobbie 2008), to invocations to "take a break from feminism" (Halley 2006), it would be reasonable to suggest that feminism is in a state of flux, or even in crisis.

This chapter considers the potential for the ethics of care to respond to the contemporary crises in feminism. While I do not offer care ethics as a panacea, or as a unified or universal feminist theory, I do suggest that it may provide a contrapuntal moral and political language that both responds to sources of unease, and offers an antidote to some of the more worrying trends in feminist theory, "popular" feminism, and "gender" policy. To this end, the chapter is divided into two main parts. First, I consider the nature of contemporary Western feminism—focusing on the state of feminist political theory, and its manifestations in global politics through the discourses and practices of "gender mainstreaming" and "gender and development." I suggest that, while sustained mourning and critical skepticism maintain a constant presence in the form of anti-essentialist post-structural and post-colonial feminist theory, perhaps the most widespread response to the post-revolutionary condition has been the re-creation of feminism as an instrumentalized movement about "empowerment" and "choice"—most often realized, it is argued, through women's individual wage-earning capacity (McRobbie 2008). This assessment is supported by scholarship in the fields of feminist international political economy and development studies, which emphasize trends in global economic governance to highlight strategies designed to increase "women's ability to compete" (Griffen 2010, 100). Discursive tropes of competition and "empowerment" dominate much popular feminist language and feminist activism; from Sheryl Sandberg's call for women to "lean in" in the workplace to Ariana Huffington's emphasis on personal well-being (through meditation, yoga and "naps"), this new brand of Western feminism is startling in its self-centered myopia (Sandberg 2013; Huffington 2014). This section will demonstrate how this language of women's empowerment emphasizes radical individualism and self-help, fitting comfortably into neoliberal governance strategies and thwarting sustained reflection on the future of care and the development of transnational solidarities among women.

Second, I consider the feminist "credentials" of the ethics of care, the debates that have surrounded care ethics, and the potential of feminist care ethics to respond to the current crises in feminism. Care ethics has been the source of much controversy and divisiveness among feminist moral, social, and political theorists. Due largely to its association—real or imagined—with maternalism and mothering, it has been attacked by feminists on "both sides," so to speak: liberal feminists have disparaged its apparent celebration of the tasks that have been the very source of women's oppression, while so-called "third wave" feminists—influenced by post-structuralist and post-colonial thought—have read care as essentialist and materialist, and thus as incompatible with a view of gender discursively produced and performatively sustained.

This section will address these critiques, and will explore a number of questions surrounding the relationship between care ethics and feminism. Is care ethics feminist? If so, what kind of feminism does it advocate; what kind of feminist politics does it entail? And on what basis does it presume to advocate anything at all? Is care ethics little more than a substantive articulation of a feminist standpoint, which offers a thick notion of gender identity as a foundation for women's caring activities? If so, would those "activities" necessarily land feminists back at the place from which they have been trying to escape?

In response to these questions, I will offer a reading of the ethics of care as the basis for a transnational feminist politics. My aim is not to defend care ethics by locating it within existing normative and epistemological debates about gender identity. Rather, I argue that, as a critical theory, care ethics can create the conditions for a new kind of feminist solidarity, but one that does not rely on fixed notions of gender identity. While it is widely known as a feminist *moral* theory, I will argue that care ethics' greatest strength lies in its ability to bring back *the political* to feminism. It does so by speaking to and with the voices of both feminist political economists—who have made great contributions to our understanding of the role and significance of women's reproductive labor—and with "cultural feminists" who offer critiques of androcentrism and hegemonic constructions of masculinity. Feminist care ethics draws our attention to the vital importance of care in everyday life, and the relations of responsibility that sustain care. In conversation with feminist political economy and feminist analysis of masculinities and violence, care ethics speaks with a voice that is both critical and transformative, offering a vision of a feminist future in which value is placed on the time and ability to care for one another.

While much feminist rhetoric today is dominated by the language of individual empowerment, care ethics represents a dissident voice which emphasizes human interdependence and vulnerability. I will suggest, along with Marian Barnes, that the expansion of the academic literature on the topic of care evidences a "hunger to develop a robust alternative to the individualizing and ultimately sterile dominance of the autonomous subject of neo-liberalism" (Barnes 2012, 183). Care ethics offers a radical politics that is, in Brown's words, "apart from left fundamentalism on one side, and apart from the refusal to reckon with deep social and economic powers entailed in liberal political pluralism on the other" (Brown 2005, 114). By foregrounding the giving and receiving of care as fundamental to the experience of being human, care ethics offers a substantive basis and a shared moral language from which to build social policy both within and across societies. Furthermore, by providing a critical lens through which to evaluate arrangements for care in societies, care ethics offers a thoroughgoing critique of existing inequalities and injustices related to gender as it intersects with race and geopolitical location.

Feminism Today

Feminist political theory has always been presented as a divided body of thought. To the undoubted relief of those "non-feminists" compelled to include it on course syllabi, feminist political theory has come packaged into neat and tidy categories—liberal, socialist, radical, "Third World," postmodern feminisms. Reducible to a shorthand of characteristics, these versions of feminism are often framed as warring factions, destined, perhaps, to obliterate one another. But across almost all of these factions has been the presence of "gender"—widely understood as the "social meaning attached to the shape of our bodies," and as a "logic," which is produced by and productive of the ways in which we understand politics (Shepherd 2010, 4–5). While gender, unlike biological sex, is not fixed or essential but socially constructed and hence always in flux, it is, for many feminists, a basis for making claims about identity. While it could be argued that the idea of gender identity could be articulated through feminist standpoint epistemology, it has also been suggested that the specific understanding of gender as an identity finds its roots in psychoanalytical traditions and, in particular, object-relations theory (Fraser 2013, 159). As Nancy Fraser puts it, "[w]ith the exception of a few holdouts, even those who rejected psychoanalysis came to understand gender as an identity or a 'cultural construction'" (2013, 159).

But even as a "cultural construction," the place and significance of "gender" in contemporary feminism is unclear. On the one hand, it has been suggested that feminists find themselves today, "beyond sex and gender" (Brown 2005). If this is the case, then it is in large measure due to the challenge of "Third World" feminism. By demonstrating their neglect of the voices of women in the global South, Third World feminists revealed Western feminism as "self-indulgent, white [and] unconnected to the real needs of most of the world's women" (111). This neglect, moreover, was no mere oversight; indeed, Western feminism was shown to be guilty of "colonization"—through the production of the "Third World Woman" as a singular monolithic subject in a number of (Western) feminist texts (Mohanty 1984, 333). This is a predominantly discursive colonization, characterized by a certain mode of appropriation and codification of "scholarship" and "knowledge" about women in the Third World (333).

Another challenge has come from within Western feminism. Post-structuralist theory has been, in Brown's words, the "final blow to the project of transforming, emancipating or eliminating gender in a revolutionary mode" (2005, 111). Brown argues:

> [G]ender is regarded (and lived) by contemporary young scholars and activists raised on poststructuralism as something that can be bent, proliferated, troubled, resignified, morphed, theatricalized, parodied, deployed, resisted, imitated, regulated . . . but not emancipated. Gender is very nearly infinitely plastic and divisible, but as a domain of subjection with no outside, it cannot be liberated in the classical sense, and the powers constituting and regulating it cannot be seized and inverted or abolished. (111–12)

According to Brown, these two intellectual developments (among others) have demonstrated both the "impossibility of circumscribing gender without participating in its construction and regulation" and the "dissociability of sex and gender from race, caste, class, nation and culture" (98). But while feminist intellectuals and academics struggle with the concept of gender, it is also widely reported today that feminism's work is done—that the feminist ideals of gender equality are now widely accepted and sit squarely in the social mainstream (Fraser 2013, 210). In a piece published in the *New York Times* in

February 2013, Stephanie Coontz argued that today the "main barriers to further progress toward gender equity no longer lie in people's personal attitudes and relationships" (Coontz 2013). In other words, we are all (in the liberal-capitalist "West") feminists today; all that is required, then, is the institutionalization of our widely accepted values.

It could be argued that this need to "institutionalize" gender finds its manifestation in the contemporary practices and policies of "gender mainstreaming." Surfacing as a concept in the early 1990s, gender mainstreaming describes efforts to "scrutinize and reinvent processes of policy formulation and implementation across all issue areas and at all levels from a gender-differentiated perspective, to address and rectify persistent and emerging disparities between men and women" (True 2003, 369). First established in the 1995 Beijing Platform for Action, and then ratified by all UN member states, gender mainstreaming has received widespread endorsement by nation-states, regional supra-state bodies, and global governance institutions (369).

But what it actually means (or should mean) to "mainstream gender" has never been entirely clear. Marisya Zalewski quotes international non-governmental organization worker Milena Vilanova, who describes her first thought when she arrived in post-conflict East Timor to work on sexual and gender-based violence: "I don't even know what gender is," Vilanova confesses (Zalewski 2010, 4). Her admission is not really surprising. There have been increasing demands for gender mainstreaming to not "only" be about women (but to also "include" men). Then there have been demands for it to not "simply" be about men and women, but to work with the complexities of transnational diversity and intersectionality (6). But as Eveline and Bacchi argue, the theoretical developments and contestations over how gender is represented take place in a parallel universe to policy developments (Eveline and Bacchi 2005, 503). Feminists "at the coal face," they argue, are confronted with the often-baffling question: "what are we mainstreaming when we mainstream gender?" (Eveline and Bacchi 2005).

But despite confusion and discord, "gender" mainstreaming itself appears to be here to stay—indeed, it is arguably one of the most visible and "successful" faces of global feminism today. Although it is marked by tensions, uneven impacts, and limitations, many experts have concluded that gender mainstreaming has had wide-ranging success (Walby 2005; Moser 2005). Indeed, Walby argues that certain forms of gender mainstreaming have provided a new basis for feminist solidarity and action at a global level (Walby 2005). This wary optimism remains evident more recently, with scholars like Jacqui True highlighting mainstreaming's transformative potential (2003). This optimism is tinged with concern, however, that gender mainstreaming is currently constrained by the hegemony of market ideology.

Indeed, while noting the "enormous progress" made in the mainstreaming of gender equality concerns into development in the last several decades, Sylvia Chant and Caroline Sweetman argue that the most visible face of gender mainstreaming today can be found in the discourses of "smart economics," which rationalizes "investing" in women and girls for more effective development outcomes (2012, 518). The thinking behind "smart economics" extends back until at least the 1980s, when it became clear that women were acting as a "buffer" to the fallout of Structural Adjustment Policies (SAPs). As restructuring slashed public-sector service provision, women picked up the slack, "cushioning" their households by providing healthcare, education, and other services. The growing consciousness of women's apparent ability to withstand economic crisis and carry on providing gave rise to the core message in the World Bank's flagship publication on gender issues in 1995. As Chant and Sweetman describe, the chapter "unashamedly entitled" "The Pay-offs to Investing in Women" professes that investing in women "speeds" economic development by promoting the more "efficient use of resources" (2012, 519).

So what is the "real" goal of gender mainstreaming here? Is the goal of female investment primarily to promote gender equality, or to facilitate development "on the cheap" and/or to promote further economic liberalization (Chant and Sweetman 2012: 521)? Indeed, the latest World Bank "Road Map" for Gender Mainstreaming has been criticized for focusing almost exclusively on economic empowerment as the sole means to achieve gender equality (Arend 2010).

What is missing, as Chant and Sweetman suggest, is a complete lack of political critique of what is wrong with the world; this results in programming which focuses solely on the agency of individual women and girls to deliver development goals (2012, 526). As long as arguments for mainstreaming have to be made in terms of "business cases" and the "efficiency gains" of human capital, they will never address the underlying normative and structural causes of gender inequality.

These strategies of gender mainstreaming are symptomatic of general trends in global economic governance. As Penny Griffen argues, "[n]eo-liberal governance strategy . . . depends on and is reproduced from a form of gendered hierarchy centred on market 'efficiency' but reproduced from heteronormative values, wherein men are perceived to labour productively and women reproductively" (2010, 101). "In seeking to socialize women, men, girls and boys, into competition-based hierarchies of economic productivity," Griffin argues, neoliberal international governmental organizations claim to advance only the "economic empowerment" of poor people (101).

It is a mistake to assume that these "gender and development" strategies are unconnected to discourses of gender, work, and neoliberalism in the global North. The discourses and policies of neoliberalism, and the norms of hegemonic masculinity which underwrite them, are at work within and across national boundaries throughout the globe. As O'Connor, Orloff, and Shaver point out, neoliberalism emerged in a period when increasing numbers of women entered into the labour market, and during which liberal feminists forcefully asserted women's personhood in law and the market (O'Connor et al. 1999, 53–4). Thus, neoliberals are "more willing to recognize women as individuals in their own right than their post-war political counterparts" (Larner 2000, 20). Hence the arguments for the "success" of feminism. At the same time, women who "opt for motherhood now find their labour devalued in a context where paid work appears to be all" (20).

Parallel to the language of "investing in women" in the development discourse is the language of women's empowerment "at work" in the global North. When Sheryl Sandberg encourages women "*everywhere*" to "lean in," so we can, "close the *ambition gap* right here, right now," questions arise (Sandberg 2011, italics added). Is the most concerning "gap" out there really an "*ambition*" gap? What happened to the wage gap? The care gap? Are the women who need to lean in really *everywhere*? If women *everywhere* "lean in" in their "careers," who is doing the care work? On Sandberg's view, women's emancipation relies on women's personal choices—their will, their drive, their ambition. "Leadership belongs to those who take it," she insists. "Leadership starts with you" (Sandberg 2011).

Sandberg notes that we (in the United States and the "developed world") feel "even more grateful when we compare our lives to those of other women around the world" (2013, 5). She goes on to list the usual atrocity statistics, referencing the sex trade, lack of education, and rape. But at no point does she suggest that women in the "developed world" may be, in some way, complicit in this injustice. Chapter 9 of her book—titled "The Myth of Doing it All"—mentions nothing of the poor women of color who are filling the care gap in the United States and many other countries around the world. It emphasizes not what social policies and institutions could be created to reduce the care gaps—in the United States and globally—but rather how women should formulate their own life goals with respect to work and care. "Instead of perfection," she suggests, "we should aim for sustainable and fulfilling" (2013, 138–9). She offers us a window on her world:

> A great day is when I rush home from the craziness of the office to have dinner with my family and then sit in the rocking chair in the corner of my daughter's room with both of my kids on my lap. We rock and read together, just a quiet (okay, not always quiet), joyful moment at the end of their day. They drift off to sleep and I drift (okay, run) back to my laptop. (138)

There is no mention of actually *cooking* the dinner (or shopping for the food, or cleaning up afterward). She is able to spend "quality time" with her children, since, apparently, there is no laundry to be done, no homework to help with, no school forms to sign, no bathroom to clean, no lunches to prepare for the following day. Just quiet moments of "good parenting"—reading and bonding.

Sandberg's book—and her wider "Lean In" Campaign—have evoked a polarized response: it has been described as "prescriptive, refreshing and perhaps even revolutionary" (Holmes 2013). Others have described it as "feminism for the 1%" (Burnham 2013). Still others, most notably Anne Marie Slaughter, have raised questions concerning the place of care. Slaughter ends her *New York Times* review of *Lean In* with the following question: "When it comes to ensuring that caregivers still have paths to the corner office, how can business lean in?" (Slaughter 2013). Susan Faludi echoes this: "[i]f you were waiting for someone to lean in for child care legislation, keep holding your breath" (Faludi 2013).

Even if women "lean in," and even if men everywhere nod in approval, this will not result in women's emancipation, or a better world. Nor can we solve the care gap just by asking men to "do their share" of housework and childcare. This simply reprivatizes social reproduction, and ensures its continued insulation from public debate. Because men (like women) will continue to work outside of the home, as well as being constrained by roles and norms of hegemonic masculinities, the result will be that this work will be done by the most marginalized individuals—women of color from income-poor countries. As Melissa Gira Grant put it recently in the *Washington Post*, "[T]here's simply no way for women to lean in without leaning on the backs of other women" (Grant 2013).

The entry of women into the labor market in income-rich countries has been facilitated, in part, by these "other women." Transnational care migration—the flow of (mainly women) caregivers from income-poor to income-rich countries in response to the increased demand for domestic and care work—has risen sharply as more women engage in paid labor outside of the home. Women in developing countries are taking up these positions in order to support their families financially. But these changing patterns of postcolonial migration do not emerge spontaneously; they are structured by the policies developed by income-rich nation-states. Migration rules construct the legal, social, and civil rights of migrants in different ways, and employment policies may serve to deregulate the economy and increase the casualization of labour. All of this, moreover, is governed by the "ongoing reconstitution of social relations of gender, care and domestic service; of hierarchies of ethnicity and nationality; and of differentiated means of, and rights to, citizenship" (Williams 2011, 21).

Focusing on the intensification of these so-called "global care chains" brings to light relations among women across spatial, class, and racial divides. As

Hochschild points out, the invisible global care chain on which the adult earner family relies often connects "three sets of care-takers—one cares for the migrant's children back home, a second cares for the children of the woman who cares for the migrant's children, and a third, the migrating mother herself, cares for the [children of] professionals in the First World" (2000, 136). Despite increasing demand for care work in affluent, income-rich countries, the value of this kind of labor has not increased. Women in the global North are encouraged to become part of the "glamorous masculine conceptual space" (Hooper 2000, 67–8) of globalization, while often illegal and under-age female migrants and domestic servants constitute the other face of globalization—the transnational regime of "sexualized, racialized labour-intimacy" (Chang and Ling 2000, 27).

How can these developments in feminism and care be explained? Like Wendy Larner, Nancy Fraser has explored the "heretical" possibility that there has been a "perverse, subterranean elective affinity between neoliberalism and second-wave feminism" (Fraser 2013, 218).

> Endowing their daily struggles with an ethical meaning, the feminist romance attracts women at both ends of the social spectrum: at one end, the female cadres of the professional middle classes, determined to crack the glass ceiling; at the other end, the female temps, part-timers, low-wage service workers, domestics, sex workers, migrants, EPZ workers, and micro-credit borrowers, seeking not only income and material security, but also dignity, self-betterment, and liberation from traditional authority. At both ends, the dream of women's emancipation is harnessed to the engine of capitalist accumulation. (221)

Neoliberalism has had a profound role not only in shaping the meaning of contemporary Western feminism, but in creating the intolerable global situation that combines increased workload, reduced work security, few or no options for adequate and affordable childcare, and often-nonexistent family and medical leave accommodations. It affects people's daily lives and, in particular, their ability to care effectively; these effects include the commodification of social life, the phenomenon of "time-poverty" and the outsourcing of intimate activities, and the gendered, racial, and geographically segregated bifurcation of people as fit for either "work" or "care." Obviously, the devastating effects of this "perfect storm," as Jody Heymann calls it, vary from country to country. But the evidence is clear about many essential points:

- Young children are being left home alone, in the care of other young children, and in grossly inadequate care.
- The health and development of all of these children are placed at risk, as is the education of the only slightly older children pulled out of school to care for them.

- The lack of decent working conditions and social supports makes it nearly impossible for millions of parents to balance caring for children well with working and prevents millions of families from exiting poverty. (Heymann 2006)

This is a world in which conversations about care have taken a back seat to the decades-long preoccupation with economic growth. Feminists, while not responsible for this preoccupation, must challenge it in a way that promotes solidarity among women, and recognizes that "emancipation" can only be achieved in and through our relationships with others.

Feminist Theory and the Ethics of Care

In the preface to the 1995 edition of the wonderful and widely misunderstood book *Maternal Thinking*, the late Sara Ruddick recalls 1980, when her first work on "maternal thinking" was published. She describes how invigorated she was by feminism at the time. "Within this context of splendid assertion," she writes, "some feminists had begun to speak of 'difference.' If women had suffered, loved, worked and reasoned distinctively, 'we'... would make that distinctiveness shine." And "if women's shining distinctiveness had also served to oppress us, then we would transform the conditions of our distinction so that women's interests would be served" (Ruddick 1995, ix).

One of those people writing about difference was Carol Gilligan. In 1982, *In a Different Voice* was published. Where Ruddick had focused on how the practices of mothering can give rise to non-violence, Gilligan wrote about how women's experiences give rise to a different moral psychology—presented as a world of relationships and psychological truths where an awareness of the connection between people gives rise to a recognition of responsibility for one another, a perception of the need for response (Gilligan 1993, 30). As Gilligan explains:

> a progressively more adequate understanding of the psychology of human relationships—an increasing differentiation of self and other and a growing comprehension of the dynamics of social interaction—informs the development of an ethic of care. This ethic, which reflects a cumulative knowledge of human relationships, revolves around a central insight, that self and other are interdependent. (1993, 74)

Gilligan became a full professor at Harvard—its first in gender studies—in 1986. Two years earlier, she was named Woman of the Year by *Ms.* magazine. But not everyone was equally enamored with the idea of a different voice for women. As Ruddick explains in her 1995 preface, from the outset, "difference" was controversial among feminists. Many argued that the very idea of "women" is hopelessly romantic, conceptually confused, and politically dangerous (1995, ix).

In 1985, political theorist Mary Dietz argued that maternal feminism reinforces an abstract split between the public and private realms that cannot or should not be maintained (1985, 250). "Maternal virtues cannot be political in the required sense," she argued, because they are connected to an activity that is special, and decidedly "unlike the activity of citizenship" (31). In 1990, Claudia Card worried that "elevating caring into an ethical ideal threatens to valorize the maintenance by carers of relationships that ought to be dissolved" (1990, 106). On these views, care ethics was seen as "anti-feminist"—valorizing women's roles in the home, and relegating them, as Onora O'Neill wrote, to the "nursery and the kitchen, to purdah and to poverty" (O'Neill 1990, 443). Identifying the different voice of women, it was argued, branded all women as "good for caring," and ignored, to the peril of women everywhere, the necessity of extending justice, rights, and citizenship to the realm of gender relations.

Almost simultaneously, care ethics was battling an onslaught of criticism from "third wave" feminists. Critics such as Elizabeth Spelman argued that Gilligan's entire theory about "women's moral voice" is based on research conducted with white, heterosexual, middle-class women in the United States, and thus that it ignores the crucial role of race and class in the psychology of morality (Spelman 1988). Thus, the ethics of care was damned on both sides—it was seen to reify and essentialize women's roles as carers, and this was wrong because, first, it was seen as rolling back the gains made by the struggle for women's rights and citizenship of "first wave" feminism, and second, it ignored or willfully washed over differences among women.

While it might legitimately be argued that care theory has been developed substantively since its earliest articulations to address many of these critiques, there remains a widespread suspicion regarding the extent to which care ethics can truly be feminist. Thus, there is a need to pose the question: can the ethics of care offer resolutions to the contradictions and debates in feminism, and antidotes to the contemporary trajectories of feminism which are dominated by the language of individual economic empowerment?

Another reason why "care" has always occupied a rather uncomfortable place within feminist theory is because it is overtly and self-consciously a theory of *ethics*. As critical theorists almost by definition, it is not surprising that many feminists have not known quite what to do with "ethics." Like the critics of the Vietnam War whom Michael Walzer (2002) describes as "reluctantly" speaking the language of morality, "second wave" feminism emerged as a struggle for women's liberation and took its place alongside other radical movements that were questioning core features of capitalist society. What they needed was the language of political economy—critical, materialist, historical—not the language of ethics—widely seen as rationalist, ideational, ahistorical. As Margaret Walker explains: "When Annette Baier asked a few years ago what women wanted in a moral theory, the answer she arrived at was that moral theory was just what women *didn't* want . . . " (1989, 139). They didn't want it because philosophical ethics—until recently almost entirely a product of some men's thinking—has completely ignored women as either the authors of ethical theories or moral agents, thus "bypassing altogether in application whole areas of life that are the province of women (voluntarily or not), such as the rearing of children" (148).

But what is so radical about the ethics of care is that it has given us a new kind of ethics—one that challenged not only the *substance* of ethics, but its *form*. No longer characterized by a distaste for politics, the ethics of care flew in the face of the "professional self-image of supposedly disinterested researchers after timeless moral truth" (Walker 1989, 148). Indeed, Ruddick's work on *Maternal Thinking* is intensely political; in tying maternal thinking to a "politics of peace," Ruddick brought into plain view the link between an ethic of attentive caring and a political stance against violence. *In a Different Voice* might be thought of as less political; it didn't take long, however, for feminist theorists (and Gilligan herself) to begin to emphasize the political implication of the devaluing and gendering of the values and practices of caring.

In her landmark book, *Moral Boundaries*, Joan Tronto challenged her readers to stop talking about "women's morality" and start talking instead about a care ethic that includes the values traditionally associated with women. At the same time, she warned us that morality is not "only morality." Moral arguments, she asserted, have to be understood in a political context. She put it simply and effectively:

> To recognize the value of care calls into question the structure of values in our society. Care is not a parochial concern of women, a type of secondary moral question, or the work of the least well off in society. Care is a central concern of human life. It is time that we began to change our political and social institutions to reflect this truth. (Tronto 1993, 180)

Importantly, Tronto's claims to certainty and truth are not grounded in a foundational moral epistemology—or moral principles derived from human rationality—but in a more ethnographic and sociological "looking" at what we do as human beings. Often, of course, we have to look hard to find care—it is hidden from view by the tidy separation of the public and the private realms. But in revealing the values and activities of care, we necessarily also reveal the political nature of care arrangements in all societies.

Joan Tronto's book was so important, I would suggest, because it gave us an *explicitly political* argument for an ethic of care. Throughout her book she insists that we need to take seriously the political context, and the inherent power relationships, within moral theories and situations (1993, 5). She critiques the narrow understandings of morality and politics found in the conventional "morality first" and "politics first" versions of the relationship between the two. Following Tronto's lead, care ethicists have argued consistently, for the past two decades, that the ethics and politics of care go hand in hand. It is in this characteristic of feminist care ethics that we find the most convincing response to the feminist critics of care.

If "care feminism" is not just an ethics, but also a set of claims about the *politics* of care—*who* cares and is cared for, and in what kind of micro and macro contexts—it becomes a viable starting point for a critical feminist theory of politics. Most importantly, it offers a basis for feminist solidarity across boundaries—of territory, race and culture, and class. Through the lens of care ethics, questions about good caring become social questions that transcend the narrow confines of individual self-actualization, nuclear-familial trade-offs or even national social policy. Indeed, the relationality of care ethics should not be limited to a simplistic understanding of the relation between "carers" and "cared for;" rather, a care perspective allows us to see politics, across multiple scales, as relational. Categories such as "strong and weak," "North and South," are relational in nature. As Barkawi and Laffey argue so convincingly, "you cannot have the North without the South. Relational processes connect the world. In so doing, they remake and interconnect spaces; they have a geographic expression" (Barkawi and Laffey 2006, 349). Care ethics recognizes the values and activities of caring as a source of *both* empowerment and oppression for all women—and that, often, the "empowerment" of some women relies on the oppression of others. "Doing" care ethics demands that we put in the spotlight those relations of power that govern attitudes, discourse, and policy surrounding care.

I would suggest that care ethics has survived its uneasy relationship with different feminisms because it is more than a valorization of mothering or an epistemological argument about women's privileged standpoint based on their universal oppression. In the end, care ethics endures, it resonates, because it speaks to a widespread sense of unease that somehow our priorities are wrong—that what really matters to us, in a deeply moral sense, has somehow been left behind. When we think further about this, we recognize that these priorities are not just the result of individual choices and preferences, but rather about the norms, structures, and institutions which guide the direction of the global political economy and the making of social policy. In other words, we are forced to confront the deep and inextricable relationship between morality and politics.

As Peta Bowden has argued, there is an "aura of invisibility" that surrounds the significance of care in everyday life (1997, 5). Marian Barnes's work shows how care is so fundamental to our capacity to live together that we simply cannot see its significance and it becomes possible to ignore it. Our task as feminists is, in Barnes's words, to lift the "cloak of invisibility that makes it possible to both disregard and devalue care" (Barnes 2012, 3). This is political work and feminist work. Care ethics is certainly about ethics—it focuses our attention on the life-sustaining value of care, and thus engages our consideration of the attributes of effective caring, including the value of patience, attentiveness, and listening. But it is not a rationalist, principled ethics that exists outside of, above, or as a corrective to politics. Rather, the critical lens of care ethics exposes the ways in which dominant norms and discourses sustain existing power relations that both hide considerations of care from public view, and lead to inequalities in the ways in which societies determine how and on what bases care will be given and received. Once we recognize this, we become empowered, as feminists, in a new, solidarist way.

The feminist question is thus not how can *I* balance *my* work and care responsibilities in a "man's world," but how can the need to care for one another in the world be recognized and addressed in ways that reveal and challenge power relations based on gender, race, class, age and ability, and citizenship? The goal must be to make care more visible, to demonstrate its crucial, life-sustaining importance to all human beings, and to challenge the norms and structures that continue to degrade, devalue, and feminize care work. Care is certainly about morality, but it is also about *governance*. A feminist future demands the creation of domestic and global social policy that challenges the unrelenting prioritization of economic growth and takes a long-term approach to a more sustainable, mutually prosperous, and equitable world.

There is no metanarrative which can ground our arguments about, for example, the moral value of good care for societies; but that does not mean that we cannot form persuasive arguments about the need to consider care as an issue of public importance. As Cressida Heyes argued in 1997, the problem-space defined by essentialism and anti-essentialism contains genuinely important epistemological and political issues. But deconstructive critique, relentlessly pursued, tends to throw the baby of political efficacy out with the bathwater of essentialism (Heyes 1997, 145). Indeed, our task as feminists is to reveal, to bring to light, the effects of feminizing and privatizing the values and activities associated with care.

It seems to me that the persuasive arguments of care ethicists—as found in the chapters of this book—provide a compelling response to Wendy Brown's challenge to feminists to "recuperate a utopian imaginary absent a revolutionary mechanism for its realization" (2005, 114). I see the ethics of care as a "new political formation" in this vein—not a revolutionary feminism, or one that is certain of its epistemological foundations or the precise future to which it will give rise. It does not advocate any particular models for organizing care in societies, but reveals the inadequacies, gender inequities, racializations, and economic and geopolitical implications of vastly different existing arrangements regarding care within and across societies. There is no recipe for a "care revolution," but only a slow, plodding journey where tiny victories are achieved each time a moment is spent listening attentively and patiently to the needs of another, where that moment spent can be recognized as deeply moral and of great personal and societal value without coming at great immediate or long-term cost, either to individuals or to society as a whole.

Embracing an ethics of care would mean bringing some hard questions to the forefront of public debate. Why is dependence on others seen as a pathology rather than an inevitable and shared human condition? Is there a way of understanding dependency and autonomy that recognizes our shared needs for care? Could we see autonomy as emerging out of relations of care, rather than being antithetical to them? What would it take to put in place a society of "working and caring citizens"? How could informal care work become more feasible for working men and women? How could formal, paid care work positions be seen as valuable, worthwhile positions in society?

We must also ask questions about gender norms. What happens when societies feminize and devalue care, and when men and masculinity are dissociated from caring activities and relationships? How does this contribute to the construction of hegemonic forms of masculinity associated with radical individualism and different types of violence? Care ethics demands consideration of the implications of the feminization of the values and activities associated with caring, and the related constructions of hegemonic masculinities which valorize characteristics seen as antithetical to caring: autonomy, aggression, and what Joan Tronto has called "privileged irresponsibility" (2011, 167).

Of course, when we think about "masculinities," we need to be careful to avoid blaming individual, poor men for the widespread crises of care. To do so is to obfuscate the way in which both women's and men's roles in care are governed by neoliberal and hegemonic masculinist assumptions regarding the nature of care and caregiving. Rather than allowing our analyses of masculinity to target specific groups of men in ways that are often raced and classed, we should consider the effects of norms of hegemonic masculinity at a more macro level: in national budgeting; in the making and implementing of legislation governing intimate violence and intimate labour, and the relationship between the two; and in the still-powerful influence of national and global cultures of militarism. Perhaps most importantly, though, we should consider the effects of not only the substance but also the form of masculinist logic on our thinking and theorizing about politics; as Kim Hutchings has argued, "if what masculinity *is* is rooted in what it does, then it is not any particular instantiation of masculinity which feminist scholarship needs to challenge, but the work of evaluation and exclusion that it accomplishes in our frameworks for understanding the world" (2008, 28–9; emphasis in original).

Conclusion

To conclude, I would like to return to the challenge posed by Wendy Brown regarding the future of feminism. What do we feminists do now, she asks—now that we know the impossibility of circumscribing gender without participating in its construction and regulation? What do we do now that we know the degree to which the construction of gender is bound up "not just with attitude, law and custom, not just with a sexual division of labor, not just with racial, caste, and class stratifications, not even just with the psychic economies of families and their deposits in gendered subjectivities, but also with myriad social norms buried in discursively organized practices ranging from motherhood to microchip assembly to the military?" (Brown 2003, 109).

What we do, I would suggest, is to speak the language of care, loud and clear—not because feminism is dead, but because it is alive and it has work to do. This work involves rethinking many of the basic assumptions which guide our thinking about care. As feminists, we should be able to assert the value of care while simultaneously challenging the norms that currently govern it. Care ethics is not a claim about women's essential nature, or about women's universal oppression. It is not an exhortation for us all to "care" more, or to be "more caring." Care ethics is a critical feminist theory that seeks to reveal the different forms of power that keep the values and activities of care hidden from "public" view, and to demonstrate the devastating effects that ensue when care is consistently devalued, sidelined, and subordinated to the higher values of profit and military power. As an antidote to the values of neoliberalism, care must be recognized as a social responsibility, an attribute of citizenship, and a basis of feminist solidarity.

A feminist ethics of care reveals the existence of multiple, diverse, and cross-cutting relations among a variety of global actors—including migrant caregivers; their husbands/partners; their children; the children for whom they care; their women employers; their male employers; their home (sending) states; the receiving states; and various social and political associations of migrant caregivers in receiving countries. Many of the relations among these actors span both physical and discursive geographical spaces; others, however, are located within one physical space (such as relations between husbands and wives and migrant caregivers in the space of the home). While some of these relations are between individual men and women, or individuals and collective actors such as states and their institutions, other relations are primarily at the level of structure and/or discourse.

The ethics of care is not a normative articulation of the moral standpoint of women. It is a set of claims about the world and about the value of certain kinds of human activity in that world. It reminds us that human beings are not just workers—as work is normally defined—but also carers. These activities—the activities of care—are often hidden from view, due to discursive and material relations of power that circumscribe our understandings of public and private, work and care. But care is not just descriptive; care is also an ethics because it makes claims about the nature of morality and about what is valuable to and for human beings. In this sense, the ethics of care offers us a critical lens through which to view existing arrangements for care in societies, and encourages the foregrounding of care as an issue of public concern and public debate.

Human beings are not wholly or even primarily rational minds that exist autonomously and judge impartially. Rather, our subjectivity and our very existence comes into being through relations with others—relations which are thick with responsibility, and must be negotiated with due regard for both the dependence and the difference of those others. As care ethicists we can make these claims not simply by invoking Kant or some other moral authority such as "human dignity" or "fundamental rights." Instead we make them by really looking at how people live their lives, and the struggles they face.

References

Arend, Elizabeth. 2010. "Critique of the World Bank's Applying Gender Action Plan Lessons: A Three-Year Road Map for Gender Mainstreaming (2011–2013)." Washington, DC: Gender Action. <http://www.genderaction.org/publications/2010/critique_road_map.pdf>

Barkawi, Tarak, and Mark Laffey. 2006. "The Postcolonial Moment in Security Studies." *Review of International Studies* 32: 329–52.

Barnes, Marian. 2012. *Care in Everyday Life: An Ethic of Care in Practice*. Bristol: The Policy Press.

Bowden, Peta. 1997. *Caring: Gender Sensitive Ethics*. London: Routledge.

Brown, Wendy. 2005. "Feminism Unbound: Revolution, Mourning, Politics." In *Edgework: Critical Essays on Knowledge and Politics*, 98–115. Princeton, NJ: Princeton University Press.

Burnham, Linda. 2013. "1% Feminism." *OpenDemocracy*, 8 April. <http://www.opendemocracy.net/5050/linda-burnham/1-feminism>

Card, Claudia. 1990. "Caring and Evil." *Hypatia* 5(1): 101–8.

Chang, Kimberly A., and L. H. M. Ling. 2000. "Globalization and Its Intimate Other: Filipina Domestic Workers in Hong Kong." In *Gender and Global Restructuring: Sightings, Sites and Resistances*, edited by Marianne Marchand and Anne Sisson Runyan, 27–43. London: Routledge.

Chant, Sylvia, and Caroline Sweetman. 2012. "Fixing Women or Fixing the World? 'Smart Economics', Efficiency Approaches and Gender Equality in Development." *Gender and Development* 20(3): 517–29.

Coontz, Stephanie. 2013. "Why Gender Equality Stalled." *New York Times*, 16 February. <http://www.nytimes.com/2013/02/17/opinion/sunday/why-gender-equality-stalled.html?pagewanted=3&_r=0>

Dietz, Mary G. 1985. "Citizenship with a Feminist Face: The Problem with Maternal Thinking." *Political Theory* 13(1): 19–37.

Eveline, J., and C. Bacchi. 2005. "What Are We Mainstreaming when We Mainstream Gender?" *International Feminist Journal of Politics* 7(4): 496–512.

Faludi, Susan. 2013. "Facebook Feminism: Like It or Not." *The Baffler*, no. 23. <http://thebaffler.com/past/facebook_feminism_like_it_or_not>

Fraser, Nancy. 2013. *Fortunes of Feminism: From State-Managed Capitalism to Neoliberal Crisis*. New York: Verso.

Gilligan, Carol. 1993. *In a Different Voice: Psychological Theory and Women's Development*. Cambridge, MA: Harvard University Press.

Gira Grant, Melissa. 2013. "Sheryl Sandberg's 'Lean In' Campaign Holds Little for Most Women." *Washington Post*, February 25.

Griffen, Penny. 2010. "Gender, Governance and the Global Political Economy." *Australian Journal of International Affairs* 64(1): 86–104.

Halley, Janet. 2006. *Split Decisions: How and Why to Take a Break from Feminism*. Princeton, NJ: Princeton University Press.

Heyes, Cressida. 1997. "Anti-essentialism in Practice: Carol Gilligan and Feminist Philosophy." *Hypatia* 12(3): 142–63.

Heymann, Jodi. 2006. *Forgotten Families: Ending the Growing Crisis Confronting Children and Working Parents in the Global Economy*. Oxford: Oxford University Press.

Hochschild, Arlie Russell. 2000. "Global Care Chains and Emotional Surplus Value." In *Global Capitalism*, edited by Will Hutton and Anthony Giddens, 130–46. New York: New Press.

Holmes, Anna. 2013. "Maybe You Should Read the Book: The Sheryl Sandberg Backlash." *The New Yorker*, 4 March.

Hooper, Charlotte. 2000. "Masculinities in Transition: The Case of Globalization." In *Gender and Global Restructuring: Sightings, Sites and Resistances*, edited by Marianne Marchand and Anne Sisson Runyan, 59–73. London: Routledge.

Huffington, Ariana. 2014. *Thrive: The Third Metric to Redefining Success and Creating a Life of Well-Being, Wisdom and Wonder*. New York: Harmony.

Hutchings, Kimberly. 2008. "Cognitive Shortcuts." In *Re-thinking the Man Question: Sex, Gender and Violence in International Relations*, edited by Jane Parpart and Marysia Zalewski, 23–46. London: Zed.

Larner, Wendy. 2000. "Neo-liberalism: Policy, Ideology, Governmentality." *Studies in Political Economy* 63: 5–25.

McRobbie, Angela. 2008. *The Aftermath of Feminism: Gender, Culture and Social Change*. London: Sage.

Mohanty, Chandra Talpade. 1984. "Under Western Eyes: Feminist Scholarship and Colonial Discourses." *Boundary 2* 12(3)/13(1): 333–58.

Moser, Caroline. 2005. "Has Gender Mainstreaming Failed?" *International Feminist Journal of Politics* 7(4): 576–90.

O'Connor, J. S., A. S. Orloff, and S. Shaver. 1999. *States, Markets, Families: Gender, Liberalism and Social Policy in Australia, Canada, Great Britain and the United States*. Cambridge: Cambridge University Press.

O'Neill, Onora. 1990. "Justice, Gender and International Boundaries." *British Journal of Political Science* 20(4): 439–59.

Ruddick, Sara. 1995. *Maternal Thinking: Toward a Politics of Peace*, 2nd ed. Boston, MA: Beacon Press.

Sandberg, Sheryl. 2011. "Commencement Address, Barnard College." New York City, 17 May. <http://barnard.edu/headlines/transcript-and-video-speech-sheryl-sandberg-chief-operating-officer-facebook>

Sandberg, Sheryl. 2013. *Lean In: Women, Work and the Will to Lead*. New York: Knopf.

Shepherd, Laura J. 2010. "Sex or Gender? Bodies in World Politics and Why Gender Matters." In *Gender Matters in Global Politics*, edited by Laura J. Shepherd, 3–16. London: Routledge.

Slaughter, Ann Marie. 2013. "Yes, You Can: Sheryl Sandberg's Lean In." *New York Times*, 7 March.

Spelman, Elizabeth. 1988. *Inessential Woman: Problems of Exclusion in Feminist Thought*. Boston, MA: Beacon Press.

Tronto, Joan. 1993. *Moral Boundaries: A Political Argument for an Ethic of Care*. New York: Routledge.

Tronto, Joan. 2011. "A Feminist Democratic Ethics of Care and Global Care Workers: Citizenship and Responsibility." In *Feminist Ethics and Social Policy: Towards a New Global Political Economy of Care*, edited by Rianne Mahon and Fiona Robinson, 162–77. Vancouver: University of British Columbia Press.

True, Jacqui. 2003. "Mainstreaming Gender in Global Public Policy." *International Feminist Journal of Politics* 5(3): 368–96.

Walby, Sylvia. 2005. "Comparative Gender Mainstreaming in a Global Era." *International Feminist Journal of Politics* 7(4): 453–70.

Walker, Margaret Urban. 1989. "Moral Understandings: Alternative 'Epistemology' for a Feminist Ethics." In *Justice and Care: Essential Readings in Feminist Ethics* edited by Virginia Held, 139–52. Boulder, CO: Westview Press.

Walzer, Michael. 2002. "The Triumph of Just War Theory (and the Dangers of Success)." *Social Research* 69(4): 925–44.

Williams, Fiona. 2011. "Towards a Transnational Analysis of the Political Economy of Care." In *Feminist Ethics and Social Policy: Towards a New Global Political Economy of Care*, edited by Rianne Mahon and Fiona Robinson, 21–38. Vancouver: University of British Columbia Press.

Zalewski, Marisya. 2010. "I Don't Even Know What Gender Is: A Discussion of the Connections between Gender, Gender Mainstreaming and Feminist Theory." *Review of International Studies* 36(1): 3–27.

Index